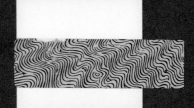

# SELF-ASSESSMENT IN HEAD AND NECK SURGERY AND ONCOLOGY

# SELF-ASSESSMENT IN HEAD AND NECK SURGERY AND ONCOLOGY

EDITORS:

## James Paul O'Neill, MD, MB, FRCSI, MMSc, MBA, ORL-HNS

Professor of Otolaryngology, Head and Neck Surgery
The Royal College of Surgeons in Ireland
St. Stephen's Green
Dublin, Ireland;
Consultant Otolaryngology Head and Neck Surgeon
Beaumont Hospital
Dublin, Ireland

## Jatin P. Shah, MD, PhD (Hon), FACS, FRCS (Hon), FDSRCS (Hon), FRACS (Hon)

Chief, Head and Neck Service
E.W. Strong Chair in Head and Neck Oncology
Memorial Sloan Kettering Cancer Center;
Professor of Surgery
Weill Cornell Medical College of Cornell University
New York, New York
United States

ASSOCIATE EDITORS:

## Ian Ganly, MD, PhD, FRCS
## Luc G. T. Morris, MD, MSc
## Snehal Patel, MD, MS, FRCS
## Ashok Shaha, MD, FACS
## Bhuvanesh Singh, MD, PhD, FACS

**ELSEVIER**
SAUNDERS

## ELSEVIER
SAUNDERS

1600 John F. Kennedy Blvd.
Ste 1800
Philadelphia, PA 19103-2899

**Library of Congress Cataloging-in-Publication Data**

Self-assessment in head and neck surgery and oncology / editors, James Paul O'Neill, Jatin P. Shah ; associate editors, Ian Ganly, Luc G.T. Morris, Snehal Patel, Ashok Shaha, Bhuvanesh Singh.
  p. ; cm.
  Includes bibliographical references and index.
  ISBN 978-0-323-26003-9 (pbk. : alk. paper)
  I. O'Neill, James Paul, editor of compilation. II. Shah, Jatin P., editor of compilation. III. Ganly, Ian, editor of compilation.
  [DNLM: 1. Head and Neck Neoplasms--surgery--Examination Questions. 2. Head--surgery--Examination Questions. 3. Neck--surgery--Examination Questions. WE 18.2]
  RC280.H4
  616.99'4910076--dc23
                                                2014004737

*Senior Content Strategist:* Belinda Kuhn
*Senior Content Development Manager:* Maureen Iannuzzi
*Publishing Services Manager:* Patricia Tannian
*Senior Project Manager:* Kristine Feeherty
*Design Direction:* Ellen Zanolle

Printed in China

Last digit is the print number:  9  8  7  6  5  4  3  2  1

Working together
to grow libraries in
developing countries

www.elsevier.com • www.bookaid.org

*To our families, for their love and support*
*To our patients, for their bravery enduring the burden of head and neck disease*

# Preface

The term "cancer of the head and neck" generally includes neoplasms arising from the mucosa of the upper aerodigestive tract, including the nasal cavity and paranasal sinuses, as well as tumors of the salivary glands, thyroid and parathyroid glands, and neoplasms arising from the skin, soft tissues, and bones of the craniofacial skeleton. Tumors of neurovascular origin and those arising in the ear canal, temporal bone, orbit, and skull base are also included in this list. Over the course of the past century, the specialty treating these tumors has evolved into a very complex multidisciplinary field requiring the expertise of head and neck surgeons, radiation oncologists, medical oncologists, maxillofacial/dental surgeons, reconstructive microsurgeons, and other allied specialists. The training programs for specializing in this complex specialty have also evolved over the course of the past 30 years, with the need to incorporate training in increasingly complex technologies, development of new skill sets, and integration of exposure to nonsurgical disciplines. An increasing number of textbooks have been published over the past 20 years, as well as a plethora of published journal articles, with emphasis on multidisciplinary treatments. Ample literature is available for the trainee and the practitioner to remain abreast of the advances made in the field.

However, no specialty or board certification examination is available in this complex field, and thus there is no measure of one's competency in the specialty. The graduates of the senior fellowship program in head and neck surgery and oncology and the faculty of the head and neck program at Memorial Sloan Kettering Cancer Center in New York have created this self-assessment compendium to measure the fundamental basic knowledge required of an individual engaged in the specialty of head and neck surgery and oncology. This book by no means is sufficient to measure competency in the specialty, nor is it intended to be sufficient to gain certification in the specialty. On the other hand, it certainly introduces the reader to the process of self-assessment of knowledge, judgment, an algorithmic thinking process, and the decision-making ability in dealing with day-to-day problems in patients with neoplasms arising in the head and neck.

Each chapter contains a topic, following the sequence of the chapters in *Jatin Shah's Head and Neck Surgery and Oncology,* Fourth Edition. The questions are presented in three categories: (1) True or False, (2) Single Best Answer, and (3) Multiple Choice combinations. Each chapter includes the basic Core Knowledge required and has a Suggested Reading list. The answers to the questions are provided at the end of each chapter. It is our hope that the reader will benefit from initially taking the examination, pursue the topic further by reviewing the Core Knowledge, and then gain further knowledge from reading the recommended textbooks. We also hope that this initial attempt at self-assessment will stimulate the reader to remain engaged in continuing medical education in order to remain current with this rapidly advancing specialty.

## Acknowledgment

We would like to express our sincere appreciation and special thanks to the faculty of the head and neck service of Memorial Sloan Kettering Cancer Center for their advice, input, guidance, and support throughout this project.

Our special thanks are also due to the editorial staff of the head and neck service who provided timely help in processing the manuscripts and numerous edits and corrections to bring about this work.

Finally, we want to thank each and every one of the contributors to this book, the faculty members of the head and neck service, former fellows of the head and neck program, and the current fellows on the service for their hard and ingenious work in developing the questions, which truly test the knowledge of the reader. We are grateful for their support.

**James Paul O'Neill, MD, MB, FRCSI, MMSc, MBA, ORL-HNS**
**Jatin P. Shah, MD, PhD (Hon), FACS, FRCS (Hon), FDSRCS (Hon), FRACS (Hon)**

# Contributors

**George C. Bohle III, DDS**
Clinical Assistant Professor
University of Oklahoma College of
    Dentistry;
Private Practice
Implant and Prosthodontic Associates
Oklahoma City, Oklahoma
United States
    *Oncological Dentistry: Maxillofacial Pros-
    thetics and Implants*

**Jeffrey Chang-Jen Liu, MD**
Assistant Professor of Otolaryngology and
    Head and Neck Surgery
Temple University School of Medicine;
Assistant Professor of Head and Neck Surgery
Fox Chase Cancer Center
Philadelphia, Pennsylvania
United States
    *Larynx and Trachea*

**Natalya Chernichenko, MD**
Assistant Professor of Otolaryngology
Chief of Head and Neck Surgery
SUNY Downstate Medical Center
Brooklyn, New York
United States
    *Neurogenic Tumors and Paragangliomas*

**Mark D. DeLacure, MD, FACS**
Chief, Division of Head and Neck Surgery
    and Oncology
Department of Otolaryngology, Head and
    Neck Surgery
Associate Professor of Plastic Surgery
Institute of Reconstructive Plastic Surgery
Department of Plastic Surgery
New York University School of Medicine
New York University Clinical Cancer Center
New York, New York
United States
    *Reconstructive Surgery*

**Matthew Fury, MD, PhD**
Assistant Member
Memorial Sloan Kettering Cancer Center;
Assistant Attending Physician
Memorial Hospital
New York, New York
United States
    *Chemotherapy*

**Ian Ganly, MD, PhD, FRCS**
Associate Professor of Otolaryngology and
    Head and Neck Surgery
Weill Cornell Medical College of Cornell
    University;
Associate Attending Surgeon
Memorial Sloan Kettering Cancer Center
New York, New York
United States
    *Lips and Oral Cavity*

**Babak Givi, MD**
Assistant Professor of Otolaryngology,
    Head and Neck Surgery
New York University School of Medicine
NYU Langone Medical Center
New York, New York
United States
    *Reconstructive Surgery*

**Allen S. Ho, MD**
Assistant Professor of Surgery
Cedars-Sinai Medical Center
Los Angeles, California
United States
    *Nutrition*

**Nora Katabi, MD**
Assistant Attending
Department of Pathology
Memorial Sloan Kettering Cancer Center
New York, New York
United States
    *Pathology*

**Nancy Lee, MD**
Attending
Department of Radiation Oncology
Memorial Sloan Kettering Cancer Center
New York, New York
United States
    *Radiation Oncology*

**Ellie Maghami, MD, FACS**
Associate Professor
Chief, Division of Otolaryngology and
    Head and Neck Surgery
City of Hope National Medical Center
Duarte, California
United States
    *Nasal Cavity and Paranasal Sinuses*

**Arash Mohebati, MD**
Attending Surgeon
John Muir Medical Center
Walnut Creek, California
United States
  *Pharynx and Esophagus*

**Luc G.T. Morris, MD, MSc**
Assistant Professor of Otolaryngology
Weill Cornell Medical College of Cornell
  University;
Assistant Attending Surgeon
Memorial Sloan Kettering Cancer Center
New York, New York
United States
  *Skin*

**Iain James Nixon, PhD**
Consultant Ear, Nose, and Throat/Head and
  Neck Surgeon
East Kent Hospitals University NHS
  Foundation Trust
Ashford, Kent
United Kingdom
  *Thyroid and Parathyroid*

**Caitriona O'Neill, PhD, BSc(Pharm),**
**MBA, Dip Stat**
Trinity College Dublin
Dublin, Ireland
  *Epidemiology and Biostatistics*

**James Paul O'Neill, MD, MB, FRCSI,**
**MMSc, MBA, ORL-HNS**
Professor of Otolaryngology, Head and
  Neck Surgery
The Royal College of Surgeons in Ireland
St. Stephen's Green
Dublin, Ireland;
Consultant Otolaryngology Head and
  Neck Surgeon
Beaumont Hospital
Dublin, Ireland
  *Skull Base; Pharynx and Esophagus; Salivary*
  *Glands; Soft Tissue Tumors; Surgical Anatomy*

**Daniel Louis Price, MD**
Assistant Professor
Department of Otolaryngology, Head and
  Neck Surgery
Mayo Clinic
Rochester, Minnesota
United States
  *Salivary Glands*

**Rahmatullah Rahmati, MD**
Assistant Professor of Otolaryngology,
  Head and Neck Surgery
Columbia University Medical Center
New York, New York
United States
  *Bone Tumors and Odontogenic Tumors*

**Nadeem Riaz, MD**
Resident Physician
Department of Radiation Oncology
Memorial Sloan Kettering Cancer Center
New York, New York
United States
  *Radiation Oncology*

**Patrick Sheahan, MD, MB, FRCSI**
**(ORL-HNS)**
Clinical Lecturer
University College Cork;
Consultant Otolaryngologist, Head and
  Neck Surgeon
South Infirmary Victoria University Hospital
Cork, Ireland
  *Cervical Lymph Nodes*

**Andrew G. Shuman, MD**
Department of Otolaryngology, Head and
  Surgery
University of Michigan Health System
Ann Arbor, Michigan
United States
  *Eyelids and Orbit*

**Hilda Stambuk, MD**
Attending Radiologist
Clinical Head of Head and Neck Imaging
Department of Radiology
Memorial Sloan Kettering Cancer Center
New York, New York
United States
  *Radiology*

**Volkert Wreesmann, MD, PhD**
Head and Neck Surgeon
Department of Otolaryngology, Head and
  Neck Surgery
Netherlands Cancer Institute
University Medical Center Utrecht
Amsterdam and Utrecht
The Netherlands
  *Molecular Oncology*

# Contents

# SELF-ASSESSMENT IN HEAD AND NECK SURGERY AND ONCOLOGY

# 1 Skin

## Questions

### TRUE/FALSE

1. Melanoma incidence is rapidly increasing in the United States and Europe. (T/F)

2. A history of blistering sunburns is a risk factor for melanoma. (T/F)

3. Skin color and hair color are risk factors for melanoma. (T/F)

4. Melanoma is more common in women than men. (T/F)

5. *NRAS* is the most commonly mutated gene in melanomas. (T/F)

6. Of all melanomas, the desmoplastic subtype has the highest incidence of lymphatic spread. (T/F)

7. All nodes with at least 10% of the count of the hottest node should be removed at the time of sentinel lymph node biopsy (SLNB). (T/F)

8. The median number of nodes removed in a sentinel lymph node (SLN) procedure is three. (T/F)

9. The Multicenter Selective Lymphadenectomy Trial (MSLT) demonstrated that SLNB for melanoma was associated with improved overall survival rate. (T/F)

10. SLNB should be performed for ulcerated melanomas, even if <1 mm in thickness. (T/F)

11. Tumor thickness >1 mm is a high-risk feature of non–melanoma skin cancers that has been incorporated into staging systems. (T/F)

12. Perineural invasion is a high-risk feature of non–melanoma skin cancers that has been incorporated into staging systems. (T/F)

13. Tumor location on an ear or the hair-bearing lip is a high-risk feature of non–melanoma skin cancers that has been incorporated into staging systems. (T/F)

14. High-grade histology is a high-risk feature of non–melanoma skin cancers that has been incorporated into staging systems. (T/F)

15. Mitotic rate >1/mm$^2$ is a high-risk feature of non–melanoma skin cancers that has been incorporated into staging systems. (T/F)

16. Tumor thickness >1 mm is a high-risk feature of cutaneous melanoma that has been incorporated into staging systems. (T/F)

17. Perineural invasion is a high-risk feature of cutaneous melanoma that has been incorporated into staging systems. (T/F)

18. Tumor location on an ear or hair-bearing lip is a high-risk feature of cutaneous melanoma that has been incorporated into staging systems. (T/F)

19. High-grade histology is a high-risk feature of cutaneous melanoma that has been incorporated into staging systems. (T/F)

20. Mitotic rate >1/mm$^2$ is a high-risk feature of cutaneous melanoma that has been incorporated into staging systems. (T/F)

21. Merkel cell carcinoma is difficult to distinguish from other neuroendocrine carcinomas. (T/F)

22. Merkel cell carcinoma has been causally linked to a paramyxovirus. (T/F)

23. Merkel cell carcinoma is considered to be a radiosensitive tumor. (T/F)

24. Merkel cell carcinoma is more appropriate for elective lymphadenectomy rather than SLNB, given its aggressive nature. (T/F)

25. Merkel cell carcinoma is associated with a poorer survival rate when lymphovascular invasion is present. (T/F)

26. The most common subtype of basal cell carcinoma (BCC) is superficial. (T/F)

27. BCC stains for low-molecular-weight cytokeratins. (T/F)

28. BCC has been causally linked to ultraviolet (UV) light exposure and radiation therapy. (T/F)

29. BCC responds to hedgehog pathway inhibitors. (T/F)

30. BCC almost never arises within oral mucosa. (T/F)

31. Sebaceous carcinoma rarely arises from hair-bearing skin. (T/F)

32. Sebaceous carcinoma most commonly arises on the eyelid. (T/F)

33. Sebaceous carcinoma may exist with a syndrome requiring colonoscopy. (T/F)

34. Sebaceous carcinoma rarely metastasizes (<5% of cases). (T/F)

35. Sebaceous carcinoma can be effectively treated with local irradiation and no surgery. (T/F)

36. Sweat gland tumors may have eccrine or apocrine differentiation. (T/F)

37. Eccrine poroma, a sweat gland tumor, is the most common skin adnexal malignancy. (T/F)

38. Sweat gland tumors, or eccrine carcinomas, rarely metastasize (<5% of cases). (T/F)

39. Sweat gland tumors are amenable to Mohs micrographic surgery. (T/F)

40. Sweat gland tumors frequently stain for epidermal growth factor receptor (EGFR). (T/F)

41. Squamous cell cancers (SCCs) of the skin rarely metastasize to lymph nodes (<5% of cases). (T/F)

42. Immunocompromised patients are at elevated risk of metastases. (T/F)

43. The degree of differentiation of cutaneous SCC has no impact on the risk of recurrence. (T/F)

44. An elective parotidectomy and neck dissection should be considered in a patient with a recurrent, 4.4-cm in diameter, 5-mm thick SCC of the cheek, despite no clinically evident nodes in the parotid gland. (T/F)

45. The presence of perineural invasion should prompt consideration of adjuvant radiation therapy to the neural pathway and the brainstem. (T/F)

46. The median survival time in patients with stage IV melanoma is 5.6 years. (T/F)

47. Vemurafenib only has benefit in patients with melanoma harboring a BRAF mutation. (T/F)

48. Ipilimumab improves survival in stage IV melanoma by inhibiting signaling through the MAPK pathway. (T/F)

49. Mucosal melanomas are more likely than cutaneous melanomas to have BRAF mutations. (T/F)

50. Patients treated with vemurafenib for melanoma have an elevated risk of developing cutaneous SCCs. (T/F)

## MULTIPLE CHOICE

51. A 76-year-old woman presents to your office with a 1 × 1-cm flat pink lesion on the right cheek, close to the lower eyelid (Figure 1-1). A full thickness biopsy is consistent with melanoma in situ.

    Which of the following is true?
    A. Melanoma in situ is also known as *lentigo maligna.*
    B. Melanoma in situ is also known as *lentigo maligna melanoma.*
    C. Melanoma in situ is also known as *Hutchinson freckle.*

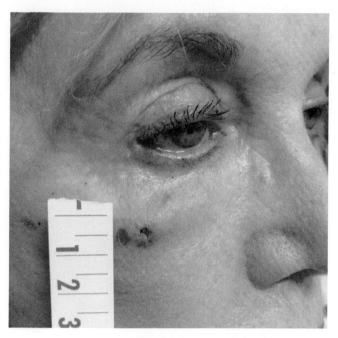

**Figure 1-1**

    D. A and C are true.
    E. B and C are true.

52. Which of the following describes the diagnosis of melanoma in situ?
    A. It normally occurs in sun-damaged skin.
    B. It is not related to sun exposure.
    C. The lesion is generally small in size and easy to diagnose with the naked eye.
    D. Shave biopsy is appropriate.
    E. Punch biopsy is appropriate.

53. Which of the following treatment options is an appropriate next step?
    A. Excision of the lesion, followed by primary closure
    B. Excision of the lesion, followed by a skin graft
    C. Wide excision with 5-mm margins, followed by a local rotational flap
    D. Wide excision with 5-mm margins and delayed closure until confirmation of margins

54. Which of the following alternative treatment options would also be appropriate?
    A. Mapping biopsies around the entire periphery of the lesion; once the results are confirmed to be negative, excision and immediate closure
    B. Wide excision with 10-mm margins, frozen-section assessment of margins, SLNB, and local flap closure if margins are negative on frozen-section analysis
    C. Wide excision with 10-mm margins, superficial parotidectomy, selective neck dissection of levels I through III, and cervicofacial rotational flap
    D. Wide excision with 20-mm margins, frozen-section assessment of margins, SLNB, and local flap closure if margins are negative on frozen-section analysis

55. The patient asks why surgery is necessary if lentigo maligna is not an invasive cancer. She asks about her risks of developing invasive melanoma.
    A. Invasive melanoma is commonly misdiagnosed as melanoma in situ.
    B. 70% to 90% of melanomas in situ evolve into invasive melanoma.
    C. 30% to 50% of melanomas in situ evolve into invasive melanoma.
    D. 3% to 5% of melanomas in situ evolve into invasive melanoma.
    E. Melanomas in situ almost never evolve into invasive melanoma.

56. Choose which type of BCC is amenable to the specified treatment modality.
    A. Small superficial BCC; topical imiquimod
    B. Small superficial BCC; photodynamic therapy
    C. Morpheaform BCC; topical 5-fluorouracil (5-FU)
    D. Large, infiltrative BCC; high-dose imiquimod

57. Choose which type of BCC is amenable to the specified treatment modality.
    A. BCC near cosmetically sensitive areas; Mohs micrographic surgery
    B. Infiltrative BCC; electrodesiccation
    C. Recurrent BCC; cryotherapy
    D. Basosquamous carcinoma; topical imiquimod

58. Choose which type of BCC is amenable to the specified treatment modality.
    A. Unresectable BCC; hedgehog inhibitors
    B. Large BCC in a patient not medically fit for excision; radiation therapy
    C. Both A and B
    D. None of the above

59. Dermatofibrosarcoma protuberans describes a tumor that
    A. Is a sarcoma.
    B. Is a carcinoma.
    C. Is a carcinosarcoma.
    D. Is a benign tumor.

60. Dermatofibrosarcoma protuberans tumors
    A. Commonly metastasize to regional nodes.
    B. Have a high risk of local recurrence after resection.
    C. Are generally lethal as a result of lung metastases.
    D. Are all of the above.

61. Dermatofibrosarcoma protuberans tumors
    A. Stain for CD34.
    B. Stain for S-100.
    C. Stain for HMB-45.
    D. Stain for cadherins.

62. Dermatofibrosarcoma protuberans tumors are
    A. Characterized by a t(17:22) translocation resulting in overexpression of platelet-derived growth factor receptor (PDGFR).
    B. Characterized by an SYT-SSX2 translocation protein.

C. Characterized by an NFIB-MYB translocation protein.
D. Both A and C.

63. The recommended treatment for dermatofibrosarcoma protuberans is
    A. Excision with wide margins or Mohs micrographic surgery, both of which are considered appropriate modalities for surgical excision.
    B. Wide local resection, with positive margins generally requiring postoperative radiation therapy.
    C. Imatinib, if recurrent tumors are unresectable.
    D. All of the above.

64. Merkel cell carcinoma excised with surgery
    A. Has low rates of local recurrence (<1%).
    B. Has intermediate rates of local recurrence (5% to 10%).
    C. Has high rates of local recurrence (25% to 30%).
    D. Has very high rates of local recurrence (>70%).

65. Merkel cell carcinoma excised with surgery
    A. Rarely, if ever, metastasizes distantly (<5%).
    B. Sometimes develops distant metastases (5% to 10%).
    C. Has high rates of distant metastases (30% to 35%).
    D. Nearly always recurs distantly (>70%).

66. The etiology of Merkel cell carcinoma is
    A. Nearly always Merkel cell polyomavirus, irrespective of UV light exposure.
    B. Usually attributable to UV exposure but can be Merkel cell polyomavirus in a minority of cases.
    C. Merkel cell polyomavirus in 25% of cases.
    D. Merkel cell polyomavirus in 80% of cases.

67. Merkel cell carcinoma is also known as
    A. Neuroendocrine melanoma.
    B. Cutaneous APUDoma.
    C. Trabecular skin carcinoma.
    D. B and C.

68. Merkel cell carcinoma
    A. Looks morphologically similar to BCC.
    B. Stains for CD20.
    C. Stains for CK-20.
    D. Is both A and C.

69. After an SLNB is performed on a patient with Merkel cell cancer, the following course(s) of action is/are appropriate:
    A. A positive SLN in the neck should prompt completion nodal dissection.
    B. Completion lymphadenectomy is strongly favored over radiation therapy to the nodal basin in cases of a positive SLN.
    C. Radiation therapy is acceptable as a treatment option when surgery is not feasible.
    D. A and C are true.

70. What is the recommended margin for wide excision of an in situ melanoma?
    A. Negative (tumor not touching the inked margin)
    B. 1 mm

C. 5 mm
D. 10 mm

71. What is the recommended margin for wide excision of a thin/intermediate-thickness melanoma?
    A. 0.7 mm in depth; 0.5-cm margin
    B. 1.0 mm; 1.0- to 2.0-cm margin
    C. 1.3 mm; 1.0- to 2.0-cm margin
    D. 2.0 mm; 2.0-cm margin

72. What is the recommended margin for wide excision of melanoma?
    A. 2.3-mm thickness, 2.0-cm margin
    B. 3.3-mm thickness, 3.0-cm margin
    C. 6.8-mm thickness, 3.0-cm margin
    D. 7.2-mm thickness, 2.0-cm margin

73. A 2.6-mm thick, ulcerated melanoma with satellitosis but no evidence of lymph node metastases or distant metastases would be staged as
    A. T2b N0 M0.
    B. T3a N0 M0.
    C. T3b N0 M0.
    D. T3b N3 M0.

74. A 0.7-mm thick, nonulcerated melanoma with one positive lymph node and no evidence of distant metastases is excised. What additional information is required to complete staging?
    A. Mitoses per mm$^2$; micrometastasis versus macrometastasis
    B. Mitoses per high-power field; micrometastasis versus macrometastasis
    C. Mitoses per mm$^2$; serum lactate dehydrogenase (LDH) level
    D. Mitoses per high-power field; positron emission tomography/computed tomography (PET/CT) imaging

75. A 2.0-mm thick, nonulcerated melanoma is excised. Nodal dissection reveals 8 of 28 positive nodes. There is no evidence of distant disease. What is the TNM staging?
    A. T3 N3 M0
    B. T2 N3 M0
    C. T2 N2b M0
    D. T2 N3a M0

76. What stage does a thick (>4.0 mm) nonulcerated melanoma with no nodal or distant disease fall into?
    A. Stage II
    B. Stage IIB
    C. Stage IIC
    D. Stage IV

77. Which of the following variables is relevant for staging melanoma and included in the TNM staging system?
    A. Age
    B. Serum LDH level in patients with distant metastases
    C. Number of mitoses in thick melanomas
    D. Bone scans in patients with distant metastases

78. An 80-year-old woman with a right cheek cutaneous SCC develops masses in the parotid gland and under the jaw and complete paralysis of all branches of the facial nerve. At the time of surgery, the main trunk of the facial nerve is observed to be red and inflamed (Figure 1-2). The appropriate treatment is

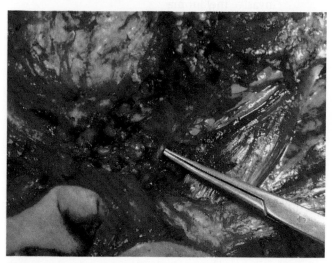

**Figure 1-2** (Courtesy of Memorial Sloan Kettering Cancer Center, New York.)

    A. Wide local excision of the primary tumor and superficial parotidectomy with preservation of the facial nerve, followed by postoperative radiation therapy to the skin, parotid bed, neck, and along the course of the facial nerve.
    B. Wide local excision, superficial parotidectomy with preservation of the facial nerve, modified radical neck dissection, and postoperative radiation therapy to the skin, parotid bed, neck, and along the course of the facial nerve.
    C. Wide local excision of the primary tumor, parotidectomy with sacrifice of the facial nerve at the stylomastoid foramen, and postoperative radiation therapy to the skin, parotid bed, neck, and along the course of the facial nerve.
    D. Wide local excision of the primary tumor, parotidectomy with the extent of facial nerve sacrifice determined by frozen-section analysis, modified radical neck dissection, and postoperative radiation therapy to the skin and parotid bed along the course of the facial nerve with concurrent chemotherapy.

79. Melanoma will usually stain positively for these antibodies on immunohistochemical analysis:
    A. HMB-45.
    B. S-100.
    C. AE1/AE3.
    D. A and B.

80. Melanoma will usually stain positively for these antibodies on immunohistochemical analysis:
    A. TTF1.
    B. MITF.
    C. Chromogranin.
    D. N-cadherin.

81. Melanoma will usually stain positively for these antibodies on immunohistochemical analysis:
    A. Melan-A/MART1.
    B. Synaptophysin.
    C. CK-20.
    D. PNL-1.

82. Which of the following interventions has been shown to improve overall survival rates in patients with melanoma?
    A. Completion lymphadenectomy after a positive SLNB
    B. Adjuvant interferon alfa
    C. Pegylated interferon
    D. None of the above

83. Which of the following interventions has been shown to improve overall survival rates in patients with melanoma?
    A. Hypofractionated radiation therapy in patients with positive margins
    B. Standard fractionation radiation therapy in patients with positive margins
    C. Accelerated fraction radiation therapy in patients with regional nodal metastasis
    D. Ipilimumab in patients with distant metastases

84. Which of the following interventions has been shown to improve overall survival rates in patients with melanoma?
    A. Dacarbazine in patients with distant metastases
    B. Vemurafenib in patients with distant metastases
    C. Biochemotherapy (cisplatin, vinblastine, dacarbazine, interleukin-2 [IL-2], and interferon) in patients with distant metastases
    D. Vemurafenib in the adjuvant setting, in patients with nodal metastases

85. Multicenter trial data from international trials run by the Intergroup, World Health Organization (WHO), and investigators in the United Kingdom, Sweden, and France have shown that the following margins achieve superior locoregional control:
    A. 1- to 2-mm thickness; 5 cm versus 2 cm.
    B. <2-mm thickness; 5 cm versus 2 cm.
    C. 1- to 4-mm thickness; 4 cm versus 2 cm.
    D. None of the above.

86. SLNs are
    A. Identified in 95% of cases.
    B. Identified in 99% of cases.
    C. Identified more successfully with Lymphazurin compared with methylene blue.
    D. None of the above.

87. SLNs are
    A. Identified more commonly in head and neck primary melanomas, followed by axilla, followed by groin.
    B. Identified less commonly in head and neck primary melanomas.
    C. More likely to be positive in older patients with thin melanomas.
    D. None of the above.

88. SLN identification rates in thin melanomas are
    A. More likely to be positive if the melanoma is ulcerated.
    B. Unrelated to ulceration or mitotic rates.
    C. More likely to be positive in melanomas with higher mitotic rates.
    D. All of the above.

89. Which of the following is true about SLN rates in thin melanomas?
    A. Melanomas <0.75 mm in thickness have a positive SLN in 15.7% of cases.
    B. Melanomas <0.75 mm in thickness have a positive SLN in 2.7% of cases.
    C. Melanomas <0.75 mm in thickness have a positive SLN in 0.7% of cases.
    D. None of the above are true.

90. Which of the following is true about thin melanomas?
    A. Melanomas 0.75 to 1.0 mm in thickness have a positive SLN in 6.2% of cases.
    B. Melanomas 0.75 to 1.0 mm in thickness have a positive SLN in 0.2% of cases.
    C. The SLN positivity rate in 0.75- to 1.0-mm thick melanomas is similar to <0.75-mm thick melanomas.
    D. The SLN positivity rate in 0.75- to 1.0-mm thick melanomas is substantially more than <0.75-mm thick melanomas.

91. Which is true about SLN rates in thick melanomas?
    A. Melanomas >4.0 mm in thickness have a positive SLN in 1% to 2% of cases.
    B. Melanomas >4.0 mm in thickness have a positive SLN in 10% of cases.
    C. Melanomas >4.0 mm in thickness have a positive SLN in 30% to 40% of cases.
    D. Melanomas >4.0 mm in thickness have a positive SLN in 85% of cases.

92. The gene mutation targeted by vemurafenib in melanoma is
    A. PIK3CA E545K.
    B. TERT promoter mutation.
    C. BRAF V600E.
    D. BRAF V599R.

93. The mutated gene targeted by ipilimumab in melanoma is
    A. BRAF.
    B. HRAS.
    C. KIT.
    D. None of the above.

94. The following is NOT a high-risk feature in cutaneous SCC:
    A. Size >2 cm.
    B. Location on the non–hair-bearing lip.
    C. High mitotic rate.
    D. Poorly differentiated histological features.

95. The following is NOT a high-risk feature in cutaneous SCC:
    A. Immunosuppressed state.

B. Perineural invasion.
C. Recurrence.
D. Thickness >1 mm.

96. The following is NOT a high-risk type of BCC:
    A. Sclerosing.
    B. Nodular.
    C. Morpheaform.
    D. Infiltrative.

97. Muir-Torre syndrome, a variant of hereditary non-polyposis colorectal cancer syndrome, should be investigated in patients found to have
    A. Sebaceous adenoma.
    B. Sebaceous carcinoma.
    C. Ceruminous adenocarcinoma.
    D. Both A and B.

98. SLNB may be useful in certain cases of
    A. Eccrine adenocarcinoma.
    B. Apocrine adenocarcinoma.
    C. Sebaceous gland carcinoma.
    D. All of the above.

99. Actinic keratoses are NOT commonly treated with
    A. Topical 5-FU.
    B. Topical imiquimod.
    C. Electrodesiccation.
    D. Electronic brachytherapy.

100. In patients with Merkel cell carcinoma, radiation therapy
    A. Has been shown to prolong survival if used in the adjuvant setting.
    B. Is rarely used, as Merkel cell cancer is not radiosensitive.
    C. Is an appropriate primary or nodal therapy if surgery cannot be done.
    D. Should only be done for palliation.

## Answers

| | | |
|---|---|---|
| 1. T | 17. F | 33. T |
| 2. T | 18. F | 34. F |
| 3. T | 19. F | 35. T |
| 4. F | 20. T | 36. T |
| 5. F | 21. T | 37. F |
| 6. F | 22. F | 38. F |
| 7. T | 23. T | 39. T |
| 8. T | 24. F | 40. T |
| 9. F | 25. T | 41. T |
| 10. T | 26. F | 42. T |
| 11. F | 27. T | 43. F |
| 12. T | 28. T | 44. T |
| 13. T | 29. T | 45. T |
| 14. T | 30. T | 46. F |
| 15. F | 31. F | 47. T |
| 16. T | 32. T | 48. F |

| | | |
|---|---|---|
| 49. F | 67. D | 85. D |
| 50. T | 68. C | 86. A |
| 51. D | 69. D | 87. B |
| 52. A | 70. C | 88. C |
| 53. D | 71. C | 89. B |
| 54. A | 72. D | 90. A |
| 55. D | 73. D | 91. C |
| 56. A | 74. A | 92. C |
| 57. A | 75. B | 93. D |
| 58. C | 76. B | 94. C |
| 59. A | 77. B | 95. D |
| 60. B | 78. D | 96. B |
| 61. A | 79. D | 97. D |
| 62. A | 80. B | 98. D |
| 63. D | 81. A | 99. D |
| 64. C | 82. D | 100. C |
| 65. C | 83. D | |
| 66. D | 84. B | |

## Core Knowledge

### MELANOMA

- The incidence of melanoma in the United States and Western Europe is rising dramatically; in the United States among men, its incidence is increasing faster than any other cancer.

- Risk factors for melanoma include family history, prior melanoma, atypical moles, dysplastic nevi, some rare genetic predisposition mutations, and sun exposure.

- Melanomas occur in any ethnic group, but individuals who have fair skin that sunburns easily and does not tan are most susceptible.

- The three most important pathological characteristics of a melanoma are Breslow tumor thickness, ulceration, and mitotic rate.

- Other predictors of survival include clinical nodal staging, the number of positive nodes, and age.

- Sentinel lymph node biopsy (SLNB) is not necessary in pure desmoplastic melanomas but is necessary in mixed desmoplastic tumors.

- Among patients undergoing SLNB, SLN status is the most important prognostic factor.

- Staging
  - Stage 0: melanoma in situ
  - Stage IA: ≤1.0 mm thick, no ulceration, mitotic rate <1/mm$^2$, and node-negative
  - Stage IB: ≤1.0 mm thick, ulceration or mitotic rate ≥1/mm$^2$; or 1.01 to 2.0 mm thick without ulceration; and node-negative

- Stage IIA: 1.01 to 2.0 mm thick with ulceration; or 2.01 to 4.0 mm thick without ulceration; and node-negative
- Stage IIB: 2.01 to 4.0 mm thick with ulceration; or >4.0 mm without ulceration; and node-negative
- Stage IIIA: any thickness, nonulcerated, with micrometastases
- Stage IIIB: any thickness, ulcerated, with micrometastases; or any thickness, nonulcerated, with macrometastases or in-transit/satellite metastases but no metastatic nodes
- Stage IIIC: any thickness, ulcerated with macrometastases
- Stage IV: distant metastases

- Margins for wide local excision
  - Melanoma in situ: 0.5 cm around visible lesion
  - Thickness 1.0 mm or less: 1.0-cm margin
  - Thickness 1.01 to 2.0 mm: 1.0- to 2.0-cm margin
  - Thickness 2.01 cm or more: 2.0-cm margin (can be modified for anatomical or cosmetic considerations in the head and neck)

- No significant tissue elevation or flap closure should be performed until margins are confirmed to be clear.

- SLNB
  - This procedure has a 95% identification rate.
  - The Multicenter Selective Lymphadenectomy Trial (MSLT)-I trial demonstrated significant improvement in disease-free survival with SLNB compared with observation (but not overall survival).
  - The role of SLNB in melanomas <1.0 mm or >4.0 mm thick is unclear.
  - SLNB should be discussed and offered to patients with thin melanomas between 0.76 and 1.0 mm thick, with ulceration or a high mitotic rate.

- Adjuvant therapy is currently limited to adjuvant interferon and radiation therapy. Neither has been shown to improve overall survival rates.

- Novel therapies include the BRAF inhibitor vemurafenib and the monoclonal antibody against cytotoxic T-lymphocyte antigen-4 (CTLA-4), ipilimumab. Both have demonstrated improved survival rates in patients with stage IV melanoma. As of 2013, neither had yet been approved for use as adjuvant therapy.

- The oncogenic kinase BRAF is targeted by vemurafenib. BRAF is mutated in 45% of metastatic melanomas and is most commonly seen as the BRAF V600E mutation.

- Non–sun-exposed melanomas are more frequently characterized by KIT mutations rather than BRAF.

## BASAL AND SQUAMOUS CELL CANCERS

- High-risk features of skin squamous cell cancers (SCCs) include
  - Size >2 cm.
  - Thickness >2 mm.
  - Clark level IV or greater.
  - Perineural invasion.
  - Primary site on the ear or non–hair-bearing lip.
  - Poorly differentiated or undifferentiated histological features.
  - Nodal metastases.

- Basal cell cancers (BCCs) and SCCs arising in the head and neck are most likely to recur.

- High-risk sites correspond to the "mask area" on the face (Figure 1-3).

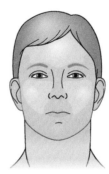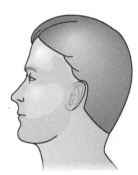

**Figure 1-3** High-risk sites for basal and squamous cell cancers correspond to the "mask area" on the face.

- BCCs and SCCs are associated with sun exposure and immunosuppression.

- BCCs with an aggressive nature include the following: micronodular, infiltrative, sclerosing, morpheaform (not nodular, superficial).

- Destructive therapies may be used in patients with multiple low-risk tumors. These include curettage, electrodesiccation, and cryotherapy.

- Imiquimod is an immune modulator sometimes used to treat small superficial BCCs.

- Skin SCC with neck nodal metastases requires neck dissection; postoperative radiation therapy is based on pathological findings.

- Skin SCC with parotid metastases generally requires both superficial parotidectomy and neck dissection.

## MERKEL CELL CARCINOMA

- Merkel cell carcinoma is a rare, aggressive neuroendocrine skin cancer.

- Local recurrence occurs in 25% to 30% of cases.

- Regional metastases develop in 50% to 60% of cases.

- Distant metastases develop in 30% to 40% of cases.

- The 5-year survival rate is 30% to 60%, although this number reflects causes of morbidity not related to Merkel cell cancer in an elderly population.

- Merkel cell polyomavirus (MCV) is detected in 50% to 100% of patient samples.

- Immunostaining should include CK-20 (positive) and TTF1 (negative) to differentiate these tumors from metastatic small-cell lung cancer.

- SLNB is indicated for clinically negative nodes.

- Positive SLNs may prompt either completion nodal dissection or radiation therapy to the involved nodal basin.

## DERMATOFIBROSARCOMA PROTUBERANS

- Dermatofibrosarcoma protuberans (DFSP) is a rare, low-grade sarcoma of fibroblast origin.

- It has very low rates of metastases.

- Low rates of local recurrence are seen after complete excision.

- DFSP is characterized by a t(17:22) translocation resulting in the overexpression of platelet-derived growth factor receptor (PDGFR).

- Imatinib is used in unresectable, recurrent, or metastatic DFSP.

## SUGGESTED READING

Balch CM, Gershenwald JE, Soong SJ, Thompson JF, Atkins MB, et al. Final version of 2009 AJCC Melanoma Staging and Classification. J Clin Oncol 2009;27:6199–206.

Ebrahimi A, Moncrieff MD, Clark JR, Shannon KF, Gao K, et al. Predicting the pattern of regional metastases from cutaneous squamous cell carcinoma of the head and neck based on location of the primary. Head Neck 2009;32:1288–94.

Fields RC, Busam KJ, Chou JF, Panageas KS, Pulitzer MP, et al. Five hundred patients with Merkel cell carcinoma evaluated at a single institution. Ann Surg 2011;254:465–73.

Morton DL, Thompson JF, Cochran AJ, Mozzillo N, Elashoff R, et al. Sentinel-node biopsy or nodal observation in melanoma. N Engl J Med 2006;355:1307–17.

National Comprehensive Cancer Network. Guidelines on basal and squamous cell carcinoma, <http://www.nccn.org/professionals/physician_gls/pdf/nmsc.pdf>; [accessed 13.01.14].

National Comprehensive Cancer Network. Guidelines on DFSP, <http://www.nccn.org/professionals/physician_gls/pdf/dfsp.pdf>; [accessed 13.01.14].

National Comprehensive Cancer Network. Guidelines on melanoma, <http://www.nccn.org/professionals/physician_gls/pdf/melanoma.pdf>; [accessed 13.01.14].

National Comprehensive Cancer Network. Guidelines on Merkel cell carcinoma, <http://www.nccn.org/professionals/physician_gls/pdf/mcc.pdf>; [accessed 13.01.14].

Pathak I, O'Brien CJ, Petersen-Schaeffer K, McNeil EB, McMahon J, et al. Do nodal metastases from cutaneous melanoma of the head and neck follow a clinically predictable pattern? Head Neck 2001;23:785–90.

## 2 Eyelids and Orbit

## Questions

**TRUE/FALSE**

1. The most important barrier to tumor spreading within the orbit is the bony skeleton. (T/F)

2. Epiphora is typically associated with overproduction of tears from the lacrimal gland. (T/F)

3. Lymphatic drainage from the medial upper eyelid is different than that from the lateral eyelid. (T/F)

4. Venous drainage of the eyelids is chiefly via the facial venous system. (T/F)

5. The lacrimal gland has two anatomically discrete lobes. (T/F)

6. The anterior and posterior ethmoidal foramina are located 24 mm and 36 mm, respectively, from the eyelids. (T/F)

7. The Tenon capsule is penetrated by the posterior components of the extraocular muscles as they attach to the annulus of Zinn at the orbital apex. (T/F)

8. The medial canthal tendon affects function of the lacrimal drainage system. (T/F)

9. Most intraorbital lesions are benign. (T/F)

10. Orbital extension from adjacent primary tumors is more common than are primary orbital malignancies. (T/F)

11. The most common pediatric intraorbital malignancy is neuroblastoma. (T/F)

12. Pleomorphic adenomas are the most common neoplasm of the lacrimal gland. (T/F)

13. Most patients given a diagnosis of retinoblastoma will have a positive family history. (T/F)

14. Rhabdomyosarcomas less than 5 cm involving the orbit are generally considered to have good prognoses. (T/F)

15. A chalazion occurs because of obstruction of a meibomian gland. (T/F)

16. Most deaths from uveal melanoma occur because of local recurrence with subsequent direct invasion of the central nervous system (CNS). (T/F)

17. Squamous cell carcinoma is the most common cutaneous malignancy occurring on the eyelid. (T/F)

18. Visual acuity should be documented when any orbital or eyelid neoplasm is evaluated. (T/F)

19. Normal orbital contents typically "light up" on positron emission tomographic (PET) scanning. (T/F)

20. Lacrimal gland neoplasms are rarely palpable. (T/F)

21. Fine-needle aspiration is an accepted modality for diagnosis of suspected metastatic disease within the orbit. (T/F)

22. Intraocular lymphoma may or may not be associated with primary CNS lymphoma. (T/F)

23. Sebaceous adenocarcinoma of the eyelid is commonly misdiagnosed as a benign entity. (T/F)

24. Rhabdomyosarcoma of the orbit will stain positive for desmin and myogenin on immunohistochemical analysis. (T/F)

25. Ocular ultrasound is contraindicated when papilledema is suspected. (T/F)

26. Asymptomatic optic gliomas may be safely observed with serial imaging. (T/F)

27. Brachytherapy is an accepted treatment modality for choroidal melanoma. (T/F)

28. Retinoblastomas less than 3 mm are best treated surgically. (T/F)

29. Corticosteroids are the treatment of choice for orbital pseudotumor. (T/F)

30. Irradiation and surgical enucleation have equivalent oncological outcomes in the management of medium-sized ocular melanomas. (T/F)

31. In general, the optic nerve can tolerate a total dose of radiation of up to 70 Gy. (T/F)

32. Pediatric patients with orbital rhabdomyosarcoma require chemotherapy. (T/F)

33. Radiation-induced vision loss will typically manifest within weeks of the initiation of treatment. (T/F)

34. Mohs surgery is contraindicated for basal cell carcinoma of the eyelids. (T/F)

35. Excision of conjunctival melanoma requires at least 1 cm margins. (T/F)

36. Surgilube is the preferred product for lubricating the eye when corneal shields are placed. (T/F)

37. Orbital rhabdomyosarcoma may present with cervical lymphatic involvement. (T/F)

38. The transcaruncular approach offers good exposure of both the medial orbit and orbital apex. (T/F)

39. Anesthesia will not significantly affect the size of the pupil. (T/F)

40. Sentinel node biopsy is contraindicated for conjunctival melanoma. (T/F)

41. Both the upper and lower eyelids have sufficient laxity to facilitate primary closure of most full-thickness defects. (T/F)

42. When the medial canthal tendon is partially resected, reconstruction requires fixation to either bone or periosteum. (T/F)

43. Lateral canthotomy is an acceptable method for increasing the length of the lower eyelid to facilitate primary closure. (T/F)

44. The Hughes flap for eyelid reconstruction is analogous to the Karapandzic flap for lip reconstruction. (T/F)

45. When sebaceous adenocarcinoma involving the medial canthus is resected, the lacrimal drainage system should be reconstructed immediately. (T/F)

## MULTIPLE CHOICE

46. What is the correct order of these orbital foramina from lateral to medial?
    A. Optic canal, inferior orbital fissure, superior orbital fissure, anterior ethmoid
    B. Inferior orbital fissure, optic canal, superior orbital fissure, anterior ethmoid
    C. Inferior orbital fissure, superior orbital fissure, optic canal, anterior ethmoid
    D. Superior orbital fissure, inferior orbital fissure, optic canal, anterior ethmoid

47. What comprises the conjunctiva?
    A. Respiratory-type epithelium
    B. Nonkeratinized stratified squamous epithelium
    C. Cuboidal epithelium
    D. Keratinized stratified squamous epithelium

48. What innervates Müller muscle?
    A. Cranial nerve (CN) III
    B. Postganglionic sympathetic fibers from the superior cervical ganglion
    C. CN IV
    D. CN VI

49. Which is NOT a bone comprising the orbit?
    A. Zygomatic
    B. Maxillary
    C. Palatine
    D. Temporal

50. What best describes the trajectory of the infraorbital nerve?
    A. Exits the inferior orbital fissure, runs along the floor of the orbit, from lateral to medial
    B. Exits the superior orbital fissure, runs along the floor of the orbit, from lateral to medial
    C. Exits the inferior orbital fissure, runs along the inferolateral wall of the orbit
    D. Exits the superior orbital fissure, runs along the inferomedial wall of the orbit

51. What is the name and function of structure A in Figure 2-1?

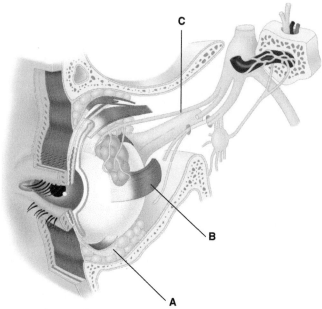

**Figure 2-1** Note: Left eye depicted from parafrontal view; left side of image is medial, right side of image is lateral. (Adapted from Shah JP, Patel SG, Singh B. Jatin Shah's head and neck: surgery and oncology. 4th ed. Philadelphia: Mosby; 2012 [Figure 4-18].)

    A. Whitnall ligament (supports globe and retracts lower lid)
    B. Lockwood ligament (supports globe and retracts lower lid)
    C. Whitnall ligament (assists with extraocular muscle function)
    D. Lockwood ligament (assists with extraocular muscle function)

52. What innervates structure B in Figure 2-1?
    A. CN III
    B. CN IV
    C. CN V
    D. CN VI

53. How would an injury to structure C in Figure 2-1 present?
    A. Epiphora
    B. Diplopia
    C. Dry eye
    D. Visual loss

54. What extraocular muscle is at most risk during transconjunctival exposure of the inferior orbital rim?
    A. Inferior rectus
    B. Medial rectus
    C. Superior oblique
    D. Inferior oblique

55. List the layers of the upper eyelid (above the tarsal plate) in order.
    A. Skin, orbicularis oculi, orbital septum, preaponeurotic fat, levator palpebrae superioris, Müller muscle, conjunctiva
    B. Skin, orbital septum, preaponeurotic fat, orbicularis oculi, levator palpebrae superioris, Müller muscle, conjunctiva
    C. Skin, orbicularis oculi, orbital septum, preaponeurotic fat, levator palpebrae superioris, conjunctiva
    D. Skin, orbicularis oculi, levator palpebrae superioris, orbital septum, preaponeurotic fat, Müller muscle, conjunctiva

56. What is true regarding sebaceous adenocarcinomas of the eyelid?
    A. Lymphatic metastases almost never occur.
    B. Multifocal extension with skip lesions is common.
    C. Outcomes are correlated with Breslow depth.
    D. Incidence is increased in patients with Gorlin syndrome.

57. From where do primary ocular melanomas frequently arise?
    A. Lens
    B. Uveal tract
    C. Conjunctiva
    D. Vitreous humor

58. What is true regarding retinoblastoma?
    A. Bilateral disease implies a germline mutation.
    B. Most cases are diagnosed in school-aged children.
    C. Unilateral disease typically presents at an earlier age than bilateral disease.
    D. Patients with retinoblastoma are at low risk of second primary malignancies.

59. What subtype of rhabdomyosarcoma is most common in the orbit?
    A. Embryonal (nonbotryoid)
    B. Alveolar
    C. Anaplastic
    D. Embryonal (botryoid)

60. An elderly patient presents with treatment-refractory uveitis, and a fundus examination reveals a yellow mass deep to the retina. What is the most likely diagnosis?
    A. Pseudotumor
    B. Lymphoma
    C. Ocular melanoma
    D. Nerve sheath tumor

61. A young patient presents with proptosis and an orbital mass. Biopsy reveals malignant lymphoid cells of myeloid origin. What is the diagnosis?
    A. Extramedullary plasmacytoma
    B. Hodgkin lymphoma
    C. Granulocytic sarcoma (i.e., chloroma)
    D. Acute lymphocytic leukemia

62. Oncological outcomes in uveal melanoma are best predicted by
    A. Mutational status of a tumor suppressor gene on chromosome 3.
    B. Breslow depth.
    C. Patient age.
    D. Size of the primary lesion.

63. A child with known neurofibromatosis presents with mild proptosis, and examination reveals edema of the optic disc. What is the most likely diagnosis?
    A. Acoustic neuroma with anterior skull base extension
    B. Neurofibroma of a cutaneous branch of CN V$_1$
    C. Optic nerve glioma
    D. Skull base meningioma

64. How does the American Joint Committee on Cancer (AJCC) stage the primary tumor in conjunctival melanoma?
    A. Depth of invasion
    B. Anatomical extent
    C. Size (in millimeters)
    D. A and B

65. An elderly patient presents with a rapidly growing hyperkeratotic mass of the lower eyelid. What is the most likely diagnosis?
    A. Keratoacanthoma
    B. Squamous cell carcinoma
    C. Basal cell carcinoma
    D. Amelanotic melanoma

66. What is the most common tumor to metastasize to the orbit?
    A. Breast
    B. Melanoma
    C. Lung
    D. Prostate

67. A patient is diagnosed with bilateral xanthelasma. What laboratory test is indicated?
    A. No testing necessary
    B. Complete blood count (CBC)
    C. Lactate dehydrogenase (LDH)
    D. Lipid panel

68. A patient presents with diplopia, ophthalmoplegia, ptosis, periorbital numbness and pain but has intact vision. The abnormality most likely involves the
    A. Orbital apex.
    B. Superior orbital fissure.
    C. Inferior orbital fissure.
    D. Cerebral cortex.

69. What characteristic would upstage an upper eyelid carcinoma from T2 to T3 according to the AJCC staging system?
    A. Perineural invasion
    B. Size greater than 2 cm
    C. Excision that requires enucleation
    D. Any of the above

70. What is the preferred imaging modality when orbital pseudotumor is suspected clinically?
    A. Magnetic resonance (MR)
    B. Positron emission tomography (PET)
    C. Computed tomography (CT)
    D. Tagged white blood cell (WBC) nuclear scan

71. A patient is given a diagnosis of von Hippel-Lindau syndrome. What is the classic ophthalmic finding associated with this condition?
    A. Plexiform neurofibroma of the eyelid
    B. Retinal capillary hemangioma
    C. Retinal astrocytoma
    D. Retinal arteriovenous malformation

72. What best describes the pathological appearance of retinoblastoma?
    A. Atypical melanocytic cells
    B. Tumor cells with an absence of calcification
    C. Malignant cells arising within immature retina
    D. Malignant cells arising within a myxoid stroma

73. What best describes chemosis?
    A. Conjunctival edema
    B. Persistent tearing
    C. Swollen optic disc
    D. Scleral erythema

74. All of the following are accepted radiation modalities for treating uveal melanoma EXCEPT
    A. Neutrons.
    B. Brachytherapy.
    C. Protons.
    D. Helium ion.

75. What is a principle of treatment of orbital rhabdomyosarcoma?
    A. Initial aggressive surgical management is typically preferred.
    B. Surgery is typically performed only for recurrent or persistent tumors.
    C. Because of its impact on vision, radiation is not part of the treatment algorithm.
    D. Chemotherapy is typically reserved for metastatic disease.

76. What structure has the lowest tolerance for radiation?
    A. Retina
    B. Optic nerve
    C. Lens
    D. Cornea

77. Which of the following are accepted adjuvant modalities in the treatment of conjunctival melanoma after local excision?
    A. Application of alcohol
    B. Cryotherapy
    C. Radiation therapy
    D. All of the above

78. What is true regarding radiation-induced corneal injury?
    A. Symptoms of corneal injury from radiation typically manifest months to years after treatment.
    B. Tungsten eye shields are preferred to protect the cornea during electron-based radiation therapy.
    C. Corneal injuries are common with a cumulative dose greater than 30 Gy.
    D. All of the above is true.

79. What is true concerning photocoagulation for retinoblastoma?
    A. It has largely replaced external beam radiation in the adjuvant setting.
    B. It is only considered for patients with bilateral disease.
    C. It is typically reserved for small, posterior tumors.
    D. None of the above is true.

80. Vincristine is commonly used to treat rhabdomyosarcoma. What is its mechanism of action?
    A. Alkylating agent
    B. Inhibits topoisomerase and interferes with DNA uncoiling
    C. Inhibits microtubule formation during M and S phases
    D. Folate antimetabolite that inhibits DNA synthesis

81. After orbitotomy for removal of a benign tumor, a patient develops a rapidly swollen, tense eye in the recovery room. What is the next step?
    A. Elevation of the head of bed
    B. Lateral canthotomy
    C. High-dose intravenous corticosteroids
    D. Administration of mannitol

82. Complete these sentences: For lesions involving the eyebrow, surgical excisions should be oriented ___(1)___. For lesions involving the eyelid, surgical excisions should be oriented ___(2)___.
    A. 1: transversely. 2: vertically.
    B. 1: vertically. 2: transversely.
    C. 1: transversely. 2: transversely.
    D. 1: vertically. 2: vertically.

83. Immediately after lateral orbitotomy for tumor resection, a patient complains of diplopia. What is the best next step?
    A. Reassurance with observation
    B. Tape the eye closed for 2 weeks
    C. Surgical reexploration
    D. Lateral canthotomy

84. Match the following procedures with their description:
    i. Removal of the eye, sparing the sclera.
    ii. Removal of the eye, including the sclera.
    iii. Removal of the orbital contents.
    A. i: Enucleation; ii: Evisceration; iii: Exenteration
    B. i: Evisceration; ii: Enucleation; iii: Exenteration
    C. i: Evisceration; ii: Exenteration; iii: Enucleation
    D. i: Exenteration; ii: Enucleation; iii: Evisceration

85. During resection of an orbital tumor, a patient experiences profound bradycardia. What is the likely explanation and recommended treatment?
    A. Vagally mediated oculocardiac reflex; treat with atropine
    B. Vagally mediated oculocardiac reflex; treat with epinephrine
    C. Sympathetically mediated oculocardiac reflex; treat with atropine
    D. Sympathetically mediated oculocardiac reflex; treat with epinephrine

86. A patient undergoes resection via orbitotomy with adjuvant radiation for a malignant tumor. Two months later, he develops painful uveitis of the contralateral eye. What is a likely explanation?
    A. Contralateral tumor recurrence
    B. Radiation-induced injury
    C. Paraneoplastic syndrome
    D. Sympathetic ophthalmia

87. What is the standard approach for removal of intraconal lacrimal tumors?
    A. Lateral orbitotomy
    B. Medial orbitotomy
    C. Combined craniofacial approach
    D. Transcaruncular approach

88. After the resection depicted in Figure 2-2, scant clear drainage from the orbital defect tests positive for β-transferrin. Which is NOT a possible explanation?

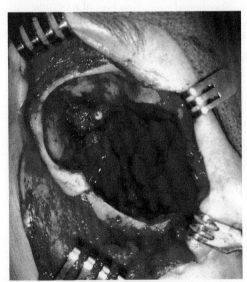

**Figure 2-2** (From Shah JP, Patel SG, Singh B. Jatin Shah's head and neck: surgery and oncology. 4th ed. Philadelphia: Mosby; 2012 [Figure 4-119].)

    A. Cerebrospinal fluid (CSF) leakage from a dural defect communicating with the anterior cranial fossa
    B. Residual vitreous humor
    C. CSF leakage from the dural sheath of an optic nerve stump
    D. All of the above

89. What best describes a relative advantage of a transconjunctival incision over a subciliary incision?

    A. Lower incidence of extraocular muscle injury
    B. Superior exposure of the inferior orbital rim
    C. Less likely to cause ectropion
    D. Less likely to cause entropion

90. A patient presents with biopsy-confirmed adenoid cystic carcinoma of the lacrimal gland. Her CT is depicted in Figure 2-3. What consideration is necessary before embarking on surgical excision?

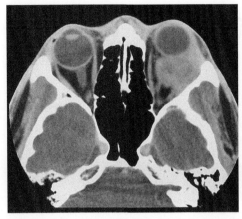

**Figure 2-3** (From Shah JP, Patel SG, Singh B. Jatin Shah's head and neck: surgery and oncology. 4th ed. Philadelphia: Mosby; 2012 [Figure 4-125].)

    A. Assess for perineural invasion into the cavernous sinus
    B. Assess the patency of nasolacrimal drainage
    C. Assess for invasion of the anterior cranial fossa via the superior orbital fissure
    D. A and C

91. Why were the skin sutures in Figure 2-4 below left long?

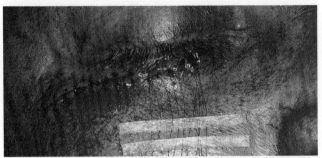

**Figure 2-4** (From Shah JP, Patel SG, Singh B. Jatin Shah's head and neck: surgery and oncology. 4th ed. Philadelphia: Mosby; 2012 [Figure 4-38].)

    A. To help prevent entropion
    B. To avoid corneal abrasion
    C. To facilitate easier removal of sutures
    D. To help prevent enophthalmos

92. What structures comprise the posterior lamella?
    A. Skin and orbicularis oculi muscle
    B. Tarsus and conjunctiva
    C. Orbicularis oculi muscle and tarsus
    D. Tarsus and orbital septum

93. A lower eyelid defect is repaired with the use of an inferiorly based advancement flap and malar skin. What is an expected complication of this technique?
    A. Entropion
    B. Ectropion
    C. Exophthalmos
    D. Enophthalmos

94. What type of reconstruction is illustrated in Figure 2-5?

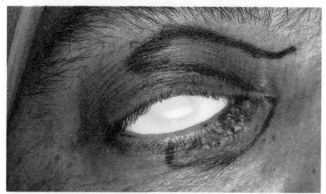

**Figure 2-5** (From Shah JP, Patel SG, Singh B. Jatin Shah's head and neck: surgery and oncology. 4th ed. Philadelphia: Mosby; 2012 [Figure 4-41].)

    A. Rotation flap
    B. Transposition flap
    C. Advancement flap
    D. Axial flap

95. What principle applies to reconstruction of the anticipated full-thickness eyelid defect depicted in Figure 2-6?

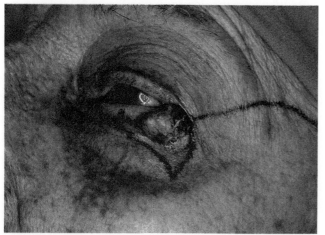

**Figure 2-6** (From Shah JP, Patel SG, Singh B. Jatin Shah's head and neck: surgery and oncology. 4th ed. Philadelphia: Mosby; 2012 [Figure 4-53].)

    A. Only the anterior lamella needs to be reconstructed.
    B. Only the posterior lamella needs to be reconstructed.
    C. Both the anterior and posterior lamella must be reconstructed, and at least one of the layers must be vascularized.
    D. Both the anterior and posterior lamella must be reconstructed, and both of the layers must be vascularized.

96. What describes the correct placement of a gold weight?
    A. Immediately under the skin
    B. On the tarsal plate, deep to the orbicularis oculi
    C. Superior to (above) the tarsal plate, deep to the orbicularis oculi
    D. Within the orbicularis oculi muscle

97. What is the most important consideration for orbital function when performing orbital-sparing maxillectomy?
    A. Integrity of the orbital floor support
    B. Sparing of the nasolacrimal system
    C. Preservation of the infraorbital nerve
    D. Avoidance of damage to the orbicularis oculi muscle

98. Which of the following is NOT an advantage of endoscopic dacryocystorhinostomy when compared with a traditional open technique?
    A. Absence of a skin incision
    B. Less disruption of the medial canthus
    C. Superior functional outcomes
    D. Ability to manage concurrent sinonasal pathology

99. An elderly man presents with cicatricial ectropion after orbit-sparing maxillectomy. What best explains the etiology of his problem?
    A. Shortened anterior lamella
    B. Shortened posterior lamella
    C. Damaged orbital septum
    D. Damaged tarsal plate

100. What surgical procedure is depicted in Figure 2-7?

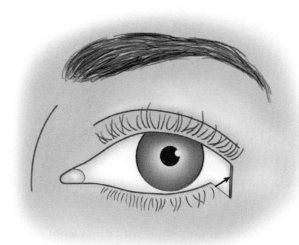

**Figure 2-7** (From Shah JP, Patel SG, Singh B. Jatin Shah's head and neck: surgery and oncology. 4th ed. Philadelphia: Mosby; 2012 [Figure 4-145].)

    A. Lateral tarsal strip
    B. Lateral canthoplasty
    C. Lateral tarsorrhaphy
    D. Lateral canthotomy

## Answers

| | | | | | |
|---|---|---|---|---|---|
| 1. | F | 35. | F | 69. | D |
| 2. | F | 36. | F | 70. | C |
| 3. | T | 37. | T | 71. | B |
| 4. | F | 38. | T | 72. | C |
| 5. | T | 39. | F | 73. | A |
| 6. | F | 40. | F | 74. | A |
| 7. | T | 41. | F | 75. | B |
| 8. | T | 42. | T | 76. | C |
| 9. | T | 43. | T | 77. | D |
| 10. | T | 44. | F | 78. | B |
| 11. | F | 45. | F | 79. | C |
| 12. | T | 46. | C | 80. | C |
| 13. | F | 47. | B | 81. | B |
| 14. | T | 48. | B | 82. | B |
| 15. | T | 49. | D | 83. | A |
| 16. | F | 50. | A | 84. | B |
| 17. | F | 51. | B | 85. | A |
| 18. | T | 52. | D | 86. | D |
| 19. | F | 53. | C | 87. | A |
| 20. | F | 54. | D | 88. | D |
| 21. | T | 55. | A | 89. | C |
| 22. | T | 56. | B | 90. | A |
| 23. | T | 57. | B | 91. | B |
| 24. | T | 58. | A | 92. | B |
| 25. | F | 59. | D | 93. | B |
| 26. | T | 60. | B | 94. | B |
| 27. | T | 61. | C | 95. | C |
| 28. | F | 62. | A | 96. | B |
| 29. | T | 63. | C | 97. | A |
| 30. | T | 64. | D | 98. | C |
| 31. | F | 65. | A | 99. | A |
| 32. | T | 66. | A | 100. | B |
| 33. | F | 67. | D | | |
| 34. | F | 68. | B | | |

## Core Knowledge

- The orbital periosteum is a critical barrier protecting against intraorbital tumor extension.

- In general, the lateral two thirds of the upper eyelid lymphatics drain to the preauricular/parotid nodes, and the medial one third drains to the perifacial nodes.

- Venous drainage of the eyelids involves both the facial venous system and the cavernous sinus via the ophthalmic vein.

- The bony orbit comprises the following bones: frontal, lacrimal, ethmoid, zygomatic, maxillary, palatine, and sphenoid.

- The anterior and posterior ethmoidal foramina are located 24 mm and 36 mm, respectively, from the anterior lacrimal crest of the orbit. The optic nerve is approximately 42 mm from the anterior lacrimal crest.

- Whitnall ligament suspends the globe superiorly and functions as an upper lid retractor. Lockwood ligament suspends the globe inferiorly and functions as a lower lid retractor.

- The inferior oblique muscle separates the inferior nasal and medial fat pads and must be carefully preserved during dissection in this region; inadvertent damage may cause diplopia. However, transient postoperative diplopia is common and typically resolves without intervention.

- The medial canthal tendon contributes to the pumping function of the lacrimal drainage system and has two components that straddle the lacrimal canaliculi before inserting on the orbital bone. The remnant medial canthal tendon should be securely fixated in order to ensure alignment and support of the lower eyelid.

- The layers of the eyelids vary based on level (i.e., above/below the tarsus), and knowledge of them is critical when ablative or reconstructive oncological surgery is performed.

- The most common benign neoplasm of the lacrimal gland is pleomorphic adenoma. The most common malignant neoplasm is adenoid cystic carcinoma.

- Primary ocular melanomas typically arise from melanocytes (of neural crest lineage) arising along scleral emissary veins of the uveal tract, most commonly within the choroid. Many radiation-based protocols have proven successful in treating uveal melanoma. In the Collaborative Ocular Melanoma Study, a randomized controlled trial, surgical enucleation and brachytherapy had similar outcomes. Uveal melanoma outcomes are strongly predicted by the mutational status of the *BAP1* tumor suppressor gene. Most deaths due to uveal melanoma are caused by distant metastases.

- Germline mutations of the *RB1* gene are associated with inherited retinoblastoma and may represent a familial or de novo mutation. They are always present in bilateral cases and are seen at an earlier age because of the "two-hit" model of pathogenesis. Generally, only advanced retinoblastoma (group D and E) may require surgery; less advanced disease (groups A-C) can often be treated nonsurgically, and intraarterial chemotherapy may be effective even for large lesions.

- Orbital rhabdomyosarcomas are, in general, considered to have good prognoses, whereas parameningeal locations have worse prognoses. Most orbital rhabdomyosarcomas are botryoid embryonal type and manifest as retrobulbar masses. Desmin, muscle-specific actin, and myogenin are immunohistochemical stains used to identify rhabdomyosarcoma. Treatment algorithms for orbital rhabdomyosarcoma are multidisciplinary and depend on the site of involvement and the extent of disease. Biopsy of lymph nodes suggestive of cancer based on clinical or radiological evidence may assist with clinical group assessment and subsequent treatment choices in rhabdomyosarcoma. In general, chemotherapy is first-line treatment, and surgery is reserved for recurrent or persistent tumors. Vincristine, dactinomycin, and cyclophosphamide (VAC) is a commonly used chemotherapy protocol for rhabdomyosarcoma.

- Lymphoma is among the most common malignant orbital tumors and typically presents with uveitis, proptosis, and/or a conjunctival mass.

- Granulocytic sarcoma (i.e., chloroma) is a manifestation of myeloid hematological cancer whose name does not correspond with its pathophysiology and may be seen before or concurrent with acute myelogenous leukemia.

- A chalazion is a chronic inflammatory condition that develops as a result of meibomian gland obstruction. A hordeolum (stye) is an acute purulent infection of otherwise similar pathophysiology.

- Conjunctival melanomas are staged based on the anatomical extent and depth of the primary tumor, as well as the presence of regional and/or distant metastases. Conjunctival melanoma has a propensity for nodal metastasis. Although not as widely accepted as it is for cutaneous disease, sentinel node biopsy may be considered. Surgical excision is first-line treatment, and surgical margins of 2 to 3 mm are generally acceptable. Adjuvant treatments are also frequently used and include application of alcohol, mitomycin C, or both, cryotherapy, and radiation therapy.

- Basal cell carcinoma is the most common cutaneous malignancy occurring on the eyelid. Eyelid carcinoma staging is based on size, anatomical extent, and surgical resectability. Surgical excisions involving the eyelid and eyebrow should take into consideration postoperative function and aesthetic outcome. Mohs surgery for nonmelanomatous cutaneous malignancies of the eyelids can facilitate preservation of critical structures and is oncologically sound.

- Superior orbital fissure syndrome (affecting cranial nerves III, IV, V$_1$, and VI) is distinguished from orbital apex syndrome by preservation of vision.

- Orbital pseudotumor is characterized on computed tomography (CT) by inflammation of the lacrimal gland (most commonly), globe, orbital fat, extraocular muscles, and/or optic nerve. Orbital pseudotumor is typically managed with steroids. Failure to respond to treatment may lead clinicians to question the diagnosis.

- Sebaceous adenocarcinoma is a highly aggressive cancer that is frequently mistaken for a benign condition such as a chalazion. Sebaceous adenocarcinomas may demonstrate lymphatic metastases in 25% of advanced primary lesions.

- All intraorbital structures are at risk from radiation, albeit with different levels of tolerance. Radiation-induced injury to the retina, lens, and optic nerve frequently take months to years to manifest. Radiation to the lens can lead to cataract development, even with very low doses (reported in patients receiving only 2 Gy). Late complications of radiation therapy (e.g., retinopathy, glaucoma, and optic nerve–related visual loss) are typically associated with total doses greater than 50 Gy.

- Postoperative orbital compartment syndrome, typically caused by intraorbital hemorrhage, is a vision-threatening emergency that requires prompt decompression.

- Evisceration refers to removal of the eye with sparing of the sclera. Enucleation involves removal of the eye, including the sclera. Exenteration refers to removal of the orbital contents, which can be accomplished in an eyelid-sparing fashion when oncologically appropriate.

- The oculocardiac reflex is a parasympathetic reaction to traction or pressure that can cause profound bradycardia. It may be prevented with the use of local anesthesia and/or minimization of intraoperative trauma; it can be treated with an anticholinergic drug (acetylcholine antagonist).

- Sympathetic ophthalmia is an autoimmune delayed hypersensitivity reaction in which ocular antigens stimulate inflammation and damage to the contralateral eye after prior surgery or trauma.

- Cicatricial ectropion is caused by vertical deficiency of the anterior lamella due to scarring. Transconjunctival approaches are less likely to cause cicatricial ectropion than are transcutaneous approaches. Lateral canthoplasty can tighten the lower eyelid and help correct ectropion.

- Various anesthetic agents can change the size of the pupil, thereby complicating intraoperative surveillance.

- The anterior lamella refers to skin and orbicularis oculi, and the posterior lamella refers to the tarsus and conjunctiva.

- Local flap closures of eyelid defects should take into account the functional consequences resulting from the trajectory of wound tension. Thus, lower eyelid lesions should recruit tissue along a transverse axis.

- Full-thickness eyelid defects require reconstruction of both anterior and posterior lamella (including conjunctiva, tarsus, and skin). For successful repair, at least one of these layers must be vascularized (such as local flaps interposed around a free cartilage graft).

- The orbital floor must be able to adequately support the orbital contents for acceptable function to be restored after maxillectomy.

- Endoscopic dacryocystorhinostomy has some favorable characteristics when compared with the open technique, although functional outcomes are similar.

- Lacrimal surgery facilitates a potential pathway for tumor spreading into the sinonasal cavity, which is a significant concern when managing infiltrative tumors with a propensity for local recurrence and extension.

- The optic canal is medial to the superior orbital fissure and is traversed by the optic nerve and ophthalmic artery.

- The conjunctiva is composed of thin, transparent, nonkeratinized, stratified squamous epithelium.

- The superior tarsal muscle (Müller muscle) is a sympathetically innervated smooth muscle that raises the upper eyelid.

- The lacrimal gland comprises discrete orbital and palpebral lobes. Function of the orbital lobe can be affected by excision of the palpebral lobe because of the position of the secretory ducts.

- The infraorbital nerve enters the orbit via the inferior orbital fissure, runs along the floor of the orbit, and exits via the infraorbital foramen at the anterior maxilla.

- The abducens nerve (sixth cranial nerve) controls the lateral rectus muscle. Abducens palsy manifests with diplopia and a medially displaced eye.

- The lacrimal gland is innervated from parasympathetic secretomotor fibers along the vidian nerve, which synapse in the pterygopalatine ganglion and join the lacrimal branch along cranial nerve V.

- Tenon capsule is a connective tissue membrane that encircles the globe (except the cornea) and the anterior parts of the extraocular muscles.

- Approximately 80% of orbital lesions are benign.

- The most common malignant lesions to extend into the orbit are skin cancers.

- The most common pediatric intraorbital malignancy is retinoblastoma.

- The most common benign neoplasm of the lacrimal gland is pleomorphic adenoma. The most common malignant neoplasm is adenoid cystic carcinoma.

- Less than 10% of patients with retinoblastoma have a positive family history.

- Optic nerve gliomas occur regularly in children with neurofibromatosis and may be slow-growing, asymptomatic, or both.

- Keratoacanthoma is an epithelial neoplasm of uncertain malignant potential occurring on sun-damaged skin that mimics squamous cell carcinoma but is notable for a rapid growth over weeks.

- Breast carcinoma commonly metastasizes to the orbit and frequently infiltrates extraocular muscles and orbital fat.

- Both visual acuity and visual fields are integral components of any evaluation of orbital pathology.

- Because normal intraorbital contents are typically not metabolically active, they are "dark" on positron emission tomographic (PET) scans.

- Most lacrimal gland neoplasms present with eyelid fullness, proptosis, and/or a palpable mass. Diplopia is a less common presentation.

- Xanthelasma are benign cholesterol-filled plaques of the eyelids associated with hyperlipidemia.

- Suspected metastatic disease within the orbit may be diagnosed with either fine-needle aspiration or open biopsy.

- Primary central nervous system lymphoma may present with ocular involvement.

- Von Hippel-Lindau syndrome is an autosomal-dominant condition associated with multiple hemangiomas, and involvement of the retina is frequent.

- Retinoblasts are malignant cells with basophilic nuclei and scant cytoplasm arising within immature retina and may demonstrate calcification and Homer Wright rosettes.

- Chemosis is a nonspecific finding of conjunctival edema.

- Ocular ultrasound is commonly used and versatile in the evaluation of benign and malignant conditions.

- Optic gliomas without significant visual symptoms or compression of adjacent structures may be observed and serially imaged.

- In select cases of intraocular melanoma, $I^{125}$ brachytherapy can be eye-sparing with similar oncological outcomes to surgery.

- In general, the corneal radiation threshold is 50 Gy, and acute injuries can be very bothersome to patients.

- Photocoagulation may be an effective primary treatment for highly selected, posterior retinoblastomas less than 6 mm in size.

- Surgilube contains chlorhexidine and is not meant for use on or near the eyes. Only ophthalmically approved products should be used.

- The transcaruncular approach offers good exposure of both the medial orbit and orbital apex, although careful dissection is required to avoid inadvertent herniation of orbital fat.

- Intraconal lacrimal tumors are best accessed via lateral orbitotomy.

- Damage to the dural sheath surrounding the optic nerve may lead to cerebral spinal fluid (CSF) leakage. Fluids other than CSF, such as perilymph and vitreous humor, contain β-transferrin.

- Adenoid cystic carcinoma has a propensity for perineural invasion. Tumor extension via the superior orbital fissure involves the middle cranial fossa.

- Corneal abrasions can occur from inadvertent injury caused by the short tails of nonabsorbable sutures.

- The upper eyelid has significantly more laxity than the lower eyelid.

- A transposition flap helps to reorient tension and is rotated over intervening normal tissue before being inset into the defect.

- Lateral canthotomy may provide up to 5 mm of additional lid advancement.

- The Hughes flap for lower eyelid reconstruction involves a staged procedure in which tissue is borrowed from the ipsilateral upper eyelid and is thus analogous to the Abbe lip-switch reconstruction.

- A gold weight should be sutured to the tarsal plate, deep to orbicularis oculi muscle.

## SUGGESTED READING

Ahmad SM, Esmaeli B. Metastatic tumors of the orbit and ocular adnexa. Curr Opin Ophthalmol 2007;18(5):405–13.

Ainbinder DJ, Esmaeli B, Groo SC, Finger PT, Brooks JP. Introduction of the 7th edition eyelid carcinoma classification system from the American Joint Committee on Cancer-International Union Against Cancer staging manual. Arch Pathol Lab Med 2009;133(8): 1256–61.

Brownstein S. Malignant melanoma of the conjunctiva. Cancer Control 2004;11(5):310–6.

Carter SR. Surgical approaches to orbital tumors. Ophthalmol Clin North Am 1999;12(2):265–78.

Czyz CN, Cahill KV, Foster JA. Reconstructive designs for the eyelids. Oper Techn Otolaryngol 2011;22:35–46.

Dutton JJ. Clinical and surgical orbital anatomy. Ophthalmol Clin North Am 1996;9(4):527–39.

Honavar SG, Singh AD. Management of advanced retinoblastoma. Ophthalmol Clin North Am 2005;18(1):65–73.

Leyvraz S, Keilholz U. Ocular melanoma: what's new? Curr Opin Oncol 2012;24(2):162–9.

Murchison AP, Walrath JD, Washington CV. Non-surgical treatments of primary, non-melanoma eyelid malignancies: a review. Clin Exp Ophthalmol 2011;39(1):65–83.

Zoumalan CI, Zoumalan RA, Cockerham KP. Surgical management of lacrimal gland tumors. Oper Techn Otolaryngol 2008;19:252–7.

# 3 Nasal Cavity and Paranasal Sinuses

## Questions

**TRUE/FALSE**

1. The majority of the tumors arising from the sinonasal cavity are malignant. (T/F)

2. The majority of cancers of the sinonasal cavity occur in the maxillary sinuses. (T/F)

3. Most sinonasal cancers are adenocarcinomas histologically. (T/F)

4. Sinonasal cancers are more common in smokers. (T/F)

5. Tumor extension into the pterygopalatine fossa worsens the prognosis. (T/F)

6. Contrast-enhanced computed tomography (CT) is preferred over magnetic resonance imaging (MRI) for determining the tumor extent and treatment plan. (T/F)

7. Most squamous cell carcinomas (SCCs) of the nasal cavity originate from the nasal septum. (T/F)

8. Inverted papillomas of the nasal cavity may coexist with an SCC counterpart. (T/F)

9. Inverted papillomas may be successfully treated with an endoscopic approach. (T/F)

10. Most adenocarcinomas originate in the ethmoid sinuses. (T/F)

11. The hallmark of adenoid cystic carcinomas is delayed distant metastasis. (T/F)

12. Radiation therapy improves the overall survival rate in mucosal melanoma. (T/F)

13. Esthesioneuroblastomas have a specific grading and staging system. (T/F)

14. Esthesioneuroblastomas are associated with a higher risk of nodal relapse than are sinonasal SCCs. (T/F)

15. Sinonasal neuroendocrine tumors are diagnosed by consistent expression of neuron-specific markers. (T/F)

16. Sinonasal undifferentiated carcinomas (SNUCs) invading the brain are treated with upfront craniofacial surgery for the best prognosis. (T/F)

17. Rhabdomyosarcomas of the maxillary sinus are treated with upfront surgery. (T/F)

18. NK/T-cell lymphomas are a common type of sinonasal lymphoma in the Western population. (T/F)

19. Sinonasal lymphomas are treated with upfront surgery followed by radiation therapy. (T/F)

20. Nasopharyngeal angiofibromas have a bimodal age distribution. (T/F)

21. Tumors of the maxillary suprastructure have a better prognosis for local control as compared with tumors of the maxillary infrastructure. (T/F)

22. Elective lymph node dissection is an essential component of surgical management of most maxillary SCCs. (T/F)

23. The Caldwell-Luc approach to biopsy of a maxillary infrastructure mass is simple, safe, and preferable to endoscopic transnasal biopsy. (T/F)

24. Definitive radiation therapy is an acceptable primary approach to treatment of maxillary sinus cancers. (T/F)

25. When the surgeon raises the cheek flap in a total maxillectomy, the skin flap is raised below the plane of the orbicularis oculi muscle. (T/F)

26. Orbital exenteration is necessary in cases in which the cancer has invaded intraorbital fat and musculature. (T/F)

27. If the eye is preserved, the orbital floor should be reconstructed to maintain function. (T/F)

28. A composite microvascular free flap is necessary for reconstruction of large midface defects if osseointegrated implants are desired for dental restoration. (T/F)

29. Postoperative epiphora and pseudotelecanthus are potential surgical complications after total maxillectomy. (T/F)

30. Trismus may be a poor prognosticator in cancers of the sinonasal cavity. (T/F)

31. Neoadjuvant chemotherapy may have a role in the treatment of locally advanced sinonasal cancers. (T/F)

32. A temporalis muscle flap is effective in covering an orbital exenteration defect. (T/F)

33. The infraorbital nerve is preserved during medial maxillectomy. (T/F)

34. Most failures after treatment of sinonasal cancers occur at the primary site.  (T/F)

35. Preoperative radiation therapy is preferable to postoperative radiation therapy for locally advanced maxillary sinus cancers.  (T/F)

36. A maxillary sinus SCC that has perforated the anterior bony antral wall into the facial musculature has a T3 designation.  (T/F)

37. A maxillary sinus SCC that has invaded the cheek skin has a T4a designation.  (T/F)

38. A maxillary sinus SCC that has invaded the anterior orbital contents has a T4a designation.  (T/F)

39. A maxillary sinus SCC that has invaded the orbital apex has a T4b designation.  (T/F)

40. An ethmoid sinus cancer with cribriform plate invasion has a T3 designation.  (T/F)

41. An ethmoid sinus cancer with dural invasion has a T4b designation.  (T/F)

42. Endoscopic piecemeal but gross resection of locally advanced cancer followed by appropriate adjuvant therapies may be appropriate for select cases to achieve local disease control.  (T/F)

43. Positron emission tomography (PET)/CT and intraoperative navigation are helpful adjuncts to salvage surgery.  (T/F)

44. There may be a beneficial role for elective upper neck radiation therapy in advanced stage maxillary sinus cancers.  (T/F)

45. Surgery for local disease control is not indicated in patients with maxillary adenoid cystic carcinoma and pulmonary metastasis.  (T/F)

46. Fibrosarcomas of the ethmoid sinus are treated with chemoradiation therapy.  (T/F)

47. Chromogranin is a pathognomonic marker for SNUC.  (T/F)

48. A Lynch incision extends the lateral rhinotomy incision below the lower lid lash line.  (T/F)

49. A midface degloving approach may be used successfully for infrastructure cancers and for cancers along the nasal floor.  (T/F)

50. The maxillary division of the trigeminal nerve is preserved during total maxillectomy.  (T/F)

## MULTIPLE CHOICE

51. A 35-year-old man has right-sided facial pressure and numbness over his right cheek for approximately 3 months. Rhinoscopy is unrevealing, except for bluish congested turbinates with mucus stranding. Facial soft tissues are without induration. No neck masses are palpable. A tuning fork examination is normal. No trismus is noted. His oral cavity is clear. He has no significant past medical history. What is the appropriate next intervention?

A. Prescribe a 1-month supply of nasal steroid spray.
B. Prescribe a 1-week course of amoxicillin.
C. Obtain plain films of the sinuses.
D. Obtain a CT scan of the sinuses.
E. Obtain an MRI of the sinuses including the skull base.

52. A 65-year-old man with a history of right-sided headaches presents with an incidental finding of an opacified right maxillary sinus on sinus plain films taken by his primary care doctor. Your examination of the patient includes nasal endoscopy, which shows slight purulence at the middle meatus but is otherwise unrevealing. He is edentulous. He has no fever. What is your next step?

A. Prescribe a weeklong course of decongestants and antibiotics.
B. Prescribe antihistamines and nasal steroid spray.
C. Perform a Caldwell-Luc approach for drainage under local anesthesia.
D. Obtain a contrast-enhanced CT scan of the sinuses.
E. Take the patient to the operating room for endoscopic sinus surgery.

53. A 56-year-old woman presents with left-sided facial pressure and left cheek numbness. Complete head and neck examination is only significant for hypoesthesia in the V2 region. A CT scan of the sinuses shows soft tissue opacification of the left maxillary sinus alone. The rest of the sinuses are completely normal. All bones are intact. No other significant findings are present on the CT scan. What is your next step?

A. Prescribe a course of antibiotics and nasal sprays.
B. Perform an office biopsy using a Caldwell-Luc approach.
C. Take the patient to the operating room for endoscopic sinus surgery.
D. Obtain a contrast-enhanced CT scan of the sinuses.
E. Obtain an MRI of the sinuses and skull base.

54. A 70-year-old woman with left-sided facial pressure and hypoesthesia of the left cheek has an MRI of the sinonasal cavities that shows enhancing tumor filling the left maxillary sinus with mild enhancement of the trigeminal nerve at the skull base. The MRI otherwise shows no significant findings. A nasal examination in clinic shows narrow passages and no obvious intranasal mass. What is your next step?

A. Perform a transoral biopsy in the clinic with a Caldwell-Luc approach.
B. Prescribe antibiotics and decongestants.
C. Schedule an endoscopic transnasal biopsy during surgery.
D. Get a consultation from a neurologist.

55. The woman in Question 54 is taken to the operating room, an antrostomy is done endoscopically, and tissue is removed and sent for pathological analysis. The histological specimen is shown in Figure 3-1. What is your diagnosis?

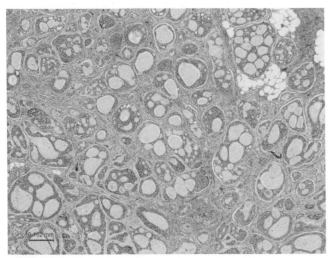

**Figure 3-1** (From Shah JP, Patel SG, Singh B. Jatin Shah's head and neck: surgery and oncology, 4th edition. Philadelphia: Mosby; 2012 [Figure 13-33].)

A. SCC
B. Adenocarcinoma
C. Mucoepidermoid carcinoma
D. Olfactory neuroblastoma
E. Adenoid cystic carcinoma

56. A 48-year-old woman has left-sided facial pressure, pain, and hypoesthesia of her left cheek. She has no visual problems. She has a tumor filling her maxillary sinus and biopsy by another ear, nose, and throat physician shows adenoid cystic carcinoma. MRI of the sinuses is shown in Figure 3-2. What are the appropriate next interventions?
A. Consult an ophthalmologist.
B. Consult a plastic surgeon.
C. Consult a prosthodontist.
D. Obtain a PET/CT scan.
E. Do all of the above.

57. The woman in Question 56 receives a normal report from the ophthalmologist. Her left eye is completely functional. Her PET scan shows two small, indeterminate nodules; each is smaller than 5 mm in the left lung field. What do you do next?
    i. Order CT-guided biopsy of the chest lesions.
    ii. Discuss defect rehabilitation options with the patient.
    iii. Discuss defect rehabilitation options with the plastic surgeon.
    iv. Discuss neoadjuvant chemotherapy options with the medical oncologist.
    v. Schedule a maxillectomy.

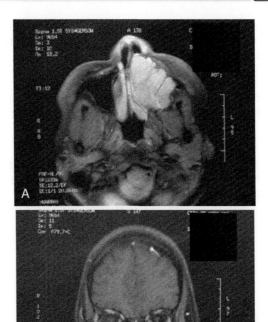

**Figure 3-2**

A. i, ii
B. ii, iii, v
C. ii, iii, iv
D. ii, iii

58. What maxillectomy approach do you recommend for the patient in Question 57?
A. Lateral rhinotomy
B. Endoscopic approach combined with an inferolateral orbitotomy
C. Weber-Ferguson incision with a Lynch extension
D. Lateral rhinotomy with a Lynch extension
E. Weber-Ferguson incision with a subciliary extension

59. You perform a total maxillectomy with removal of the orbital floor. The periorbita was sampled, and results were negative on frozen-section analysis. You spare the eye. What are acceptable reconstructive options?
A. Affix a palatal prosthetic and close the facial incisions.
B. Plate Medpor to reconstruct the orbital floor, affix the palatal prosthetic, and close all incisions.
C. Plate across the orbital floor defect, affix the palatal prosthetic, and close the incisions.
D. Use a temporalis flap to support the eye soft tissues, affix the palatal prosthetic, and then close all incisions.
E. Use a composite microvascular free flap with or without a palatal prosthetic to reconstruct the orbital floor and palatal defect.

60. What are important considerations in maintaining a functioning left eye postoperatively and maintaining good eye symmetry?
    A. Dacryocystorhinostomy
    B. Refixation of the medial canthus
    C. Provision of rigid support to the orbital floor
    D. Coverage of all free bone grafts and alloplastic material with vascularized tissue
    E. All of the above

61. The patient completes surgery and has a satisfactory postoperative course. What are your next appropriate interventions for this patient?
    i. Refer the patient to oral surgery for osseointegrated implants.
    ii. Refer the patient to plastic surgery for flap debulking and contour revision.
    iii. Refer the patient to rehabilitation for jaw motion exercises.
    iv. Refer the patient to radiation oncology for adjuvant radiation therapy.
    v. Refer the patient to medical oncology for adjuvant chemotherapy.
    A. iii, iv
    B. i, ii
    C. i, ii, iii
    D. iii, iv, v

62. Which of the following is an indication for orbital exenteration in a patient with SCC?
    A. The cancer involves the posterior ethmoid air cells.
    B. The cancer involves the orbital bony floor.
    C. The cancer involves the periorbita adjacent to the lacrimal sac.
    D. The cancer involves the lacrimal gland.
    E. The cancer involves the orbital apex soft tissues.

63. Which of the following statements are false?
    A. A lateral rhinotomy incision with lip-split and eyebrow extensions is adequate for a total maxillectomy procedure.
    B. SCC is the most common malignancy of the sinonasal tract and most commonly involves the maxillary sinus.
    C. Adenocarcinoma is the second most common malignancy of the sinonasal cavities and most commonly involves the ethmoid sinus.
    D. With current techniques of craniofacial resection, the salvage rate for locally recurrent adenoid cystic carcinoma exceeds 30%.

64. Which of the following statements about adenoid cystic carcinoma is correct?
    A. There is a strong association between adenoid cystic carcinoma and exposure to tobacco smoke.
    B. Adenoid cystic carcinoma has a high rate of systemic disease at initial presentation.
    C. Chemoradiation therapy is the preferred primary treatment for adenoid cystic carcinoma invading the orbit.
    D. Lymphatic spreading to regional nodes is the main route of metastasis for this cancer.
    E. Perineural spreading to the skull base is a hallmark of adenoid cystic carcinoma.

65. Which of the following statements about sinonasal adenocarcinoma is false?
    A. Adenocarcinoma occurs most frequently in the ethmoid sinus.
    B. There is a higher association in woodworkers exposed to hardwood dust.
    C. In this disease, tumor grade has prognostic significance.
    D. Intestinal-type adenocarcinoma is CK20 positive and associated with a better prognosis than other variants.
    E. Nonintestinal variants are CK20 negative but CK7 positive.

66. Which statement about a midfacial degloving approach is incorrect?
    A. This approach requires a complete transfixion incision of the membranous septum connected to bilateral intercartilaginous incisions within the nasal cavities.
    B. This approach requires bilateral gingivobuccal incisions to the maxillary tuberosities on both sides.
    C. This approach can be combined with Le Fort I osteotomies for access to the nasopharynx and clivus.
    D. This approach is ideally suited to cancers of the superolateral aspect of the maxillary antrum at the zygomatic recess.
    E. This incision avoids facial incisions and is well-suited to tumors of the nasal cavity involving the inferomedial walls of both maxillary sinuses.
    F. A unilateral Le Fort I combined with a paramedian osteotomy of the palate may provide better exposure to the nasopharynx compared with bilateral Le Fort I osteotomies.

67. For assessment of the skull base and intracranial extension of cancer, which combination of studies is most informative?
    A. PET and CT
    B. CT and MRI
    C. PET and MRI
    D. MRI and MR angiography
    E. PET/CT and MRI

68. For SCC of the sinonasal cavity with skull base invasion, which statement is false?
    A. Endoscopic skull base approaches may be combined with transfacial approaches to obtain better tumor visualization and resection.
    B. Neoadjuvant chemotherapy may have a role in the management of this disease with extensive skull base invasion and is recommended on protocol.
    C. Proton beam radiation therapy alone has equivalent local control rates compared with conventional surgery and adjuvant intensity-modulated radiation therapy (IMRT) techniques and can be safely substituted.
    D. Invasion of the dura is not a relative contraindication to craniofacial resection.
    E. Periorbital invasion is not a contraindication to orbital preservation as long as the periorbital fat has not been invaded.

69. Which statement is false?
    A. MRI affords better visualization of orbital soft tissue contents.
    B. MRI affords better visualization of neural tumor invasion and tracking toward the skull base.
    C. MRI affords better distinction of tumor recurrence versus inflammatory sinonasal disease.
    D. MRI allows better delineation of brain metastasis.
    E. MRI affords better delineation of cribriform plate invasion as compared with a CT scan of the sinuses.

70. Which statement is false?
    A. The infraorbital nerve can be followed through a transfacial approach all the way to the foramen rotundum.
    B. Invasion of the cavernous sinus with SCC is a contraindication to surgery.
    C. Invasion of the optic chiasm is a contraindication to surgery.
    D. Invasion of brain parenchyma in SNUC is a contraindication to upfront surgery.
    E. Invasion of the orbit with SNUC is a contraindication to primary surgery, even if there are no systemic metastases.

71. Which of the following histological types is not within the differential diagnosis of a small blue cell tumor of the sinonasal cavity?
    A. SNUC
    B. Sinonasal neuroendocrine carcinoma
    C. Mucoepidermoid carcinoma
    D. Olfactory neuroblastoma
    E. Rhabdomyosarcoma
    F. Lymphoma
    G. Malignant melanoma

72. Which one the following tumors is treated with upfront craniofacial resection?
    A. NK/T-cell lymphoma
    B. Embryonal rhabdomyosarcoma
    C. Multiple myeloma
    D. Adenocarcinoma of the ethmoid sinus
    E. SNUC with brain invasion

73. A 48-year-old man presented with right-sided proptosis and diplopia. His monocular vision was intact bilaterally. A biopsy of the mass showed small blue cell tumor cells in rosette formation in a neurofibrillary background with no necrosis (Figures 3-3 and 3-4). The cells had indistinct borders with scant cytoplasm and "salt and pepper" chromatin. What is the most likely diagnosis?
    A. Intestinal-type adenocarcinoma
    B. Adenoid cystic carcinoma
    C. B-cell lymphoma
    D. Olfactory neuroblastoma
    E. SCC

74. A patient underwent craniofacial resection through a Weber-Ferguson incision with Lynch and glabellar extensions. The periorbita and dura margins were positive on frozen-section analysis.

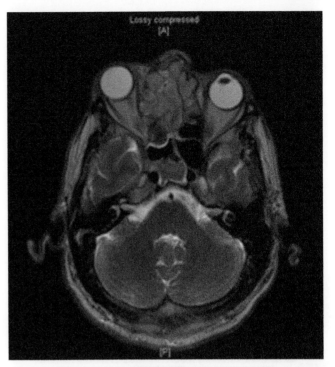

**Figure 3-3**

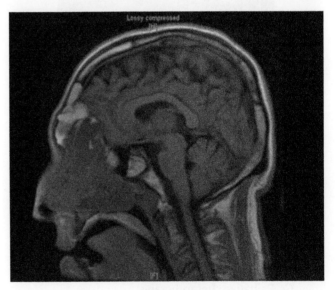

**Figure 3-4**

The periorbital fat and brain parenchyma were uninvolved. Involved periorbita and dura were resected. Duraplasty was performed by the neurosurgical service. A pericranial flap and bone cement were used to reinforce the duraplasty. The patient was then referred for postoperative adjuvant chemoradiation therapy consultation. The neck was not electively treated. Figure 3-5 is a surveillance MRI taken a year after the patient completed multimodality treatment. No evidence of local recurrence was present. Eighteen months later, the patient developed bilateral submandibular cervical masses. Fine-needle aspiration of the right submandibular mass delivered a small blue cell tumor that was positive for synaptophysin and chromogranin, consistent with metastatic esthesioneuroblastoma. The patient had no evidence of local recurrence or systemic disease. What do you recommend be done?

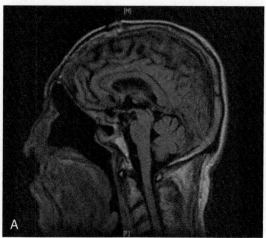

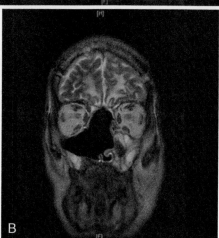

**Figure 3-5**

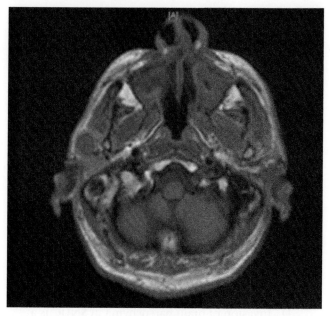

**Figure 3-6**

76. Pathological analysis revealed a 1.5-cm focus of metastatic esthesioneuroblastoma with negative resection margins. The radiation oncologist felt that additional radiation therapy could not be safely delivered. The patient is being watchfully observed at this time. There has been no further evidence of disease since the parotidectomy 6 months ago. The case in Question 74 illustrates the following important facts regarding esthesioneuroblastoma except
    A. There is a significant risk of nodal relapse in esthesioneuroblastoma.
    B. The nodal relapse in esthesioneuroblastoma may be delayed.
    C. Elective radiation therapy of the neck should be considered for advanced stage disease.
    D. Ongoing surveillance is important in this disease.
    E. Chemotherapy has a significant role in management of nodal relapse.

77. Which statements are false?
    A. The ophthalmic division of the trigeminal nerve travels through the superior orbital fissure.
    B. The orbit is composed of six different bones.
    C. The oculocardiac reflex can be prevented by injection of lidocaine into the orbital apex soft tissues during exenteration.
    D. S100, HMB-45, and Melan A are all useful markers for conjunctival melanoma.
    E. Periorbital invasion by cancer is a definite indication for exenteration.

78. Which statements are true?
    A. c-kit expression distinguishes adenoid cystic carcinoma from polymorphous low-grade adenocarcinoma.
    B. Positivity for pancytokeratin is useful in differentiating SNUC from other small blue cell tumors of the sinonasal cavity.

A. Radiation therapy to both sides of the neck
B. Concurrent chemoradiation therapy
C. Palliative chemotherapy
D. Bilateral modified radical neck dissection alone
E. Bilateral neck dissection and adjuvant radiation therapy

75. The patient in Question 74 develops a right-sided parotid mass 7 months after his neck salvage treatment (Figure 3-6). A whole-body scan shows no evidence of tumor recurrence in the primary site, treated neck, or at distant sites. What is your plan?
    A. Stereotactic radiation therapy to the parotid bed
    B. Palliative chemotherapy
    C. Chemoradiation therapy
    D. Superficial parotidectomy

C. Epstein-Barr virus (EBV)–encoded RNA (EBER) positivity is a useful marker for differentiating SNUC from nasopharyngeal undifferentiated carcinoma.

D. NK/T-cell lymphoma is the most common type of lymphoma affecting the sinonasal tract.

E. All of the above are true.

79. Which statement is false?
    A. EBER expression can help distinguish NK/T-cell lymphoma of the sinonasal cavities from Wegener granulomatosis.
    B. NUT midline carcinoma has been recently described in the sinonasal tract and is uniquely characterized by 15q14 chromosomal translocation.
    C. Sinonasal renal cell-like adenocarcinoma can be distinguished from metastatic renal clear cell carcinoma by lack of vimentin and renal cell antigen.
    D. Inverted papilloma is the most common benign sinonasal tumor within the pediatric population.

80. For treatment of a T2N0M0 SCC of the maxillary sinus, which of the following factors is/are not important in decision making?
    A. Tumor stage
    B. Tumor grade
    C. Invasion of the orbital floor
    D. Patient's medical comorbidities
    E. Surgeon's experience

81. Which structure does not course through the fissure shown by the arrow in Figure 3-7?

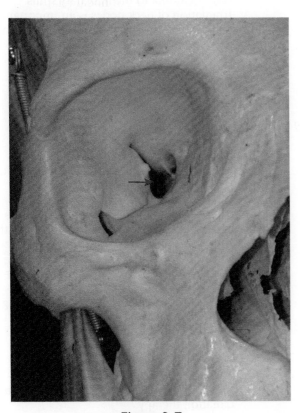

**Figure 3-7**

A. Optic nerve
B. Lacrimal nerve
C. Frontal nerve
D. Oculomotor nerve
E. Abducens nerve

82. Which bone is not part of the orbit?
    A. Sphenoid bone
    B. Frontal bone
    C. Maxillary bone
    D. Ethmoid bone
    E. Lacrimal bone
    F. Temporal bone
    G. Zygomatic bone

83. Place the following lesions in the correct order of deteriorating 5-year survival rates (from highest to lowest survival rate):
    A. SCC, SNUC, melanoma, adenocarcinoma.
    B. Adenocarcinoma, SCC, melanoma, SNUC.
    C. Melanoma, adenocarcinoma, SCC, SNUC.
    D. Adenocarcinoma, melanoma, SCC, SNUC.

84. Place the following cancer subsites in the correct order of deteriorating outcomes (from best to worst outcomes):
    A. Ethmoid sinus, maxillary sinus, nasal cavity.
    B. Nasal cavity, ethmoid sinus, maxillary cavity.
    C. Maxillary cavity, ethmoid sinus, nasal cavity.
    D. Nasal cavity, maxillary sinus, ethmoid sinus.

85. Adjuvant radiation therapy is indicated for
    A. Advanced stage disease.
    B. Close surgical margins.
    C. High-grade histological type.
    D. Perineural invasion.
    E. Vascular invasion.
    F. All of the above.

86. Which statements are true?
    A. A maxillary swing operation requires a Weber-Ferguson incision with subciliary extension and allows access to the infratemporal fossa.
    B. Local failure is the most common pattern of failure after treatment of sinonasal cancers.
    C. IMRT allows careful dose painting and maximal sparing of normal structures.
    D. There may be a beneficial role for neoadjuvant chemotherapy for locally extensive tumors of the sinonasal cavity with significant intracranial extension.
    E. All of the above are true.

87. Which of the following statements about inverted papilloma are correct?
    i. It commonly arises from the nasal septum.
    ii. Human papillomavirus (HPV) is the main causative factor for its occurrence.
    iii. It is more common in women than men.
    iv. It may be effectively resected with endoscopic techniques.
    v. It can be lined by ciliated respiratory columnar epithelium.
    vi. It can degenerate into SCC.
    vii. It can occur in the sinuses without nasal involvement.

A. i, ii, iv
B. ii, iv, v
C. iii, iv, vi, vii
D. iv, vi, vii

88. Which of the following statements about adenocarcinoma are correct?
    i. It mostly occurs in the maxillary sinuses.
    ii. It is associated with hardwood dust exposure.
    iii. Its prognosis is independent of grade.
    iv. The intestinal type is considered well-differentiated.
    v. The intestinal type is distinguished by being CK20 positive.
    A. ii, iii, v
    B. ii, v
    C. ii, iv, v
    D. iii, iv

89. Which of the following statements about adenoid cystic carcinoma are correct?
    i. It is notorious for perineural spreading to the skull base.
    ii. Lymphatic spreading to nodes occurs in more than 20% of cases.
    iii. Local recurrent disease is often treated effectively with repeated surgery.
    iv. Delayed systemic metastasis requires long-term follow-up.
    v. Unresectable cases can be treated with neutron beam radiation therapy.
    A. i, iv, v
    B. i, iii, iv
    C. ii, iii
    D. iv, v

90. Which of the following statements about mucosal melanoma are correct?
    i. Two thirds of patients have a relapse of disease at 1 year.
    ii. It is more common in the nose than in the sinuses.
    iii. Melan A is a useful diagnostic marker in nonpigmented lesions.
    iv. Adjuvant radiation therapy improves the survival rate.
    v. Neoadjuvant chemotherapy is a mainstay of treatment.
    A. i, ii
    B. i, ii, iii
    C. ii, iii, iv
    D. ii, iv

91. Which of the following statements about esthesioneuroblastoma are correct?
    i. Nodal metastasis is associated with a worse outcome.
    ii. The Kadish grading system affects the prognosis.
    iii. The Hyams staging system affects the prognosis.
    iv. It has a better outcome than other cancer types with skull base invasion.

    v. Mitosis and necrosis are common features on immunohistochemical analysis.
    A. i, iv
    B. i, ii
    C. iii, iv, v
    D. iii, iv

92. Which of the following statements about sinonasal neuroectodermal cancer are correct?
    i. It stains for chromogranin, synaptophysin, and cytokeratins.
    ii. Small cell cancer is an indolent variant.
    iii. It behaves similarly to esthesioneuroblastoma.
    iv. It is more commonly encountered in women.
    v. It may produce adrenocorticotropic hormone (ACTH), calcitonin, and antidiuretic hormone (ADH).
    A. i, ii
    B. ii, iii, iv
    C. i, v
    D. ii, iv, v

93. Which statements are false?
    i. SNUC with limited brain invasion is best treated with upfront surgery.
    ii. NK/T-cell lymphomas are more common than B-cell lymphomas in the Western population.
    iii. Sinonasal rhabdomyosarcomas are treated with surgery followed by adjuvant radiation therapy.
    iv. Surgery is advocated as the best palliation for patients with isolated metastatic renal cell carcinoma to the maxillary sinus.
    v. Irradiation of neck nodes is an important component of treatment in sinonasal rhabdomyosarcomas.
    A. i, ii, iii, iv
    B. i, ii, v
    C. i, ii, iii
    D. ii, iv, v

94. A 63-year-old man presents with an ulcerative lesion involving the left side of his hard palate. He has difficulty opening his mouth. He has numbness involving the skin over his left cheek. The patient also has left-sided ptosis and ophthalmoplegia with double vision on left lateral gaze. He has an MRI, and representative images are depicted in Figure 3-8. Transoral biopsy of the palate shows SCC. Which of the following statements are true?
    i. The patient has involvement of the pterygopalatine fossa.
    ii. The patient has perineural invasion along the trigeminal nerve.
    iii. The patient has tumor tracking into the cavernous sinus.
    iv. The patient has T4b disease.
    v. The patient should have a total maxillectomy and orbital exenteration followed by radiation therapy.

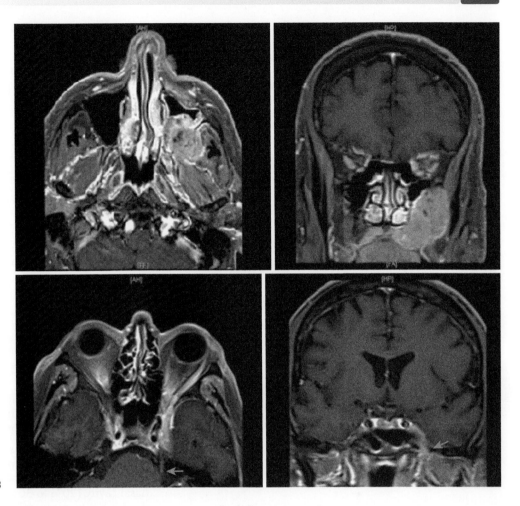

**Figure 3-8**

A. i, ii, iii
B. ii, iii, v
C. i, ii, iii, iv
D. ii, iii, iv

95. Which of the following statements are incorrect?
    i. T/NK-cell lymphoma of the nasal cavity is treated with partial rhinectomy followed by radiation therapy.
    ii. Chondrosarcomas of the nasal cavity are the most common type of sarcoma in this location.
    iii. Olfactory neuroblastoma may be seen with anosmia.
    iv. Adenocarcinomas are most commonly encountered in the nasal cavity.
    v. Inverted papillomas may be associated with SCC in 30% of recurrent cases.
  A. i, ii, iii
  B. i, ii, iii, iv
  C. i, ii, iv, v
  D. i, ii, iii, iv, v

96. Chemoradiation therapy is appropriate upfront treatment for
    i. Rhabdomyosarcoma of the sphenoid sinus.
    ii. B-cell lymphoma of the maxillary sinus.
    iii. Kadish B esthesioneuroblastoma.
    iv. Carcinoid tumor of the nasal cavity.
    v. Adenoid cystic carcinoma with involvement of the cheek and eyelid skin.

A. i, ii
B. i, ii, iii
C. ii, iii
D. ii, iii, iv
E. iv, v

97. Which of the following are relative contraindications to surgery for SCC of the maxillary sinus?
    i. Involvement of the orbital apex
    ii. Involvement of the pterygopalatine fossa
    iii. Involvement of the soft tissues of the cheek
    iv. Abducens palsy
    v. Eustachian obstruction
  A. i, ii, iv
  B. ii, iii, iv
  C. ii, v
  D. i, ii, iv, v

98. Which of the following histological types are associated with delayed metastasis?
    i. Melanoma
    ii. Adenoid cystic carcinoma
    iii. Esthesioneuroblastoma
    iv. SCC
    v. Juvenile angiofibroma
  A. i, ii
  B. i, ii, iii
  C. ii, iii
  D. ii, iii, iv

99. Which of the following statements are true?
    i. Neoadjuvant chemotherapy may be an option for patients with locally advanced disease before surgery.
    ii. IMRT allows careful dose painting and sparing of critical normal structures.
    iii. Fibrosarcomas are treated with chemoradiation therapy.
    iv. Intestinal-type adenocarcinomas are relatively indolent in comparison with SCC.
    v. Sinonasal neuroendocrine carcinomas stain positive for cytokeratin and neuron-specific markers.
    A. i, ii, iii
    B. i, ii, iv, v
    C. i, ii, v
    D. ii, iii
    E. iii, iv

100. For sinonasal cancers, which of the following are independent prognosticators for disease specific survival?
    i. Intracranial extension
    ii. Orbital invasion
    iii. Tumor histological type
    iv. Margin status
    v. Previous radiation therapy
    A. i, ii, iii
    B. i, iii, iv
    C. ii, iii
    D. ii, iii, v
    E. ii, iv, v

## Answers

| | | |
|---|---|---|
| 1. T | 20. F | 39. T |
| 2. T | 21. F | 40. T |
| 3. F | 22. F | 41. T |
| 4. F | 23. F | 42. T |
| 5. T | 24. F | 43. T |
| 6. F | 25. F | 44. T |
| 7. F | 26. T | 45. F |
| 8. T | 27. T | 46. F |
| 9. T | 28. T | 47. F |
| 10. T | 29. T | 48. F |
| 11. T | 30. T | 49. T |
| 12. F | 31. T | 50. F |
| 13. T | 32. T | 51. E |
| 14. T | 33. T | 52. D |
| 15. T | 34. T | 53. E |
| 16. F | 35. F | 54. C |
| 17. F | 36. T | 55. E |
| 18. F | 37. T | 56. E |
| 19. F | 38. T | 57. B |

| | | |
|---|---|---|
| 58. E | 73. D | 88. B |
| 59. E | 74. E | 89. A |
| 60. E | 75. D | 90. B |
| 61. A | 76. E | 91. A |
| 62. E | 77. E | 92. C |
| 63. D | 78. E | 93. C |
| 64. E | 79. D | 94. C |
| 65. D | 80. B | 95. C |
| 66. D | 81. A | 96. A |
| 67. B | 82. F | 97. D |
| 68. C | 83. B | 98. B |
| 69. E | 84. D | 99. C |
| 70. E | 85. F | 100. B |
| 71. C | 86. E | |
| 72. D | 87. D | |

## Core Knowledge

- Industrial exposure to nickel, leather, wood dust, textile dust, chromium, formaldehyde, and asbestos are causative factors for sinonasal oncogenesis.

- Of tumors in the sinonasal region, 75% are malignant. The majority of cancers in this region arise from the maxillary sinus (60% to 70%), followed by the nasal cavity (20% to 30%) and ethmoid sinuses (10% to 15%). Squamous cell carcinoma (SCC) (60% to 70%) and adenocarcinoma (10% to 20%) comprise the majority of these cancers.

- Inverted papilloma is a rare but locally aggressive benign tumor that may recur after surgical resection and is occasionally associated with SCC. Inverted papillomas characteristically arise from the lateral nasal wall in the region of the middle turbinate or ethmoid recesses and often extend secondarily into the adjacent sinuses. Inverted papillomas are composed almost exclusively of hyperplastic ribbons of basement membrane–enclosed nonkeratinizing squamous or respiratory epithelium that grow endophytically into the underlying stroma. Approximately 10% of benign sinonasal inverted papillomas degenerate into SCCs. There are no definitive markers indicative of malignant transformation. Recently, the trend has been toward the use of endoscopic surgical techniques in the management of these tumors, in contrast to the extensive open procedures recommended previously. The extent of disease should be the primary determinant in the choice of surgical approach, although previous treatment, individual patient factors, and surgical expertise are other important determinants.

- Adenocarcinoma represents the second most common malignancy of the sinonasal cavities. It most commonly involves the ethmoid sinuses. A significantly higher incidence of adenocarcinomas is seen in workers exposed to hardwood dust particles. Unlike SCCs, the tumor grade has prognostic significance: high-grade neoplasms have a dismal prognosis, in that approximately 20% have a 3-year survival rate. All intestinal-type adenocarcinomas are considered high grade; however, the papillary variant behaves more indolently. All primary intestinal-type adenocarcinomas are reactive to CK20, but all nonintestinal-type tumors are negative for CK20 and positive for CK7. Coordinate analyses of CK7 and CK20 reactivity may aid the differential diagnosis of adenocarcinoma in the sinonasal tract.

- Adenoid cystic carcinoma (ACC) accounts for 5% to 15% of sinonasal malignancies and is notorious for local, slow, relentless progression. Although lymphatic spreading of ACC is uncommon, both local recurrence and distant metastases may occur with a latency of up to 20 years after treatment of the primary tumor. Perineural spreading to the skull base is a hallmark of ACC. In a retrospective review of 35 patients with ACC of the sinonasal tract treated with surgery and radiation therapy at the University of Pittsburgh Medical Center, the disease-free survival rate was 46.4%, at a median follow-up of 40 months. Local recurrence of tumors after surgery and radiation therapy was observed in 36% of the patients. Local recurrences were treated with salvage surgical excision, and, despite aggressive management, only 1 of 17 patients with local recurrence was considered cured at 24 months. Neutron beam radiation therapy has proven effective for patients with locally advanced ACC whose disease is unresectable or in whom surgical resection will cause significant morbidity.

- Melanomas constitute about 3.5% of all neoplasms in the sinonasal tract. The nasal cavity is more commonly affected than the paranasal sinuses. Melanin may be absent in these tumors. Mucosal melanoma is often best confirmed with immunohistochemical analysis. Melan-A can be positive in cases that are S-100 or HMB-45 negative; hence it is a useful component in the immunohistochemistry panel. Surgery is the treatment of choice. Radiation therapy should be used postoperatively; however, its addition does not affect overall survival. Radiation is also useful for local disease control in inoperable cases. Significant prognostic factors for disease-specific survival on multivariate analysis include advanced clinical stage, tumor thickness greater than 5 mm, vascular invasion, and distant metastasis. Prognosis is poor: both local recurrence and distant metastasis occur in up to two thirds of patients within 1 year.

- Esthesioneuroblastoma is a tumor of neural crest origin derived from olfactory epithelium. These tumors have no gender predilection and have a bimodal age distribution with peaks in the second and sixth decades of life. The neoplastic cells have uniform small, round nuclei with scant cytoplasm and dispersed ("salt and pepper") chromatin. Nuclear pleomorphism, mitotic activity, and necrosis are usually absent. The cells lack distinct borders and are arranged in rosette pattern surrounded by a neurofibrillary matrix. Hyams proposed a histological grading system in which grade I tumors have an excellent prognosis and grade IV tumors are uniformly fatal. The Kadish staging system categorizes these tumors to stage A if the tumor is confined to the nasal cavity, stage B if the tumor extends to the paranasal sinuses, and stage C if more advanced local disease or distant metastasis is present. Both the Hyams grading system and the Kadish staging system are independent predictors of outcome. Nodal metastasis is also an important negative prognosticator of outcome and has been proposed as Kadish stage D.

- Sinonasal neuroendocrine carcinomas (SNECs) are extremely uncommon and aggressive tumors. They usually occur in the fifth to sixth decade of life and have no sex predilection. They include typical and atypical carcinoids and small cell carcinomas. Lack of neurofibrillary stroma, high mitotic rate, and necrosis are hallmarks of small cell carcinoma. Rare tumors produce adrenocorticotropic hormone (ACTH), antidiuretic hormone (ADH), and calcitonin. Diagnosis is occasionally delayed by the lack of pathognomonic antigenic profiles that can specifically distinguish these tumors from esthesioneuroblastomas. In a recent immunohistochemical analysis of neuroectodermal tumors, coexpression of neuronal markers (NSE, S-100, synaptophysin, chromogranin, and neurofilaments) and cytokeratins was proven in all cases of SNEC but in only 50% of esthesioneuroblastomas. Prognosis of small cell carcinomas of sinonasal origin is poor: frequent local recurrences and distant metastases occur despite multimodality therapy.

- Sinonasal undifferentiated cancers (SNUCs) have a propensity for extensive local invasion. In an analysis of 25 cases, the median survival was only 18 months. Gorelick et al advocate radical resection as part of the initial combined therapy for patients who present with locally advanced, nonmetastatic disease but suggest reserving surgery for patients with early brain invasion until there has been a radiographically proven central nervous system response to neoadjuvant therapy. The 2-year survival for 10 patients treated by craniofacial resection with curative intent was 64%. Patients with advanced and inoperable disease may benefit from palliative chemoradiation therapy.

- While sinonasal lymphomas are relatively rare in Western countries, they are the second most frequent group of extranodal lymphomas in Asian populations, after gastrointestinal lymphomas. B-cell lymphomas are typically located in the paranasal sinuses and have a slight predominance in Western countries, whereas T/NK-cell lymphomas are typically located in the nasal cavity and are more common in Asian and South American countries. Sinonasal T/NK-cell lymphomas have an angioinvasive growth pattern that often results in tissue necrosis and bony erosion. In the past, these tumors have been included under the descriptive and nonspecific name *lethal midline diseases*. Extranodal lymphomas are generally treated with a combination of local irradiation and chemotherapy using an anthracycline-based regimen. In a review of patients treated during a 10-year period in Nottingham, United Kingdom, the overall 5-year survival rate was 40%.

- The most common sinonasal histological sarcoma types are fibrosarcoma, rhabdomyosarcoma, and osteogenic sarcoma. Leiomyosarcoma, Ewing sarcoma, chondrosarcoma, malignant fibrous histiocytoma, and angiosarcoma are other less commonly encountered histological types. Histological diagnosis is frequently challenging, often requiring the aid of immunohisto-chemical analysis. Treatment of nonrhabdomyosarco-mas is predominantly surgical, and wide local excision is used when en bloc resection is feasible. Radiation therapy plays an important adjunctive role in management, especially for tumors in which en bloc resection with margin control is not possible. Adjuvant chemotherapy regimens are primarily designed to improve local control. Survival is predicted by both local recurrence and distant metastasis. For sinonasal rhabdomyosarcoma, a combination of chemotherapy and radiation therapy may provide the best means of locoregional control. The risk of regional disease is high and requires radiation therapy to the neck in addition to the primary site. Surgical resection is reserved for patients with residual disease after chemoradiation therapy. Chemotherapy for more than 1 year is associated with an improved survival rate as a result of decreased incidence of metastatic disease.

- Metastasis from other body sites should also be considered in the differential diagnosis of sinonasal tumors. Colonic adenocarcinoma, renal cell carcinoma, and endometrial carcinoma are among such tumors with reports of distant metastasis to the sinonasal area. Surgical excision, when possible, offers the best hope for long-term survival, and it reduces the disfigurement and other associated morbidities from the expanding tumor.

- Malignant tumors of the paranasal sinuses are usually asymptomatic until a late stage, when the tumor has filled the cavity and extended into adjacent structures. Unilateral symptoms should always raise concern for a neoplasm. Beware of unilateral sinonasal obstruction and epistaxis.

- Only 10% of malignant tumors of the paranasal sinuses present are seen with neck nodal metastasis. Nearly all patients with nodal disease have locally advanced disease.

- Endoscopic evaluation of the nasal cavity is critical. Fiberoptic or rigid scopes may be used with appropriate topical analgesia and decongestant.

- Imaging is essential in determining the extent of disease. Contrast-enhanced axial and coronal computed tomographic (CT) images work well for assessing tumor destruction of bone and penetration into adjacent structures. Gadolinium-enhanced magnetic resonance imaging (MRI) with fat suppression presents excellent soft tissue delineation of tumor in three-dimensional space. MR angiography provides information on tumor vascularity. Positron emission tomography (PET)/CT allows more accurate assessment

of tumor persistence or recurrence after multimodality therapies.
  - The Öhngren line is an imaginary line from the medial canthus to the angle of the mandible. It divides the maxillary cavity into a suprastructure that is posterosuperior and an infrastructure that is antero-inferior. Tumors of the maxillary suprastructure are seen late and often extend to difficult areas such as the pterygopalatine fossa, infratemporal fossa, skull base, and anterior and middle cranial fossa and thus have less potential for a cure.

- Tissue biopsy is mandatory for diagnosis and must be performed before an attempted removal of sinonasal tumors. The Caldwell-Luc approach to biopsy of a maxillary infrastructure mass should be avoided because it can lead to cancer seeding of cheek soft tissues and complicate subsequent definitive surgery. Endoscopic debulking of gross disease should not be done because it may confuse the surgical margins necessary for definitive treatment.

- Surgery is the mainstay of therapy for tumors of the nose and paranasal sinuses. Radiation therapy is generally not used as the initial treatment because of the bony confines of this region and proximity to critical structures such as the orbit and the brain. Surgery alone is sufficient treatment for benign tumors and early stage malignant cancers with comfortable clearance. Radiation therapy is used after surgery for more advanced stages of cancer. Chemoradiation protocols are prescribed when adequate surgical resection cannot be achieved. Published reports have shown concomitant chemotherapy and radiation therapy with delayed accelerated fractionation to be effective in this setting. Relative contraindications to upfront surgery include trismus, implicating advanced disease involving the pterygopalatine and masticator spaces, and invasion of the orbital apex, cavernous sinus, skull base, brain, and carotid artery.

- A dental evaluation is mandatory. Septic teeth may need to be extracted. Loose teeth should be left within a tumor-bearing alveolus; they will be removed with the specimen at the time of maxillectomy. A prosthodontist will take a presurgical dental impression for the patient. The surgeon will communicate the maxillectomy extent for fabrication of a palatal obturator to be affixed after tumor resection at the time of surgery. If a portion of the soft palate is to be resected, the prosthesis may be lengthened posteriorly to fill the anticipated defect so that the patient can have effective speech and swallow function postoperatively without a need for a feeding tube.

- A neurosurgeon should be consulted if the skull base is involved and a craniofacial resection is anticipated. Broad-spectrum antibiotics and steroids are used to prevent infection and reduce inflammation and edema perioperatively.

- A reconstructive surgeon is necessary if an extensive composite resection with significant removal of facial bone and soft tissues is anticipated. Reconstruction with microvascular free tissue transfer has extended the scope of safe surgical resection. Perioperative photography is necessary for documentation.

- The patient may be intubated transorally or transnasally depending on the surgical approach needed. It is best to draw proposed incisions in advance so that the tube will not distort the facial tissues. The eyes should be protected. A fine nylon tarsorrhaphy suture may be used instead of corneal shields. Patient positioning and draping should be done to the satisfaction of all surgeons participating.

- Peroral partial maxillectomy can be satisfactory for limited cancers of the upper alveolar ridge, palate, and maxillary floor. Nasotracheal intubation through the opposite nasal cavity and muscle relaxants is recommended for optimal exposure.

- Larger lesions may require a transfacial approach. Surgical incisions used for transfacial access of tumors of the nasal cavity and paranasal sinuses include the following, as shown in Figure 3-9:
  - Lateral rhinotomy (no lip-split)
  - Weber-Ferguson (lip-split added)
  - Weber-Ferguson with Lynch extension
  - Weber-Ferguson with lateral subciliary extension
  - Weber-Ferguson with subciliary and supraciliary extension

- A lateral rhinotomy provides excellent exposure for tumors of the lower nasal cavity that may not lend themselves to adequate exposure and complete removal by endoscopic techniques.

- A Weber-Ferguson incision with a Lynch extension provides excellent exposure to the superior antrum and ethmoid sinuses. Subciliary and supraciliary extensions are used when orbital invasion is present and exenteration is necessary.

- Medial maxillectomy is indicated for removal of tumors of the lateral nasal wall or medial wall of the maxillary antrum. A lateral rhinotomy or Weber-Ferguson incision can be used depending on the tumor location and extent. A Lynch extension allows for optimal exposure of the ethmoid complex. The surgeon should be aware of the inferior orbital nerve as the cheek flap is elevated. Entry through the anterior maxillary sinus wall is best made with a high-speed drill and burr. The opening should be large enough to see everything in the maxillary antrum. The periorbita is incised along the medial orbital rim and elevated with a periosteal dissector. The medial canthal ligament is detached and laterally reflected. It can be marked with a fine silk suture for later identification and reapproximation to the nasal bone. A malleable retractor allows gentle retraction of orbital contents to allow the lacrimal sac and duct to be exposed. The sac and duct should be elevated from the lacrimal fossa, and the duct should be transected obliquely. This releases

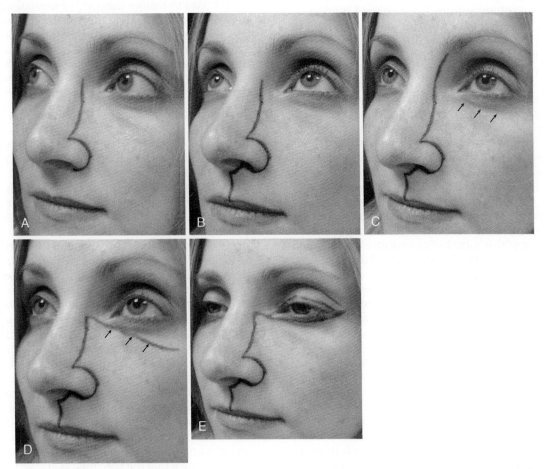

**Figure 3-9** (From Shah JP, Patel SG, Singh B. Jatin Shah's head and neck: surgery and oncology, 4th edition. Philadelphia: Mosby; 2012 [Figure 5-37].)

the periorbita and allows for easy lateral retraction of orbital contents and exposure of the entire medial orbital wall. During this maneuver, the anterior and posterior ethmoid arteries are identified and ligated or electrocoagulated. The nasal cavity should be entered next. A curved osteotome is used to divide the medial wall of the maxillary antrum along the nasal floor. The anterior bony cuts are gently made with an osteotome encompassing the medial maxillary and orbital walls up to the nasofrontal suture. Gentle rocking of the specimen mobilizes the ethmoid complex. Finally, angled scissors are used to make the final posterior cut through the nasal choana, and the specimen is released. Bleeding should be controlled, and sharp bone edges should be made smooth. A nasolacrimal stent can be placed through the upper and lower lacrimal puncta and tied up in the nasal cavity. Alternatively, a dacryocystorhinostomy can be performed along the residual lateral nasal wall. A skin graft is not necessary because mucus forms over and covers the defect. Bismuth tribromophenate (Xeroform) strip gauze is used to pack the antrum and the nasal cavity. The strip is brought out through the nares. The medial canthus is anchored to the nasal bone with the use of nonabsorbable sutures that match up with the opposite side. The skin is again meticulously closed in layers. The nasal packing is removed in 5 to 6 days, and nasal irrigations are begun in the patient for cleansing.

- Total maxillectomy is necessary when the tumor fills the entire maxillary antrum. The preferred surgical approach is a modified Weber-Ferguson incision with subciliary extension along the lower eyelid. The subciliary extension is necessary in a total maxillectomy so that the posterolateral maxillary antral wall and the pterygomaxillary fissure are optimally exposed. The subciliary incision is usually extended about a centimeter lateral to the lateral canthus so that sufficient exposure is provided. The skin incision is connected to a gingivolabial and gingivobuccal incision to the maxillary tuberosity. This allows for elevation of a full-thickness cheek flap. The lower eyelid incision should be placed very superficially because the skin here is very thin. In raising this eyelid skin flap, the surgeon should use a fine tip cautery at low voltage and remain superficial to the orbicularis oculi muscle to prevent denervation of this muscle. Subperiosteal dissection of the orbital contents along the orbital floor will allow for exposure and resection of the orbital plate of the maxilla as the superior limit of the resection. The attachment of the masseter muscle to the zygoma is released next with electrocautery. The focus then shifts to the oral cavity where a mouth gag and tongue depressor will allow for optimal exposure. While a needle-tip electrocautery is used to minimize bleeding, a mucosal incision is made between the lateral incisor and canine through the gingiva down to the alveolar bone. This will designate the anterior line of resection. The incision is then extended to the midline of the hard palate anteriorly and then extended all the way back to the junction of the hard and soft palates, at which point it turns laterally toward the maxillary

tubercle and into the gingivobuccal sulcus. The incision is deepened through the medial pterygoid musculature for release of the maxilla. The hard palate incision is deepened all the way down to the bone. The nasal vestibule is entered through the pyriform recess, and the nasal process of the maxilla is exposed. Next are the bone cuts of the total maxillectomy:
- Nasal process of the maxilla
- Maxillary zygomatic buttress
- Alveolar ridge and hard palate
- Orbital plate
- Pterygomaxillary separation

The bone cuts are completed with a high-speed saw and osteotomes, and then posterior soft tissue attachments are released with heavy Mayo scissors. The specimen is removed in a monobloc fashion. Bleeding should be controlled. The wound is irrigated with bacitracin solution, and a split-thickness skin graft is harvested to reline the raw areas of the defect. Interrupted catgut sutures are used to secure the skin graft, and bismuth tribromophenate gauze packing is applied to bolster the skin graft. A prefabricated palatal prosthetic is applied and wired around the remaining teeth to keep the bolster in place and allow for postoperative speech and peroral nutrition. In edentulous patients, the prosthetic can be suspended with screws in the remaining palatal shelf or with wires. The lip-and-cheek skin incision is closed in two layers, and care should be taken in the realignment of the vermillion border of the lip. A 3-0 chromic suture is used to realign the divided musculature, and 5-0 nylon is used to realign the epidermis. The subciliary incision is closed with a single, running, fine plain gut suture. The postoperative care is similar to that for partial maxillectomy. Bolus extension of the final palatal obturator into the maxillary defect allows for obliteration of the airspace and improved voice quality.

- Total maxillectomy with orbital exenteration is indicated when the cancer of the sinonasal cavity extends through the orbital periosteum. A functioning eye is only justifiably removed if there is a chance of cure with the exenteration. The operation essentially is an extension of the total maxillectomy approach with a supraciliary incision around the palpebral fissure. The subciliary and supraciliary incisions are connected at the medial and lateral canthi. The thin skin flaps are elevated above the plane of the orbicularis oculi muscle all the way to the orbital bony rims. Superiorly, the orbital rim is exposed, and the attachment of the orbital periosteum to the rim is incised. A Freer periosteal elevator is used to develop the supraperiosteal plane all the way to the orbital apex, which completely exposes the bony orbital roof. The musculature at the orbital apex is divided with electrocautery. The optic nerve and ophthalmic artery are clamped with a right-angle dissector, and all attachments at the orbital apex are divided. The nerve and artery are tied off, and vessels still bleeding are cauterized. Elevation of the periosteum medially or inferiorly should be avoided if the tumor has penetrated through the medial wall or the floor of the orbit, respectively. The remaining steps are identical to a total maxillectomy with the caveat that the specimen is allowed to remain in continuity with the orbital contents, inasmuch as tumor location and adequacy of margins are respected. A large defect is left and can be addressed in one of two ways: either a microvascular composite free flap can be tailored to the defect to separate the oral cavity and provide soft tissue coverage or the defect can be rehabilitated with skin grafting followed by application of a dental prosthetic in combination with a facial prosthetic. The choice is individualized based on a variety of considerations that include tumor recurrence risk, patient comorbidities, and wishes. A preoperative detailed assessment and discussion with the patient are essential in this decision. A microvascular free-flap reconstruction will become necessary if extensive soft tissues of the cheek and overlying skin are resected. Multiple skin paddles may be necessary in flap design; furthermore, the choice of soft tissue or composite free flap in reconstruction is complex and beyond the scope of this chapter.

- Tumor extension into the periorbita does not necessarily condemn the eye to exenteration. In a retrospective consecutive review of 66 patients undergoing surgical treatment for sinonasal malignancy encroaching on the orbit, Imola and Schramm preserved the orbit in 54 patients with tumor extension up to and including resectable periorbita. Eye-sparing surgery was associated with local recurrence at the original site of orbital involvement in only 7.8% of cases (4 of 54). Overall eye function was graded as functional without impairment in 54% of patients (29 of 54), functional with impairment in 37% (20 of 54), and nonfunctional in 9% (5 of 54). The most common abnormality (34 of 54 patients) was globe malposition associated with the lack of adequate rigid reconstruction of the orbital floor. A globe that has been preserved without the support of the orbital floor is unlikely to retain significant function, especially if radiation therapy is used. Radiation therapy increased the risk of ocular complications, in particular, optic atrophy, cataract formation, excessive dryness, and ectropion. My approach is to resect involved periorbita and preserve the orbital contents in cases in which there is no invasion of orbital fat, orbital musculature, or involvement of the orbital apex. The invasion of any of these structures is an indication for orbital exenteration. I emphasize the necessity for orbital floor reconstruction in cases with orbital preservation. However, orbital preservation should not come at the potential cost of decreased local disease control and survival.

- Nasal exenteration and partial or total rhinectomy are surgeries suited to nasal cavity tumors. If a tumor is intranasal, a nasal exenteration can be done through a lateral rhinotomy approach, either unilaterally or bilaterally. However, if nasal skin is involved, then a partial or total rhinectomy may be necessary, depending on the extent. A monobloc resection is executed. Choice of defect rehabilitation again depends on the extent and configuration of the defect. Local tissue flaps or microvascular free flaps can be used. Depending on whether a septectomy was performed, a composite flap may be necessary to provide nasal support. A total rhinectomy defect is frequently rehabilitated with a nasal prosthesis. If patient tissues are used for reconstruction, revision surgeries or staged surgeries for refinement are often necessary.

- Nasopharyngeal angiofibromas are benign, highly vascular tumors usually occurring in teenage boys. Nasal obstruction, epistaxis, aural fullness, and conductive hearing loss are the usual presenting symptoms. These tumors may grow and involve the sinonasal cavities, skull base, and adjacent fossa. They may even extend intracranially. CT and MRI scans are helpful in combination for assessing the tumor extent. In addition, angiography is mandatory for studying the blood supply and preoperative embolization. Limited tumors can be resected through a transpalatal approach. For larger tumors filling the paranasal sinuses, a wider exposure through a Weber-Ferguson incision is necessary.

- Localized skull base invasion does not necessarily preclude surgery because these tumors may still be resectable by combined craniofacial approaches. In a recent multiinstitutional collaborative study, a series of 209 patients who had undergone craniofacial resection for sinonasal neoplasia with up to 17 years' follow-up was analyzed. For malignant tumors, the 5-year actuarial survival rate was 44%, falling to 32% at 10 years. Statistical analysis identified three factors that independently affected outcome and survival: tumor histology, brain involvement, and positive margins of resection. The improved survival rate and minimal morbidity and mortality associated with craniofacial resection make it the optimal approach for locally advanced sinonasal tumors. Massive parenchymal brain invasion, extensive skull base invasion, massive tumor volume with trismus, and carotid artery invasion are contraindications to surgical resection.

- Endoscopic techniques have created the potential for approaching the intranasal aspect of skull base lesions without external incisions while still allowing en bloc tumor resection. A large retrospective study from two Belgian institutions of 78 patients who underwent minimally invasive endoscopic management for malignant sinonasal tumors has been recently published. All patients were treated primarily for a cure. A total of 66 patients were operated on by a purely endoscopic technique, while 9 patients had a simultaneous neurosurgical and endoscopic approach, and 3 had a limited orbital approach. Twenty-three patients (29.5%) presented with local recurrence. The overall 5-year survival rate was 52.3%. Morbidity was minimal, and the local control and survival rates were comparable with literature data. Bogaerts et al reported on 44 patients with primary ethmoid adenocarcinoma treated with endoscopic surgery and radiation therapy (50 to 70 Gy, 5 weeks postoperatively). Patients with dural, orbital, and brain invasion were excluded. The 5-year overall survival and disease-specific survival rates were 53% and 83%, respectively. The local control rate was reported at 62%. Although I do not consider this approach a replacement for the traditional anterior craniofacial resection, it is an important adjunct in the skull base surgeon's armamentarium.

- Several different factors affect treatment decisions in the neck, including tumor histology and TNM stage. For SCC, clinically positive metastatic disease in the neck is managed with some form of neck dissection. Postoperative radiation therapy to the neck is indicated for multiple positive nodes, any single node greater than 3 cm in size, or extracapsular spreading. The management of a patient whose neck is clinical stage N0 is debatable. Traditional guidelines have not indicated a need for prophylactic neck treatment unless the sinonasal tumor encroaches on areas of increased risk of lymphatic spreading, such as the nasopharynx or soft palate. Our center's approach is to not treat the N0 neck electively in cases of sinonasal SCC. The impact of elective nodal irradiation (ENI) in locally advanced SCC of the maxillary sinus is unclear. Jeremic et al advocate this approach and report that a total dose of 50 Gy, delivered in standard fractionation, can achieve locoregional control in about 95% of all cases with low toxicity. The pattern of nodal failure in their patients suggested limiting the radiation field to the ipsilateral submandibular and jugulodigastric areas. However, this issue needs to be further studied. Management of the neck in cases of esthesioneuroblastoma is equally controversial. Substantial evidence shows that this disease is associated with a significant (20% to 25%) incidence of cervical metastasis that may not become apparent for some time (2 to 8 years). In a 21-year update on the University of Virginia experience with esthesioneuroblastomas, 25% of patients ultimately developed cervical metastasis. Only one third of patients with delayed nodal metastasis were candidates for salvage therapy, despite local disease control, probably because of a higher incidence of distant metastases in these patients.

- The majority of patients with malignant tumors of the sinonasal cavity present with an advanced stage of disease. Cure rates depend on the stage of disease. The 5-year survival rates for stage I, II, III, and IV SCC are 100%, 86%, 39%, and 25%, respectively. A total of 62% of patients experience treatment failure after surgery. Local failure is most common for SCCs of the maxillary sinus. Regional failure is rare and occurs in only 3% to 20% of cases. Adjuvant radiation therapy improves locoregional control rates. Intensity-modulated radiation therapy (IMRT) can be safely delivered in a spatial conformal fashion while sparing critical healthy surrounding structures such as the skin, orbit, brain, and salivary glands. Distant failure rates are reported to be approximately 17% to 25%.

- Combination treatments using multimodality strategies are being explored to improve control and cure rates for sinonasal cancers. There is presently sufficient evidence to support chemotherapy as a fundamental component of multimodality treatment for sinonasal lymphomas and sarcomas. However, the existing evidence for the beneficial use of systemic chemotherapy outside the palliative treatment setting for other tumor histological types is little more than anecdotal and awaits a more thorough assessment. Samant et al studied 19 patients with advanced paranasal sinus cancer. Intraarterial cisplatin was delivered two to

three times per week. Simultaneous radiation therapy (50 Gy every 5 weeks) was administered. Craniofacial resection was done 8 weeks later. The actuarial overall survival rates at 2 and 5 years were 68% and 53%, respectively. Lee et al reported excellent long-term outcome in locoregionally advanced paranasal sinus cancer treated with induction chemotherapy and surgery, followed by concomitant chemoradiation therapy. These results are encouraging and appear superior to the survival rates achieved with surgery and radiation therapy alone. However, further validation is warranted. New molecular targeting strategies also show promise going into the future. The hope is to improve curability while maintaining high functionality.

## Seventh Edition American Joint Committee on Cancer Primary Tumor Staging for Maxillary Sinus Cancer

| T1 | Tumor limited to maxillary sinus mucosa with no erosion or destruction of bone |
| --- | --- |
| T2 | Tumor causing bone erosion or destruction including extension into the hard palate and/or middle nasal meatus, except extension to the posterior wall of the maxillary sinus and pterygoid plates |
| T3 | Tumor invades any of the following: bone of the posterior wall of the maxillary sinus, subcutaneous tissues, floor or medial wall of the orbit, pterygoid fossa, ethmoid sinuses |
| T4a | Moderately advanced local disease<br>Tumor invades the anterior orbital contents, skin of the cheek, pterygoid plates, infratemporal fossa, cribriform plate, sphenoid or frontal sinuses |
| T4b | Very advanced local disease<br>Tumor invades any of the following: orbital apex, dura, brain, middle cranial fossa, cranial nerves other than the maxillary division of the trigeminal nerve (V2), nasopharynx, or clivus |

*Adapted from AJCC: Paranasal sinus and nasal cavity. In: Edge SB, Byrd DR, Compton CC, Fritz AG, Greene FL, et al, editors. AJCC cancer staging manual. 7th ed. New York: Springer; 2010.*

## Seventh Edition American Joint Committee on Cancer Primary Tumor Staging for Nasal Cavity and Ethmoid Sinus

| T1 | Tumor restricted to any one subsite, with or without bone invasion |
| --- | --- |
| T2 | Tumor invading two subsites in a single region or extending to involve an adjacent region within the nasoethmoidal complex, with or without bony invasion |
| T3 | Tumor extends to involve the medial wall or floor of the orbit, maxillary sinus, palate, or cribriform plate |
| T4a | Moderately advanced local disease<br>Tumor invades any of the following: anterior orbital contents, skin of the nose or cheek, minimal extension to the anterior cranial fossa, pterygoid plates, sphenoid or frontal sinuses |
| T4b | Very advanced local disease<br>Tumor invades any of the following: orbital apex, dura, brain, middle cranial fossa, cranial nerves other than maxillary division of the trigeminal nerve (V2), nasopharynx, or clivus |

*Adapted from AJCC: Paranasal sinus and nasal cavity. In: Edge SB, Byrd DR, Compton CC, Fritz AG, Greene FL, et al, editors. AJCC cancer staging manual. 7th ed. New York: Springer; 2010.*

## Seventh Edition American Joint Committee on Cancer Sinonasal Cancer Stage Grouping

| | | | |
|---|---|---|---|
| 0 | Tis | N0 | M0 |
| I | T1 | N0 | M0 |
| II | T2 | N0 | M0 |
| III | T3 | N0 | M0 |
| | T1-3 | N1 | M0 |
| IVA | T4a | N0 | M0 |
| | T4a | N1 | M0 |
| | T1-4a | N2 | M0 |
| IVB | T4b | Any N | M0 |
| | Any T | N3 | M0 |
| IVC | Any T | Any N | M1 |

*Adapted from AJCC: Paranasal sinus and nasal cavity. In: Edge SB, Byrd DR, Compton CC, Fritz AG, Greene FL, et al, editors. AJCC cancer staging manual. 7th ed. New York: Springer; 2010.*

## SUGGESTED READING

Bogaerts S, Vander Poorten V, Nuyts S, Van den Bogaert W, Jorissen M. Results of endoscopic resection followed by radiotherapy for primarily diagnosed adenocarcinomas of the paranasal sinuses. Head Neck 2008;30(6):728–36.

Bridge JA, Bowen JM, Smith RB. The small round blue cell tumors of the sinonasal area. Head Neck Pathol 2010;4(1):84–93.

Chen AM, Sreeraman R, Mathai M, Vijayakumar S, Purdy JA. Potential of helical tomotherapy to reduce dose to the ocular structures for patients treated for unresectable sinonasal cancer. Am J Clin Oncol 2010;33(6):595–8.

Day TA, Beas RA, Schlosser RJ, Woodworth BA, Barredo J, et al. Management of paranasal sinus malignancy. Curr Treat Options Oncol 2005;6(1):3–18.

Dirix P, Vanstraelen B, Jorissen M, Vander Poorten V, Nuyts S. Intensity-modulated radiotherapy for sinonasal cancer: improved outcome compared to conventional radiotherapy. Int J Radiat Oncol Biol Phys 2010;78(4):998–1004.

Duprez F, Madani I, Morbee L, Bonte K, Deron P, et al. IMRT for sinonasal tumors minimizes severe late ocular toxicity and preserves disease control and survival. Int J Radiat Oncol Biol Phys 2012;83(1):252–9.

Eggesbo HB. Imaging of sinonasal tumours. Cancer Imaging 2012;12:136–52.

Gorelick J, Ross D, Marentette L, Blaivas M. Sinonasal undifferentiated carcinoma: case series and review of the literature. Neurosurgery 2000;47(3):750–4.

Hanna E, DeMonte F, Ibrahim S, Roberts D, Levine N, et al. Endoscopic resection of sinonasal cancers with and without craniotomy: oncologic results. Arch Otolaryngol Head Neck Surg 2009;135(12):1219–24.

Harvey RJ, Gallagher RM, Sacks R. Extended endoscopic techniques for sinonasal resections. Otolaryngol Clin North Am 2010;43(3):613–38, x.

Imola MJ, Schramm Jr VL. Orbital preservation in surgical management of sinonasal malignancy. Laryngoscope 2002;112(8 Pt 1):1357–65.

Jeremic B, Nguyen-Tan PF, Bamberg M. Elective neck irradiation in locally advanced squamous cell carcinoma of the maxillary sinus: a review. J Cancer Res Clin Oncol 2002;128(5):235–8.

Kim DY, Hong SL, Lee CH, Jin HR, Kang JM, et al. Inverted papilloma of the nasal cavity and paranasal sinuses: a Korean multicenter study. Laryngoscope 2012;122(3):487–94.

Lombardi D, Tomenzoli D, Butta L, Bizzoni A, Farina D, et al. Limitations and complications of endoscopic surgery for treatment for sinonasal inverted papilloma: a reassessment after 212 cases. Head Neck 2011;33(8):1154–61.

Lund VJ, Chisholm EJ, Takes RP, Suárez C, Mendenhall WM, et al. Evidence for treatment strategies in sinonasal adenocarcinoma. Head Neck 2012;34(8):1168–78.

Lupinetti AD, Roberts DB, Williams MD, Kupferman ME, Rosenthal DI, et al. Sinonasal adenoid cystic carcinoma: the M. D. Anderson Cancer Center experience. Cancer 2007;110(12):2726–31.

Madani G, Beale TJ, Lund VJ. Imaging of sinonasal tumors. Semin Ultrasound CT MR 2009;30(1):25–38.

Maghami E, Kraus DH. Cancer of the nasal cavity and paranasal sinuses. Expert Rev Anticancer Ther 2004;4(3):411–24.

Mine S, Saeki N, Horiguchi K, Hanazawa T, Okamoto Y. Craniofacial resection for sinonasal malignant tumors: statistical analysis of surgical outcome over 17 years at a single institution. Skull Base 2011;21(4):243–8.

Mirghani H, Hartl D, Mortuaire G, Armas GL, Aupérin A, et al. Nodal recurrence of sinonasal cancer: Does the risk of cervical relapse justify a prophylactic neck treatment? Oral Oncol 2013;49(4):374–80.

Nicolai P, Battaglia P, Bignami M, Bolzoni Villaret A, Delù G, et al. Endoscopic surgery for malignant tumors of the sinonasal tract and adjacent skull base: a 10-year experience. Am J Rhinol 2008;22(3):308–16.

Pantvaidya GH, Vaidya AD, Metgudmath R, Kane SV, D'Cruz AK. Minor salivary gland tumors of the sinonasal region: results of a retrospective analysis with review of literature. Head Neck 2012;34(12):1704–10.

Rajapurkar M, Thankappan K, Sampathirao LM, Kuriakose MA, Iyer S. Oncologic and functional outcome of the preserved eye in malignant sinonasal tumors. Head Neck 2013;35(10):1379–84.

Reiersen DA, Pahilan ME, Devaiah AK. Meta-analysis of treatment outcomes for sinonasal undifferentiated carcinoma. Otolaryngol Head Neck Surg 2012;147(1):7–14.

Rischin D, Coleman A. Sinonasal malignancies of neuroendocrine origin. Hematol Oncol Clin North Am 2008;22(6):1297–316, xi.

Robbins KT, Ferlito A, Silver CE, Takes RP, Strojan P, et al. Contemporary management of sinonasal cancer. Head Neck 2011;33(9):1352–65.

Samant S, Robbins KT, Vang M, Wan J, Robertson J. Intra-arterial cisplatin and concomitant radiation therapy followed by surgery for advanced paranasal sinus cancer. Arch Otolaryngol Head Neck Surg 2004;130(8):948–55.

Slootweg PJ, Ferlito A, Cardesa A, Thompson LD, Hunt JL, et al. Sinonasal tumors: a clinicopathologic update of selected tumors. Eur Arch Otorhinolaryngol 2013;270(1):5–20.

Suarez C, Ferlito A, Lund VJ, Silver CE, Fagan JJ, et al. Management of the orbit in malignant sinonasal tumors. Head Neck 2008;30(2):242–50.

Suarez C, Llorente JL, Fernandez De Leon R, Maseda E, Lopez A. Prognostic factors in sinonasal tumors involving the anterior skull base. Head Neck 2004;26(2):136–44.

Turner JH, Reh DD. Incidence and survival in patients with sinonasal cancer: a historical analysis of population-based data. Head Neck 2012;34(6):877–85.

# 4 Skull Base

## Questions

### TRUE/FALSE

1. Esthesioneuroblastoma is an uncommon malignant neoplasm of the nasal vault believed to arise from olfactory epithelium. (T/F)

2. Basal cells within the olfactory epithelium are progenitors to esthesioneuroblastoma tumors. (T/F)

3. In esthesioneuroblastoma, Kadish C tumors may have cervical lymph nodal metastases. (T/F)

4. Flexner-Wintersteiner rosettes are characteristic histopathological features of well-differentiated esthesioneuroblastomas. (T/F)

5. Distant metastases are seen in approximately 8% of patients with esthesioneuroblastoma. (T/F)

6. When a craniofacial resection is performed, the facial exposure is usually obtained through a modified Weber-Ferguson incision. (T/F)

7. A scalp flap is elevated in a plane deep to the galea aponeurotica and the pericranium in a craniofacial resection. (T/F)

8. A bifrontal coronal skin incision is made when a craniotomy is performed as part of an anterior craniofacial resection. (T/F)

9. Cerebrospinal fluid (CSF) removal allows for brain decompression and improved exposure of the posterior part of the cribriform plate and the planum sphenoidale in a craniofacial resection. (T/F)

10. The bone plate in a bifrontal craniotomy contains only the frontal bone in a craniofacial resection. (T/F)

11. Hemangiopericytomas are highly vascular benign tumors of the anterior cranial fossa. (T/F)

12. A hemangiopericytoma is a soft tissue sarcoma originating in the pericytes in the walls of capillaries. (T/F)

13. Hemangiopericytomas are associated with low rates of local recurrence. (T/F)

14. With hemangiopericytoma, gross total resection followed by adjuvant radiation therapy provides patients with the highest probability of an increased recurrence-free interval and overall survival. (T/F)

15. Metastases may develop years after initial treatment of hemangiopericytoma. (T/F)

16. Paragangliomas are rare highly vascular neuroendocrine tumors. (T/F)

17. Up to 80% of paragangliomas secrete catecholamines. (T/F)

18. Individual paraganglioma cells are polygonal to oval and are arranged in distinctive cell balls, called Zellballen. (T/F)

19. A vagal paraganglioma is the least common head and neck paraganglioma. (T/F)

20. Less than 5% of paragangliomas cause distant metastases. (T/F)

21. The scalp has four individual layers. (T/F)

22. The galea aponeurotica extends from the frontalis muscle anteriorly to the occipitalis posteriorly lying deep to the pericranial layer. (T/F)

23. The scalp derives its blood supply from the internal and external carotid arteries. (T/F)

24. Lymph nodes lie within the loose areolar tissue layer of the scalp. (T/F)

25. The posterior-based pericranial flap may be used for anterior craniofacial reconstruction. (T/F)

26. The inferior border of the infratemporal fossa is the medial pterygoid muscle. (T/F)

27. The terminal branch of the 16 branches of the internal maxillary artery is the sphenopalatine artery. (T/F)

28. The medial border of the infratemporal fossa is the pterygomaxillary fissure. (T/F)

29. The mandibular nerve enters the infratemporal fossa by passing through the foramen ovale in the middle cranial fossa. (T/F)

30. The superior aspect of the infratemporal fossa is defined by the greater wing of sphenoid below the infratemporal crest. (T/F)

31. The risk of infection is not increased with endonasal skull base surgery. (T/F)

32. Hot water irrigation may be used for hemostasis in endoscopic skull base surgery. (T/F)

33. The nasoseptal flap is based on the greater palatine artery. (T/F)

34. Tumor-free margins cannot be achieved with endoscopic techniques in endoscopic skull base surgery. (T/F)

35. Anatomical limits to endonasal skull base surgery are vessels and nerves. (T/F)

36. The dura mater is the innermost layer of the meninges. (T/F)

37. The three layers of meninges are arachnoid, pia mater, and dura mater. (T/F)

38. The dura mater has two layers: the endocranium and the actual dura mater. (T/F)

39. The rupture of bridging veins (which puncture the dura mater) causes a subdural hematoma resulting in blood between the dura mater and the arachnoid layer. (T/F)

40. The anterior ethmoidal artery contributes to the dura mater vascular supply. (T/F)

41. The internal carotid artery (ICA) lies behind and lateral to the external carotid. (T/F)

42. The ophthalmic branch of the ICA gives rise to the anterior but not the posterior ethmoidal artery. (T/F)

43. There are seven ICA segments according to the Bouthillier classification. (T/F)

44. The ICA does not branch in the neck. (T/F)

45. The ICA passes through the foramen lacerum. (T/F)

46. Trigeminal schwannomas arise in the majority of cases from postganglionic divisions. (T/F)

47. Trigeminal schwannomas are highly vascular and bright on T2-weighted magnetic resonance imaging (MRI). (T/F)

48. The majority of trigeminal schwannomas arise sporadically. (T/F)

49. The majority of trigeminal schwannomas are seen with trigeminal nerve dysfunction, which recovers after excision. (T/F)

50. The most important factor predicting recurrence of trigeminal schwannomas is completeness of surgical resection. (T/F)

**MULTIPLE CHOICE**

51. Which of the following anatomical structures are found within the anterior skull base?
    i. Planum sphenoidale
    ii. Posterior wall of the frontal sinus
    iii. Posterior clinoid process
    iv. Cribriform plate
    v. Crista galli
    vi. Sella turcica
    vii. Lesser wing of the sphenoid
    A. i, iv, v, vi, vii
    B. i, iii, v, vi, vii
    C. i, ii, iv, v, vi

D. i, ii, iii, v, vii
E. i, iii, v, vi
F. ii, iv, v, vii

52. From the following options (i-vii), choose the single most likely diagnosis for each of the scenarios given. Each option may be used once, more than once, or not at all.
    i. Chondrosarcoma
    ii. Chondroma
    iii. Squamous cell carcinoma
    iv. Glomus jugulare
    v. Craniopharyngioma
    vi. Meningioma
    vii. Pituitary macroadenoma
    (a). An amenorrheic 26-year-old woman with a 2.3-cm benign tumor with suprasellar extension
    (b). A 55-year-old woman with a mutation of the succinate dehydrogenase gene (SDHD)
    (c). A 44-year-old man with neurofibromatosis type II
    (d). A 52-year-old with a tumor that most commonly originates from the petrooccipital synchondrosis
    (e). A slow-growing malignant mesenchymal tumor

53. Which of the following anatomical structures are found within the middle cranial fossa?
    i. Posterior clinoid process
    ii. Arcuate eminence
    iii. Sella turcica
    iv. Planum sphenoidale
    v. Olfactory grooves
    vi. Foramen ovale
    vii. Cavernous sinus
    viii. Tegmen tympani
    A. i, iii, vii, viii
    B. i, iii, iv, vi, viii
    C. i, ii, iii, vi, vii, viii
    D. i, ii, iii, vi, viii
    E. i, ii, iii, vi, vii

54. Which of the following statements regarding malignant tumors of the skull base are correct?
    i. Approximately 10% of tumors that arise in the sinonasal tract originate in the ethmoid sinus and/or frontal sinus and are likely to involve the anterior cranial base.
    ii. Computed tomography (CT) is superior to MRI in defining the extent of bony invasion.
    iii. MRI is usually reserved for patients seen with invasion of soft tissue, notably of the brain and orbit.
    iv. Human papillomavirus (HPV)-positive squamous cell carcinoma confers a survival advantage.
    v. Osteoradionecrosis of the skull base secondary to radiation therapy is rarely, if ever, seen in dosages less than 60 Gy.
    A. ii, iii, v
    B. i, ii, iii
    C. ii, iii, iv, v
    D. i, ii, iii, v
    E. i, ii, iii, iv, v

55. Which of the following statements regarding the ICA are correct?
   i. The internal maxillary artery is the final branch before entry into the skull.
   ii. The ICA lies behind and lateral to the external carotid artery.
   iii. The ICA passes through the superior non-fibrocartilaginous portion of the foramen lacerum.
   iv. C1 extends from the carotid bifurcation to the foramen lacerum.
   v. C2 is the petrous segment with three sections: the vertical, the genu, and the horizontal components.
   A. ii, iii, v
   B. i, ii, iv, v
   C. ii, iv, v
   D. i, iii, iv, v
   E. i, iii, iv

56. Which of the following statements regarding CSF are correct?
   i. The majority of CSF is produced by modified ependymal cells within the choroid plexus.
   ii. The choroid plexus produces approximately 1.5 L CSF per day.
   iii. CSF occupies the subdural space around the brain and spinal cord.
   iv. CSF allows for hemostatic regulation of the central nervous system through the blood–brain barrier.
   v. Beta-2 transferrin in otorrhea would be suggestive of either a perilymphatic or CSF leak.
   A. i, ii, iv
   B. i, ii, iv, v
   C. ii, iv
   D. i, ii, iii
   E. i, iv, v

57. Which of the following anatomical structures are found within the cavernous sinus?
   i. Oculomotor nerve
   ii. Trochlear nerve
   iii. $V_1$
   iv. Ophthalmic nerve
   v. ICA
   vi. Optic nerve
   vii. $V_2$
   viii. Abducens nerve
   A. i, ii, iii, iv, v, vii, viii
   B. i, ii, iii, v, vii, viii
   C. i, ii, iii, v, vi, viii
   D. i, iii, v, vii, viii
   E. i, ii, iv, v, vii, viii

58. Which nerve is transmitted through the skull base foramen shown in Figure 4-1?
   A. Vidian nerve
   B. Mandibular nerve
   C. Maxillary nerve
   D. Optic nerve
   E. Alveolar nerve

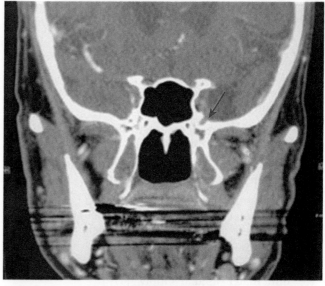

**Figure 4-1**

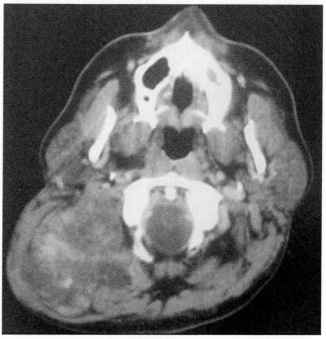

**Figure 4-2**

59. Which of the following statements is correct regarding malignant peripheral nerve sheath tumors (MPNST) as shown in Figure 4-2?
   A. MPNSTs account for approximately 40% of all soft tissue sarcomas.
   B. MPNSTs are commonly found in the head and neck.
   C. MPNSTs are more commonly seen in pediatric age groups.
   D. *MPNST* is a relatively new term for tumors formerly called *malignant schwannoma, neurofibrosarcoma,* or *neurogenic sarcoma.*
   E. Neoadjuvant cisplatin/5-fluorouracil therapy is broadly recommended for offsetting the risk of lung metastases.

60. Which of the following statements is correct regarding craniofacial resections as shown in Figure 4-3?

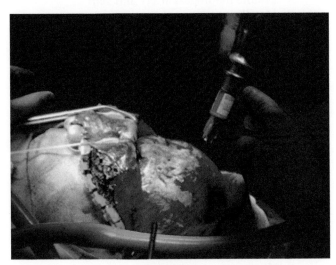

**Figure 4-3**

  i. All calvarial defects require reconstruction to protect the brain.
 ii. Elevation of the galeal pericranial flap requires sharp dissection between the subcutaneous tissue and the galea.
iii. The blood supply to the galeal pericranial flap comes from the superficial temporal artery.
 iv. A spinal catheter may be required to remove CSF before bone cuts through the floor of the anterior cranial fossa.
  v. The facial approach may be made using a Weber-Ferguson or lateral rhinotomy incision.
   A. i, iv, v
   B. i, ii, iv
   C. i, iii, v
   D. ii, iv, v
   E. ii, iii, v

61. A clival chordoma is
   A. A destructive tumor on the lateral margin of the clivus with high T2 signal intensity.
   B. A destructive midline tumor centered on the clivus with high T2 signal intensity.
   C. A destructive tumor on the lateral margin of the clivus with low T2 intensity.
   D. A destructive midline tumor centered on the clivus with low T2 signal intensity.

62. A clival chordoma
   A. Is a highly vascular tumor.
   B. Is an avascular mass.
   C. Is a solid vascular tumor with central necrosis.
   D. Has flow voids as a characteristic feature.

63. Clival chordomas show a
   A. High T2 signal secondary to high fluid content of vacuolated cellular components.
   B. High T2 signal due to increased vascularity and flow voids.

   C. Low T2 signal secondary to high fluid content of vacuolated cellular components.
   D. Low T2 signal due to increased vascularity and flow voids.

64. Which statement regarding chondrosarcomas is incorrect?
   A. Chondrosarcomas have MR T1 and T2 characteristics similar to clival chordomas.
   B. Chondroid calcifications are present in 50% of tumors.
   C. Chondrosarcomas have midline axial pathological features.
   D. Chondrosarcomas are tumors seen in the petrooccipital fissure.

65. Which statement regarding chondrosarcomas is incorrect?
   A. Chondrosarcomas are seen along the lateral aspect of the clivus.
   B. Chondrosarcomas are cartilaginous in origin.
   C. Chondrosarcomas are predominantly low-grade tumors in the head and neck.
   D. The T2 signal intensity of chondrosarcomas is low to intermediate.

66. The MR findings of glomus jugulare paraganglioma include a
   A. T1 and T2 "salt and pepper" appearance.
   B. T1 and T2 "ground glass" appearance.
   C. T1 and T2 high signal for cystic necrosis.
   D. T1 and T2 high signal within the petromastoid air cells.

67. In the phrase *MR T1 and T2 salt and pepper appearance,*
   A. *Salt* means hypointense foci representing hemorrhage or slow flow, and *pepper* means hyperintense foci representing high velocity arterial flow voids.
   B. *Salt* means hyperintense foci representing hemorrhage or slow flow, and *pepper* means hypointense foci representing high velocity arterial flow voids.
   C. *Salt* means hypointense foci representing central necrosis, and *pepper* means hyperintense foci representing venous flow voids.
   D. *Salt* means hyperintense foci representing central necrosis, and *pepper* means hypointense foci representing venous flow voids.

68. The *MR T1 and T2 salt and pepper appearance* is seen in
   A. All paragangliomas.
   B. No paragangliomas; it is not a radiological feature of these tumors.
   C. Paragangliomas greater than 4 cm.
   D. Paragangliomas greater than 2 cm.

69. A jugular foramen schwannoma
   A. Has no "pepper" flow voids, even if it is a large tumor.
   B. Has characteristic flow voids.
   C. Is a benign tumor of sympathetic nerves in the jugular foramen.
   D. Has a high T1 signal.

70. The jugular foramen schwannoma differential includes the following, except
    A. Glomus jugulare paraganglioma.
    B. Jugular foramen meningioma.
    C. Jugular foramen granuloma.
    D. Acoustic schwannoma.

71. Giant cell tumors of the skull base are also known as
    A. Plasmacytomas.
    B. Osteoid myelomas.
    C. Osteoclastomas.
    D. Osteolytic metastases.

72. The classic imaging finding in clival meningioma is
    A. "Dural tails."
    B. Flow voids.
    C. Central calcification.
    D. Peripheral necrosis.

73. Fibrous dysplasia of the skull base is best described as
    A. Progressive replacement of normal cancellous bone by Langerhans-type histiocytes.
    B. Progressive replacement of normal cancellous bone by fibrous tissue and immature woven bone.
    C. Progressive replacement of normal cancellous bone by multinucleated giant cells.
    D. Progressive replacement of normal cancellous bone by monoclonal plasma cells.

74. The classic CT appearance of fibrous dysplasia of the skull base includes
    A. Pagetoid mixed pattern.
    B. Sclerotic pattern.
    C. Cystic pattern.
    D. All of the above.

75. Langerhans histiocytosis of the skull base has also been known as
    A. Hand-Schüller-Christian disease.
    B. O'Neill-Morris-Wreesman syndrome.
    C. Schüller Siwe syndrome.
    D. Delkargios syndrome.

76. All of the following structures extend through the foramen ovale except the
    A. Mandibular nerve.
    B. Cranial nerve (CN) V₃.
    C. Meningeal branch of the mandibular nerve.
    D. Accessory meningeal artery.

77. All of the following structures extend through the superior orbital fissure except the
    A. Ophthalmic artery.
    B. Oculomotor nerve.
    C. Abducens nerve.
    D. Superior ophthalmic vein.

78. All of the following structures extend through the jugular foramen except the
    A. Inferior petrosal sinus.
    B. Glossopharyngeal nerve.
    C. Middle meningeal artery.
    D. Sigmoid sinus.

79. Which of the following structures extend through the foramen rotundum?
    A. Middle meningeal artery and vein
    B. Maxillary nerve
    C. Occasionally, the lesser petrosal nerve
    D. Mandibular nerve

80. All of the following structures extend through the optic canal except the
    A. Optic nerve.
    B. Superior ophthalmic vein.
    C. Ophthalmic artery.
    D. CN II.

81. All of the following structures extend through the foramen magnum except the
    A. Meninges.
    B. Vertebral arteries.
    C. Posterior meningeal artery.
    D. Medulla oblongata.

82. The carotid passes through
    A. The foramen ovale.
    B. The foramen lacerum.
    C. The jugular foramen.
    D. None of the above.

83. The foramen cecum contains the
    A. Accessory meningeal artery.
    B. Emissary vein to the superior sagittal sinus.
    C. Emissary vein to the inferior sagittal sinus.
    D. Emissary vein to the middle sagittal sinus.

84. The internal acoustic meatus contains
    A. CN VII.
    B. CN VIII.
    C. The labyrinthine artery.
    D. All of the above.

85. The sella turcica is in the
    A. Anterior cranial fossa.
    B. Middle cranial fossa.
    C. Posterior cranial fossa.
    D. Occipital bone.

86. The agger nasi air cell is
    A. The largest and most consistent ethmoid air cell.
    B. Positioned anterior to the insertion of the inferior turbinate.
    C. Positioned anterior to the insertion of the middle turbinate.
    D. Consistently pneumatized.

87. The uncinate process may be attached to any of the following except the
    A. Skull base.
    B. Lamina papyracea.
    C. Nasal septum.
    D. Middle turbinate.

88. Any of the following may narrow the frontal recess except
    A. Inferior turbinate pneumatization.
    B. The agger nasi air cell.
    C. The ethmoid bulla.
    D. The frontoethmoid air cells.

89. Normally, the natural maxillary ostium cannot be visualized at endoscopy because it is
    A. Hidden by the uncinate process.
    B. Absent in the majority of the population but is a major cause of nasal outflow obstruction.
    C. Hidden by the middle turbinate.
    D. Hidden by the ethmoid bulla.

90. The inferior turbinate is
    A. Part of the ethmoid complex.
    B. Considered a separate bone and is not part of the ethmoid complex.
    C. Considered a separate bone and is part of the maxilla.
    D. Considered a separate bone and is part of the sphenoid bone.

91. On a coronal CT scan, the ethmoid roof is noted to be 7 mm above the cribriform plate, which makes this a Keros type
    A. I.
    B. II.
    C. III.
    D. IV.

92. The most common Keros type is
    A. I.
    B. II.
    C. III.
    D. IV.

93. The following are all characteristics of Kuhn type 3 cells except
    A. Type 3 cells extend into the frontal sinus by less than 50% of the sinus height.
    B. Type 3 cells are single cells in the frontal recess with pneumatization in the frontal sinus.
    C. Type 3 cells extend into the frontal sinus by more than 50% of the sinus height.
    D. Type 3 cells' posterior walls are part of the frontal recess.

94. The sphenoid sinus ostium is generally located
    A. Superior to the superior turbinate 1 to 1.5 cm above the roof of the choana.
    B. Inferior to the superior turbinate 1 to 1.5 cm above the roof of the choana.
    C. Medial to the superior turbinate 1 to 1.5 cm above the roof of the choana.
    D. Lateral to the superior turbinate 1 to 1.5 cm above the roof of the choana.

95. Which of the following statements about mandibular swing is correct?
    A. This approach is for lesions in the parapharyngeal space, pterygomandibular space, and infratemporal fossa.
    B. This approach is only for lesions in the pterygomandibular space.
    C. This approach is only for lesions in the infratemporal fossa.
    D. This approach is only for lesions in the pterygomandibular space and infratemporal fossa.

96. Mandibular swing should not be performed alone when
    A. The tumor is lateral to the ICA.
    B. The tumor extends beyond the floor of the middle cranial fossa.
    C. The tumor involves intracranial structures.
    D. Any of the above is true.

97. Technical variations of skull base defect reconstruction include
    A. Nerve grafting.
    B. The galeal pericranial flap.
    C. A split-thickness skin graft (STSG).
    D. All of the above.

98. Technical variations of facial reconstruction include
    A. None.
    B. A prosthesis.
    C. A composite free flap.
    D. All of the above.

99. Technical variations of a craniotomy include
    A. A single large frontal burr hole.
    B. Bifrontal craniotomy.
    C. Parasagittal burr holes.
    D. All of the above.

100. When should composite free-flap reconstruction of the skull base be avoided?
    A. In patient with a low risk of recurrence
    B. In patients with a high risk of recurrence
    C. In patients with a high risk of recurrence and the possibility of successful salvage surgery
    D. In patients with a high risk of recurrence and no possibility of successful salvage surgery

## Answers

| | | |
|---|---|---|
| 1. T | 18. T | 35. T |
| 2. T | 19. T | 36. F |
| 3. F | 20. T | 37. T |
| 4. T | 21. F | 38. T |
| 5. T | 22. F | 39. T |
| 6. T | 23. T | 40. T |
| 7. F | 24. F | 41. T |
| 8. T | 25. F | 42. F |
| 9. T | 26. T | 43. T |
| 10. F | 27. T | 44. T |
| 11. F | 28. F | 45. F |
| 12. T | 29. T | 46. F |
| 13. F | 30. T | 47. F |
| 14. T | 31. T | 48. T |
| 15. T | 32. T | 49. F |
| 16. T | 33. F | 50. T |
| 17. F | 34. F | 51. C |

| 52. (a) vii, (b) iv, (c) vi, (d) i, (e) i | 67. B | 84. D |
|---|---|---|
| | 68. D | 85. B |
| 53. C | 69. A | 86. C |
| 54. D | 70. C | 87. C |
| 55. A | 71. C | 88. A |
| 56. E | 72. A | 89. A |
| 57. A | 73. B | 90. B |
| 58. C | 74. D | 91. B |
| 59. D | 75. A | 92. B |
| 60. D | 76. C | 93. C |
| 61. B | 77. A | 94. C |
| 62. B | 78. C | 95. A |
| 63. A | 79. B | 96. D |
| 64. C | 80. B | 97. D |
| 65. D | 81. C | 98. D |
| 66. A | 82. D | 99. D |
| | 83. B | 100. C |

## Core Knowledge

- The anterior skull base is formed by the frontal, ethmoid, and sphenoid bones. The anterior boundary is the posterior wall of the frontal sinus. The posterior boundaries are the anterior clinoid processes and the planum sphenoidale (roof of the sphenoid sinus). The frontal bone forms the lateral boundaries. The central floor of the anterior skull base is the cribriform plate (horizontal lamina), which is part of the ethmoid bone. The olfactory tracts pass through the cribriform plate, which is made of thin bone. The lateral lamella of the cribriform plate is thin bone continuing laterally as the fovea ethmoidalis (thick bone). This is of relevance during endoscopic approaches to the skull base. The Keros classification measures the depth of the lateral lamellae of the cribriform plate (olfactory fossa): type I, 1 to 3 mm; type II, 4 to 7 mm; and type III, 8 to 16 mm.

- The middle cranial fossa is bounded in front by the posterior margins of the lesser wing of the sphenoid, the anterior clinoid processes, and the ridge forming the anterior margin of the chiasmatic groove. The lateral boundary is the squamous portion of the temporal bones, the sphenoidal angles of the parietal bone, and the greater wing of the sphenoid. Its posterior boundary is the superior angles of the petrous portions of the temporal bones and the dorsum sellae.

- The following are anterior cranial fossa foramina: foramen cecum (including the emissary vein to the superior sagittal sinus), foramina of the cribriform plate (including olfactory bundles), anterior ethmoidal foramen (including the anterior ethmoid nerve, artery, and vein), and the posterior ethmoidal foramen (including the posterior ethmoid nerve, artery, and vein).

- Middle cranial fossa foramina include the superior orbital fissure (cranial nerves III, IV, $V_1$ [lacrimal, frontal, and nasociliary], and VI [superior ophthalmic vein]), foramen rotundum ($V_2$), foramen ovale ($V_3$ and, intermittently, the lesser petrosal nerve and the accessory meningeal artery), foramen spinosum (the meningeal branch of $V_3$ and the middle meningeal artery), and foramen lacerum (vidian nerve [greater superficial parasympathetic nerve and the deep petrosal sympathetic nerve] and vidian artery [one of the terminal branches of the ascending pharyngeal artery and emissary veins connecting the cavernous sinus with the extracranial pterygoid plexus]).

- Of note, the internal carotid artery (ICA) does not pass through the foramen lacerum.

- The ICA, according to the 1996 Bouthillier classification, is divided into the following alphanumeric segments: C1, cervical; C2, petrous; C3, lacerum; C4, cavernous; C5, clinoid; C6, ophthalmic; and C7, communicating. The ICA passes through the superior part of the foramen lacerum on its way to the cavernous sinus. It does not traverse the skull through these foramina.

- The scalp has five layers: S, skin; C, connective tissue; A, galea aponeurotica (fibrous tissue attaching from the frontalis muscle anteriorly to the occipitalis posteriorly); L, loose areolar tissue; and P, pericranium. The pericranial flap is vascularized by the deep branches of the supraorbital and supratrochlear arteries and veins that course between the galea frontalis muscle layer and the pericranium.

- The majority of tumors of the anterior cranial fossa arise extracranially with secondary extension to the skull base. The most common benign tumors are angiofibromas, chondromas, and neurovascular tumors. The most common epithelial malignant tumors are squamous cell carcinomas, minor salivary gland carcinomas, esthesioneuroblastomas, sinonasal undifferentiated carcinomas, neuroendocrine carcinomas, and melanomas. Chondrosarcomas and osteosarcomas are the most frequently encountered bone tumors.

- The majority of patients with primary malignant tumors involving the central anterior skull base require either an open craniofacial resection or an endoscopic endonasal resection. An open craniofacial resection involves a bicoronal incision made from tragus to tragus, providing wide exposure for a bifrontal craniotomy. The scalp is incised through its subcutaneous tissue up to a plane superficial to the galea aponeurotica and the pericranium. A limited craniotomy is required for a subcranial approach to the cribriform plate. The bone flap is removed without injury to the underlying dura. The next step is cranialization of the frontal sinus and removal of the bony septa with a rongeur. Sharp bony spicules are smoothed with a high-speed burr, and all mucosa must be removed with the use of a curette and a burr. The dura is elevated and, if torn, repaired (4-0 nylon [Nurolon] sutures); however, if a tumor is present, it must also be removed in continuity with the specimen. The crista galli is then excised. Cerebro-spinal fluid (CSF) may then be aspirated from a spinal catheter to facilitate exposure of the cribriform plate and planum sphenoidale. A high-speed burr is used to make the necessary bony cuts. The facial approach begins with either a lateral rhinotomy or a Weber-Ferguson incision, and the necessary paranasal sinus ablative excision is tailored to the tumor's orientation.

- Middle cranial fossa tumors are most commonly of neurovascular, soft tissue or bony origin. A schwannoma is a benign neurogenic, nerve sheath tumor. Trigeminal schwannomas are rare intracranial tumors. Jefferson defined three types of trigeminal schwannomas: type A, located mainly in the middle fossa; type B, located mainly in the posterior fossa; and type C, having significant components in both the middle fossa and the posterior fossa. Symptoms and signs of these lesions depend on the site of the tumor, which may compress the nerve of origin or adjacent nerves.

- Treatment requires multidisciplinary discussion. Tumor control rates (94%) for trigeminal schwannomas are excellent when stereotactic radiation therapy and fractionated stereotactic radiation therapy are used; the treatment has minimal toxicity. For a large symptomatic trigeminal schwannoma causing mass effect, surgical removal is the preferred initial management strategy. When a tumor cannot be excised completely and the residual tumor is less than 3 cm in diameter, radiosurgery is an excellent adjunctive strategy. Patients who have asymptomatic primary, residual, or recurrent tumors smaller than 3 cm in diameter may be offered the option of radiosurgery instead of resection.

- Malignant sinonasal neoplasms with skull base involvement can be safely resected in accordance with sound oncological principles and with the use of the endoscopic endonasal technique. In the literature, however, long-term follow-up data are currently lacking. The endoscopic approach includes debulking the intranasal tumor portion, which provides visualization of the tumor extent and margin definition, and opening uninvolved sinuses to facilitate safe margins and identify key anatomical landmarks. Margins normally required are the posterior wall of the frontal sinus, medial orbit wall(s), superior nasal septum, and sphenoid roof. Bone removal extends from the crista galli to the planum sphenoidale and to the medial orbital border. Reconstruction firstly involves an inlay fascial graft followed by a nasal septal flap. This flap is based on the sphenopalatine artery (the terminal branch of the internal maxillary artery—itself the terminal branch of the external carotid artery) and was first described by the Pittsburgh group. This flap can cover the full anterior cranial fossa, provided that the nasal mucosa on the ipsilateral side is free of disease.

- Esthesioneuroblastomas are uncommon malignant neoplasms of the nasal vault, believed to arise from olfactory epithelium–cribriform plate, superior nasal concha, medial nasal concha, and upper part of the septum. These tumors can be visualized as obstructing, red, firm nasal polyps (70% cases), epistaxis (50% cases), or both. The bimodal peak is in the second and third decade and sixth and seventh decade of life. These tumors have varying malignant potential, ranging from indolent to highly aggressive behavior.

- The Kadish staging system (1976) is as follows: A, the tumor is confined to the nasal cavity; B, the tumor extends into the paranasal sinuses; C, the tumor has spread beyond the nasal cavity and paranasal sinuses; and D, the tumor has caused metastasis to cervical nodes or distant sites.

- The University of California Los Angeles (UCLA) staging system for esthesioneuroblastoma is as follows: T1, represents nasal/paranasal disease; T2, includes the sphenoid bone and/or extension to the cribriform plate; T3, indicates orbital or anterior cranial fossa invasion without dural invasion; T4, indicates dural invasion; N0, indicates a lack of cervical lymph node metastasis; N1, indicates cervical lymph node metastasis; M0, indicates a lack of metastasis; and M1, indicates distant metastasis.

- The UCLA system may be more accurate prognostically because early involvement of the cribriform plate is recognized in the T2 stage, and intracranial but extradural tumors are separated from those with true brain involvement. The initial stage of presentation is highly predictive of survival. Combined modality therapy is required, and craniofacial resection, either open or endoscopic, is the gold standard in management. Almost 20% of patients have nodal metastases, and controversy exists as to the elective management of the neck as a result of delayed presentation of cervical nodal metastases.

- Craniopharyngiomas are epithelial neoplasms arising from the sellar and suprasellar regions. The sella turcica is bounded anteriorly by the tuberculum sella and posteriorly by the dorsum sella. Laterally are the anterior clinoid processes of the lesser wing of the sphenoid. The floor is the roof of the sphenoid sinus. Craniopharyngiomas very rarely may also be identified within the nasopharynx, cerebellopontine angle, and paranasal sinuses. They are nearly always benign and are found in two age peaks: childhood and older adults. Survival rates in the literature vary between 83% and 93% at 10 years. Surgery with or without adjuvant radiation therapy is the treatment of choice. Microsurgical dissection of these tumors is extremely challenging and requires the combined expertise of physicians in the head and neck and neurosurgery specialties.

- Osteosarcomas are rare head, neck, and skull base tumors. They are most commonly found in relation to the mandible and have the capability of metastasizing to the neck. The major concern, as with all sarcomas, is distant metastases to the lungs. Surgical excision is the mainstay of treatment. Neoadjuvant therapy for osteosarcomas is commonly used because of three main advantages: reduction of micrometastases to the lungs; determination of the degree of necrosis in the tumor specimen, which helps guide adjuvant chemotherapy; and preemptive treatment because of the reality of probable positive microscopic margins from giant osteosarcoma tumors with intimate anatomical proximity to vital structures. The benefits, however, are largely extrapolated from the pediatric and adult extremity osteosarcoma experience. A threefold improvement in pediatric osteosarcoma survival rates can be related to neoadjuvant chemotherapy, and up to 80% of extremity osteosarcomas have lung micrometastases on presentation.

- A malignant peripheral nerve sheath tumor (MPNST), also known as malignant schwannoma, neurofibrosarcoma, and neurosarcoma, is a sarcoma. These tumors are strongly linked to neurofibromatosis. MPNST is a markedly metastatic, aggressive, poor-prognosis tumor.

## SUGGESTED READING

Chiu ES, Kraus D, Bui DT, Mehrara BJ, Disa JJ, et al. Anterior and middle cranial fossa skull base reconstruction using microvascular free tissue techniques: surgical complications and functional outcomes. Ann Plast Surg 2008;60(5):514–20.

Ganly I, Patel SG, Singh B, Kraus DH, Cantu G, et al. Craniofacial resection for malignant tumors involving the skull base in the elderly: an international collaborative study. Cancer 2011;117(3):563–71.

Gil Z, Patel SG, Cantu G, Fliss DM, Kowalski LP, et al. Outcome of craniofacial surgery in children and adolescents with malignant tumors involving the skull base: an international collaborative study. Head Neck 2009;31(3):308–17.

Ketcham A, Chretien P, Van Buren J, Hoye R, Beazley R, et al. The ethmoid sinuses: a re-evaluation of surgical resection. Am J Surg 1973;126:469–76.

Ketcham AS, Wilkins RH, Van Buren JM, Smith R. A combined intracranial facial approach to the paranasal sinuses. Am J Surg 1963;106:698–703.

O'Neill JP, Bilsky MH, Kraus D. Head and neck sarcomas: epidemiology, pathology, and management. Neurosurg Clin N Am 2013;24(1):67–78.

Paluzzi A, Gardner P, Fernandez-Miranda JC, Snyderman C. The expanding role of endoscopic skull base surgery. Br J Neurosurg 2012;26(5):649–61.

Shah JP. Quality of life after skull base surgery: the patient's predicament. Skull Base 2010;20(1):3–4.

Shah JP, Galicich JH. Craniofacial resection for malignant tumors of ethmoid and anterior skull base. Arch Otolaryngol 1977;103:514–7.

Snyderman CH, Carrau RL, Kassam AB, Zanation A, Prevedello D, et al. Endoscopic skull base surgery: principles of endonasal oncological surgery. J Surg Oncol 2008;97(8):658–64.

# 5 Lips and Oral Cavity

## Questions

### TRUE/FALSE

1. The upper lip drains first into buccal and parotid lymph nodes. (T/F)

2. The most common cause of lower lip squamous cell carcinoma (SCC) is carcinogens related to smoking. (T/F)

3. Muscles of the lower lip are supplied by the marginal mandibular nerve of the facial nerve and those of the upper lip and orbicularis oris by the buccal branch of the facial nerve. (T/F)

4. The parotid (Stenson duct) opens on a papilla opposite the first upper molar. (T/F)

5. The region overlying the ascending ramus of the mandible from the level of the last molar to the apex superiorly adjacent to the tuberosity of the maxilla is the retromolar trigone region. (T/F)

6. Cancers of the buccal mucosa do not metastasize to the facial lymph nodes. (T/F)

7. Tumors of the lower jaw are less likely to metastasize than tumors of the upper jaw. (T/F)

8. Elective neck dissection is recommended for cancers of the upper alveolus. (T/F)

9. Cancers of the floor of the mouth may mimic salivary gland obstruction. (T/F)

10. The most common site in the oral cavity for minor salivary gland cancers is the hard palate. (T/F)

11. Cancers of the hard palate metastasize to the retropharyngeal lymph nodes. (T/F)

12. The posterior hard palate is supplied by the greater palatine nerve and the anterior premaxillary region by the nasopalatine nerves. (T/F)

13. The most common cancer of the oral cavity is cancer of the floor of the mouth. (T/F)

14. The cancer of the oral cavity with the poorest outcome is buccal cancer. (T/F)

15. Cancers of the oral cavity are frequently treated with definitive chemoradiation therapy. (T/F)

16. The two most important factors predictive of local recurrence in cancer of the oral tongue are close or positive margins and perineural invasion. (T/F)

17. The most important predictor of neck metastases in early oral tongue cancer is the tumor thickness. (T/F)

18. Occult metastases incidence increases with the tumor thickness. (T/F)

19. The presence of positive lymph nodes reduces the survival rate by 25%. (T/F)

20. The main muscle of the tongue is the genioglossus. (T/F)

21. The hypoglossal nerve supplies all the muscles of the tongue except for the palatoglossus, which is supplied by the pharyngeal plexus. (T/F)

22. The lingual nerve mediates sensation while the chorda tympani supplies taste to the oral tongue. (T/F)

23. Human papillomavirus is a common cause of oral cavity cancer. (T/F)

24. Cancer of the oral tongue is increasing in young adult men. (T/F)

25. Young patients (younger than 20 years) with oral tongue cancer have a poorer outcome than older patients. (T/F)

26. Verrucous carcinoma of the oral cavity spreads via invasive islands. (T/F)

27. Approximately 40% to 50% of minor salivary gland cancers of the oral cavity are malignant. (T/F)

28. A computed tomographic (CT) scan is more accurate at assessing mandibular invasion than clinical examination. (T/F)

29. Mandibular invasion is more common in patients with dentate mandibles than in patients with edentulous mandibles. (T/F)

30. Invasion of the mandibular canal is more common in older patients. (T/F)

31. Marginal mandibulectomy is safe in patients who have received previous radiation to the oral cavity. (T/F)

32. The incidence of occult metastases from cancers of the oral cavity is 20% to 30%. (T/F)

33. Sentinel node biopsy is the standard of care for staging of clinically negative neck nodes. (T/F)

34. Sentinel node biopsy is defined as the first-echelon lymph node to which cancer spreads. (T/F)

35. The overall sensitivity of sentinel node biopsy in patients with clinically N0 neck nodes is 94%. (T/F)

36. 13-cis-Retinoic acid can reverse epithelial dysplasia and reduce the risk of a second primary cancer. (T/F)

37. Aneuploidy decreases the risk of malignant transformation of oral dysplasia. (T/F)

38. The occurrence of a second primary head and neck cancer exists at a constant rate of 4% to 7% per year. (T/F)

39. Oral submucous fibrosis is associated with the development of hypertrophic epithelium. (T/F)

40. Verrucous carcinoma is associated with a high incidence of local recurrence. (T/F)

41. Verrucous carcinoma is associated with human papillomavirus infection. (T/F)

42. Oral tongue cancer is more common in young women than in young men. (T/F)

43. Smokeless tobacco is associated with development of buccal mucosa cancer. (T/F)

44. Ameloblastoma is a malignant tumor of the mandible. (T/F)

45. Skip metastases to level IV of the neck are most commonly associated with cancer of the anterior floor of the mouth. (T/F)

46. The probability of metastases to the neck in T4 tumors is 40%. (T/F)

47. SCC of the lower gum is less common than SCC of the upper gum. (T/F)

48. The rate of occult metastases increases as the depth of invasion of the primary tumor increases. (T/F)

49. Dental caries within the radiation field is the prime initiator of osteoradionecrosis. (T/F)

50. The 5-year survival rate of patients with a T1N0 oral tongue SCC is 75%. (T/F)

## MULTIPLE CHOICE

51. The patient shown in Figure 5-1 has an SCC of the middle third of the lower lip. What are the most common lymph nodes at risk?
    A. Submandibular lymph nodes
    B. Submental nodes
    C. Level II nodes
    D. Level III nodes
    E. Level IV nodes

52. The defect after resection is shown in Figure 5-2. This is best repaired by a
    A. Skin graft.
    B. Free radial forearm flap.
    C. V-Y advancement flap.
    D. Abbe-Estlander flap.
    E. Bilateral Karapandzic flaps.

53. The most common minor salivary gland cancer is
    A. Mucoepidermoid cancer.
    B. Acinic cell cancer.
    C. Adenoid cystic cancer.
    D. Polymorphous low-grade adenocarcinoma.
    E. Salivary duct carcinoma.

54. The patient in Figure 5-3 has an adenoid cystic cancer of the hard palate. Which of the following is false regarding adenoid cystic cancer?
    A. High incidence of local recurrence
    B. Characteristic perineural invasion
    C. Metastasizes to regional lymph nodes
    D. Metastasizes to the lung
    E. Classified by histology into cribriform, solid, and tubular subtypes

55. Figure 5-4 shows a CT scan of the patient in Question 54. The patient should be managed by
    A. Local resection and secondary intention.
    B. Composite resection and an obturator prosthesis.
    C. Composite resection and a local flap.

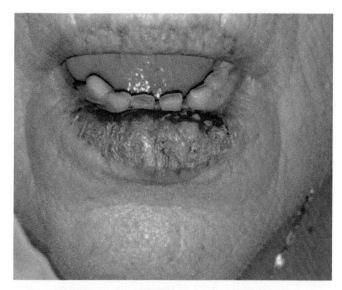

**Figure 5-1**

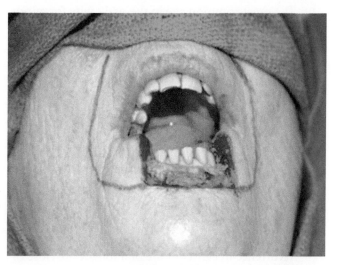

**Figure 5-2**

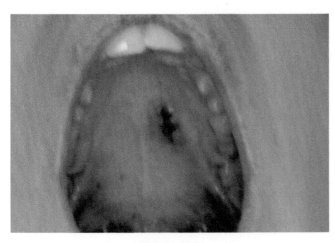

**Figure 5-3**

D. Soft tissue resection and a skin graft.
E. Local resection and a rotation flap.

56. Postoperative treatment should be
    A. Observation.
    B. Postoperative radiation therapy (PORT) to the primary resection site.
    C. PORT to the primary resection site and levels II to IV nodes and retropharyngeal nodes.
    D. PORT to the primary resection site and the course of the maxillary nerve bilaterally to the trigeminal ganglion bilaterally.
    E. Postoperative chemoradiation therapy.

57. The premalignant lesion at highest risk of malignant transformation is
    A. Homogeneous leukoplakia.
    B. Erythroplakia.
    C. Nonhomogeneous leukoplakia.
    D. Oral lichen planus.
    E. Oral submucous fibrosis.

58. Which risk factor is not associated with an increased risk of transformation?
    A. Leukoplakia in nonsmokers
    B. Nonhomogeneous subtype
    C. Presence of dysplasia
    D. Size less than 2 cm
    E. Female gender

59. Which of the following about tobacco and oral cancer are true?
    i. History of smoking in 60% of patients with oral cancer
    ii. Dose–response relationship
    iii. Synergistic interaction with alcohol
    iv. Associated with mutations in p53 gene
    v. No association with smokeless tobacco
    A. i, ii, iii, iv
    B. ii, iii, iv
    C. ii, iii, iv, v
    D. i, iii, iv, v
    E. All the above

60. Which of the following is not a risk factor for oral cancer?
    A. Tobacco
    B. Alcohol
    C. Fanconi anemia
    D. Herpes simplex virus
    E. Human immunodeficiency virus (HIV) infection

61. Which of the following is false about the epidemiology of oral cancer?
    A. More common in men
    B. Increases with age
    C. More common in developing countries
    D. Association with betel nut chewing
    E. Poorer prognosis in patients younger than 40 years

62. Which subsite of the oral cavity has the highest frequency of oral cancer?
    A. Buccal mucosa
    B. Hard palate
    C. Oral tongue
    D. Lower gum
    E. Upper gum

63. Which subsite of the oral cavity has the lowest frequency of oral cancer?
    A. Buccal mucosa
    B. Hard palate
    C. Oral tongue
    D. Lower gum
    E. Upper gum

64. Which oral cancer subsite is associated with oral submucous fibrosis?
    A. Buccal mucosa

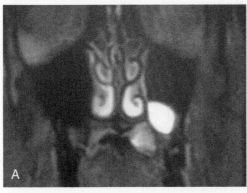

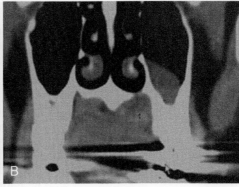

**Figure 5-4** (Courtesy of Memorial Sloan Kettering Cancer Center, New York.)

B. Hard palate
C. Oral tongue
D. Lower gum
E. Upper gum

65. Which is true about Gorlin syndrome?
    i. Associated with SCC of the skin
    ii. Associated with basal cell cancer of the skin
    iii. Associated with ameloblastoma
    iv. Associated with odontogenic keratocysts
    v. Associated with *PTCH1* mutations
    A. i, ii, iv, v
    B. ii, iii, v
    C. ii, iv, v
    D. ii, iv
    E. All of the above

66. Which of the following is not associated with oral submucous fibrosis?
    A. Malignant transformation potential of 10%
    B. Trismus
    C. Betel nut chewing
    D. Buccal cancer
    E. Gum cancer

67. Which of the following is not associated with Fanconi anemia?
    A. Associated with oral tongue cancer
    B. Associated with leukemia
    C. Associated with short stature
    D. Adverse response to radiation
    E. Typical survival to age 60

68. The inheritance pattern of Fanconi anemia is
    A. Autosomal dominant with high penetrance.
    B. Autosomal recessive.
    C. X-linked recessive.
    D. X-linked dominant.
    E. Autosomal dominant with low penetrance.

69. The patient in Figure 5-5 has an SCC of the lateral border of the oral tongue. The tumor measures 3 cm × 2 cm. A CT scan shows no enlarged lymph nodes. The stage of the patient is

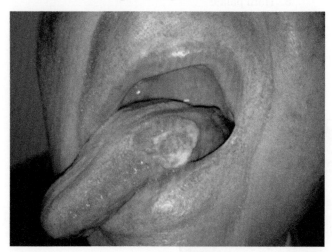

**Figure 5-5**

A. I.
B. II.

C. III.
D. IVa.
E. IVb.

70. Elective treatment of the neck in this case involves dissection of levels
    A. I, II, III.
    B. I, II, III, IV.
    C. II, III, IV.
    D. I, II.
    E. I, II, III, IV, V.

71. In patients who have occult metastases, which of the following is false?
    A. The rate is not dependent on T stage.
    B. The risk of recurrence after neck dissection is 10% to 25%.
    C. Postoperative radiation therapy reduces the risk of recurrence.
    D. The possibility increases with tumor thickness more than 4 mm.
    E. The incidence is 25% to 30%.

72. The two most important factors predictive of local recurrence in cancer of the oral tongue are
    A. Close/positive margins and perineural invasion.
    B. Close/positive margins and grade.
    C. Tumor thickness and close/positive margins.
    D. T stage and tumor thickness.
    E. T stage and close/positive margins.

73. Resection of cancers of more than one third of the oral tongue are best managed by
    A. Primary closure.
    B. Skin graft.
    C. Alloderm graft.
    D. Free radial forearm flap.
    E. Secondary intention.

74. An absolute indication for postoperative radiation therapy is
    A. Positive margins.
    B. Perineural invasion.
    C. Tumor thickness more than 4 mm.
    D. T2 stage tumor.
    E. Vascular invasion.

75. Postoperative chemoradiation therapy is indicated in patients with
    A. Positive neck nodes.
    B. Vascular invasion.
    C. Perineural invasion.
    D. T4 tumors.
    E. Extracapsular lymph node spreading.

76. In patients with oral tongue SCC with metastatic SCC to level II of the neck, which neck dissection gives the best regional control?
    A. Selective neck dissection levels I, II, III
    B. Selective neck dissection levels I, II, III, IV
    C. Modified radical neck dissection, type I
    D. Modified neck dissection, type III
    E. Radical neck dissection

77. The patient in Figure 5-6 has osteoradionecrosis of the mandible. Which of the following are true about osteoradionecrosis?
    i. Associated with dental caries
    ii. Associated with radiation doses greater than 65 Gy
    iii. Painless
    iv. Reversed with hyperbaric oxygen
    v. Requires specialist dental care
    A. i, ii, v
    B. i, ii, iii, v
    C. i, iv, v
    D. i, iii, iv, v
    E. All of the above

78. Optimal management of the osteoradionecrosis shown in Figure 5-6 is

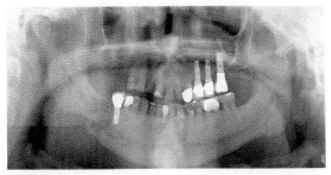

**Figure 5-6** (Courtesy of Memorial Sloan Kettering Cancer Center, New York.)

    A. Curettage and antibiotics.
    B. Hyperbaric oxygen.
    C. Hemimandibulectomy and free fibula flap reconstruction.
    D. Hemimandibulectomy and primary closure.
    E. Hemimandibulectomy and a free rectus flap.

79. The patient in Figure 5-7 has SCC of the left lower gum. Assessment of the mandible is best done by

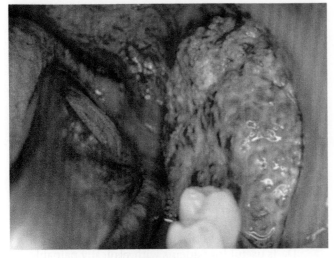

**Figure 5-7**

    A. CT scan.
    B. Magnetic resonance imaging.
    C. Clinical examination.
    D. Positron emission tomography.
    E. Orthopantomogram.

80. The primary tumor in Figure 5-7 measures 5 cm × 3 cm. A CT scan shows erosion of the cortex of the mandible. Two enlarged lymph nodes with central necrosis are shown in level 1b. One lymph node measures 4 × 2 cm and the other 1.5 × 2 cm. Under the TNM staging system, this patient's tumor is classified as
    A. T3N2a.
    B. T3N2b.
    C. T2N2b.
    D. T4N2b.
    E. T4N2a.

81. Optimum treatment of the primary tumor for this patient is
    A. Chemoradiation therapy.
    B. Wide local resection with a split-thickness skin graft.
    C. Wide local resection with marginal mandibulectomy.
    D. Wide local resection with segmental mandibulectomy.
    E. Wide local resection with buccal fat pad flap.

82. Optimal reconstruction in this patient is by
    A. Split-thickness skin graft.
    B. Free radial forearm flap.
    C. Free rectus abdominis flap.
    D. Free fibula flap.
    E. Pectoralis major flap.

83. Pathological examination shows a 4-cm moderately differentiated SCC with perineural invasion and vascular invasion. All margins are negative for cancer. There are 2 of 43 lymph nodes with metastatic disease. No extracapsular spreading is present. Adjuvant therapy
    A. Is not necessary.
    B. Should consist of postoperative primary and ipsilateral neck irradiation.
    C. Should consist of postoperative chemoradiation therapy.
    D. Should consist of postoperative ipsilateral neck irradiation only.
    E. Should consist of postoperative primary and bilateral neck irradiation.

84. Pathological examination shows a 4-cm moderately differentiated SCC with perineural invasion and vascular invasion. All margins are close (<5 mm) for cancer. There are 2 of 43 lymph nodes with metastatic disease. Extracapsular spreading to one lymph node is seen. Adjuvant therapy
    A. Is not necessary.
    B. Should consist of postoperative primary and ipsilateral neck irradiation.
    C. Should consist of postoperative chemoradiation therapy.
    D. Should consist of postoperative ipsilateral neck irradiation only.
    E. Should consist of postoperative primary and bilateral neck irradiation.

85. Cancer of the buccal mucosa is not associated with which of the following?
    A. Occult metastases of 30%
    B. Oral submucous fibrosis
    C. Betel nut chewing
    D. Metastases to facial lymph nodes
    E. Neck metastases associated with thickness of the tumor

86. A 50-year-old man presents with a painless swelling on the right side of the floor of his mouth. The mass is submucosal in nature. The differential diagnosis includes
    i. Adenoid cystic cancer.
    ii. Ranula.
    iii. Sialolithiasis.
    iv. Lymphoma.
    v. Schwannoma.
    A. i, ii, iii
    B. i, ii
    C. i, iii, v
    D. i, ii, iv
    E. All of the above

87. Which of the following oral cancer subsites has the worst prognosis?
    A. Buccal mucosa
    B. Hard palate
    C. Oral tongue
    D. Lower gum
    E. Upper gum

88. A 45-year-old man presents with a painless submucosal swelling of the hard palate. The differential diagnosis includes
    i. Adenoid cystic cancer.
    ii. Pleomorphic adenoma.
    iii. Lymphoma.
    iv. Melanoma.
    v. Metastases.
    A. i, ii, iii
    B. i, ii
    C. i, iii, v
    D. i, ii, iv
    E. All of the above

89. Which of the following is false about ameloblastoma of the mandible?
    A. Locally aggressive
    B. Can be unilocular and multilocular
    C. More common in the maxilla than in the mandible
    D. Of epithelial origin
    E. Painless swelling

90. A 40-year-old man is referred with a cystic mass in the ramus of the mandible. The patient is asymptomatic. Which of the following is not in the differential diagnosis?
    A. Odontogenic keratocyst
    B. Calcifying odontogenic cyst
    C. Ameloblastoma
    D. Dentigerous cyst
    E. Periapical cyst

91. A 60-year-old woman presents with a 2.5- × 1-cm ulcerated lesion on the left upper gum adjacent to the first molar. The lesion is fixed to the underlying bone. A biopsy shows SCC. A CT scan shows slight erosion of the cortex of the upper alveolus. No radiologically enlarged lymph nodes are present. The stage of this patient is
    A. I.
    B. II.
    C. III.
    D. IVa.
    E. IVb.

92. A 35-year-old Indian man with a history of betel nut chewing presents with trismus and pain. Examination shows an interincisor distance of 2 cm. An exophytic tumor of the buccal mucosa measures 5 cm × 3 cm. A biopsy shows SCC. The clinical T stage of this patient is most likely to be
    A. T1.
    B. T2.
    C. T3.
    D. T4a.
    E. T4b.

93. A 60-year-old man presents with a 2- × 3-cm cancer of the left lower gum. A CT scan shows a 4- × 2-cm left level Ib lymph node. A smaller lymph node in level II measures 1.5 × 2 cm. The clinical stage of the neck is
    A. N1.
    B. N2a.
    C. N2b.
    D. N2c.
    E. N3.

94. The overall stage of this patient in Question 93 is
    A. I.
    B. II.
    C. III.
    D. IVa.
    E. IVb.

95. Which of the following statements is false regarding marginal mandibulectomy?
    A. Dependent on the vertical height of the body of the mandible
    B. Contraindicated in the edentulous patient
    C. May require a fixation plate
    D. Unsafe in the irradiated mandible
    E. Contraindicated if the tumor is through the cortical bone

96. Which of the following is false with regard to sentinel node biopsy?
    A. Requires preoperative lymphoscintigraphy
    B. Is a procedure that defines the sentinel node as the first-echelon lymph node to which cancer spreads
    C. May be useful in the staging of the neck
    D. Is useful for patients with clinically palpable lymph nodes
    E. Identifies patients who require a neck dissection

97. A 65-year-old woman (Figure 5-8) presents with an ulcerated lesion of the left upper gum measuring 3 × 2 cm. A staging CT scan shows erosion of the bone of the upper alveolus with extension into the maxillary sinus. No enlarged cervical lymph nodes were present. The stage of the cancer in this patient is

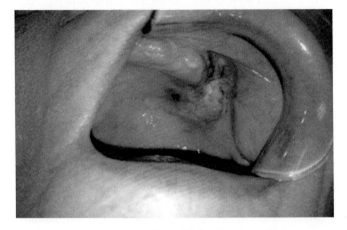

**Figure 5-8**

   A. I.
   B. II.
   C. III.
   D. IVa.
   E. IVb.

98. Management of the primary tumor is by
   A. Chemoradiation therapy.
   B. Upper alveolectomy with a split-thickness skin graft.
   C. Upper alveolectomy and an obturator prosthesis.
   D. Subtotal maxillectomy with an obturator prosthesis.
   E. Total maxillectomy with a rectus flap.

99. Which oral cancer subsite is associated with the highest rate of occult neck metastases?
   A. Buccal mucosa
   B. Hard palate
   C. Oral tongue
   D. Lower gum
   E. Upper gum

100. Which is not an indication for segmental mandibulectomy?
   A. Osteosarcoma of the mandible
   B. Metastases to the mandible
   C. Gross invasion of the mandible by SCC
   D. Invasion of the mandibular canal and inferior alveolar nerve
   E. Odontogenic keratocyst

## Answers

| | | |
|---|---|---|
| 1. T | 4. F | 7. F |
| 2. T | 5. T | 8. T |
| 3. T | 6. F | 9. T |

| | | |
|---|---|---|
| 10. T | 41. T | 72. A |
| 11. T | 42. F | 73. D |
| 12. T | 43. T | 74. A |
| 13. F | 44. F | 75. E |
| 14. T | 45. F | 76. E |
| 15. F | 46. T | 77. A |
| 16. T | 47. F | 78. C |
| 17. T | 48. T | 79. C |
| 18. T | 49. T | 80. D |
| 19. F | 50. T | 81. D |
| 20. T | 51. B | 82. D |
| 21. T | 52. E | 83. E |
| 22. T | 53. C | 84. C |
| 23. F | 54. C | 85. A |
| 24. T | 55. B | 86. E |
| 25. F | 56. D | 87. A |
| 26. F | 57. B | 88. E |
| 27. T | 58. D | 89. C |
| 28. F | 59. B | 90. E |
| 29. F | 60. D | 91. B |
| 30. T | 61. E | 92. D |
| 31. F | 62. C | 93. C |
| 32. T | 63. B | 94. D |
| 33. F | 64. A | 95. B |
| 34. T | 65. C | 96. D |
| 35. T | 66. A | 97. D |
| 36. T | 67. E | 98. D |
| 37. T | 68. B | 99. C |
| 38. T | 69. B | 100. E |
| 39. F | 70. B | |
| 40. F | 71. A | |

## Core Knowledge

- Squamous cell carcinomas account for more than 90% of malignant tumors of the oral cavity. Other tumors include minor salivary gland tumors, melanoma, and lymphoma. Minor salivary gland tumors are most common in the hard palate. Approximately 50% of intraoral minor salivary gland tumors are malignant. The most common carcinomas are adenoid cystic carcinoma (35.4%), adenocarcinoma (21.5%), and mucoepidermoid carcinoma (15.5%). Cervical nodal metastases are present in 22% of minor salivary gland cancers predominantly by small cell carcinomas, malignant mixed tumors, and high grade mucoepidermoid tumors.

Adenoid cystic carcinomas present with cervical nodal metastases in <10% of cases. Distant metastases are observed most often in patients with adenoid cystic carcinoma (39.7%). Mean survival for a patient with adenoid cystic carcinoma lung metastases is 3 years reflecting the relatively indolent activity of the tumor.

- Epithelial precursor lesions can be classified into leukoplakia (white plaques) and erythroplakia (red patch). Both conditions are associated with smoking and alcohol. Leukoplakia can be subdivided into a homogeneous type (i.e., flat, thin, and uniformly white) and a nonhomogeneous type. The homogeneous type is the most common and appears as a homogeneous white area broken up by longitudinal fissures. The lesions are generally hyperorthokeratotic. Nonhomogeneous leukoplakia can be nodular, speckled, or verrucous. Nodular and speckled lesions are usually associated with severe epithelial dysplasia. Approximately 1% of leukoplakias undergo malignant transformation annually. This figure is much higher for nonhomogeneous leukoplakia. The factors that carry a statistically significant risk of malignant transformation are female gender, long duration of leukoplakia, location on the tongue or floor of the mouth, leukoplakia in nonsmokers, size greater than 2 cm, nonhomogeneous type, and presence of dysplasia.

- Erythroplakia is a bright red velvety patch that histologically shows at least some degree of dysplasia and often even carcinoma in situ. These lesions have a very high rate of aneuploidy (68%), and if present, the majority develop into cancer. As such, all erythroplakia lesions should be treated aggressively by wide surgical excision.

- Other premalignant lesions are oral lichen planus, which has an extremely low malignant transformation rate of less than 1%. Oral submucous fibrosis is caused by the chewing of areca and betel quid. Clinically, this condition is characterized by extreme sensitivity to spicy and hot foods, fibrosis and stiffening of the oral mucosa, and the development of trismus. Histologically, fibrosis of the lamina propria is seen with atrophy of the overlying epithelium. This atrophied epithelium predisposes to the development of squamous cell carcinoma. The annual malignant transformation rate is approximately 0.5%.

- Worldwide, an estimated 405,000 new cases of oral cancer are diagnosed each year, and two thirds occur in developing countries. The incidence increases with age, and 85% of cases occur after the fifth decade. The disease is more common in men. When oral cancer rates are analyzed by age group, the rates have halved for men older than 80 years, have remained stable for men 60 to 70 years of age, but have increased markedly in men between 40 and 60 years.

- Smoking and alcohol drinking are the major risk factors in the white population, whereas betel nut and tobacco consumption have been associated with oral cancer in the Asian population. Other etiological factors are a diet deficient in vitamin A, chronic irritation from poor dental hygiene, syphilis, chronic use of mouthwash, and marijuana smoking. Types 2, 11, and 16 of the human papillomavirus have also been associated with oral cancer, as well as immunosuppression associated with kidney transplantation, bone marrow transplantation, and human immunodeficiency virus (HIV) infection. Genetic factors associated with increased risk include mutagen sensitivity, which reflects a defect in DNA repair seen in conditions like xeroderma pigmentosum, Fanconi anemia, and ataxia telangiectasia.

- Lymphatic spreading in oral cancer into the neck follows a stepwise, orderly fashion. The patient with clinically negative neck nodes is at highest risk of metastasis to levels I to III. Skip metastases to level IV do occur (skipping levels II and III) and are more commonly associated with cancer of the anterior tongue. The probability of lymph node metastases is directly related to T stage. This understanding determines the type of neck dissection required for patients with oral cancer.

- Tumors of the lower and upper gum drain into levels I to III. Lower gum cancers metastasize more frequently than those of the upper gum. Tumors of the floor of the mouth drain initially to the submental and submandibular nodes and 12% to 30% of early (T1 to T2) lesions will have occult metastases, depending on the thickness of the lesion. The incidence of lymph node metastases in larger lesions (T3 to T4) is between 47% and 53%. Carcinoma of the oral tongue has the greatest propensity among all oral cancers for metastasis to the neck. The primary echelon of drainage is level II. The rate of occult metastases is 25% to 30%. The depth of invasion and tumor thickness seem to be significant predictors of lymph node metastasis. Only 10% of patients with buccal cancer have clinically significant neck nodes at presentation. The primary echelons are levels I and II. Buccal cancer has a recognized risk for metastatic spreading to the facial and prevascular facial lymph nodes. As such, careful attention should be paid to these lymph nodes so that adequate removal is ensured during a neck dissection. Tumor thickness is a significant prognostic factor.

- The mainstay of treatment is surgery with or without postoperative radiation or chemoradiation therapy. Surgery involves resection of the primary tumor, either transorally or using a cheek flap or mandibulotomy to improve access. For more advanced tumors with bone invasion, mandibulectomy or maxillectomy may be required. Elective supraomohyoid neck dissection (SOHND) (levels I to III) is usually done, and an extended SOHND (levels I to IV) is performed for cancer of the oral tongue.

- The mechanism of invasion of the mandible has been established by work done by MacGregor and MacDonald. The periosteum acts as a deterrent to mandibular invasion. In the dentate mandible, tumor creeps up from the gingiva, through the dental socket, into the cancellous bone. In the edentulous mandible, invasion of the cancellous bone occurs more easily through the dental pores of the alveolar process.

- Clinical evaluation has been shown to be reliable in the assessment of early bony invasion. The accuracy of conventional radiography with an orthopantomogram (OPG) in detecting early invasion is limited by the fact that 30% to 50% mineral loss must occur before the changes are radiologically apparent. A computed tomographic (CT) scan can be limited by artifacts produced by irregular dental sockets or other dental artifacts. Magnetic resonance imaging (MRI) is useful for evaluation of invasion of the medullary space and perineural invasion of the inferior alveolar nerve.

- The understanding of tumor invasion into the mandible enables the use of marginal resection of bone based on the observation that the cortical part of the bone containing the mandibular canal lies inferior to the dental roots and remains relatively uninvolved in early stage disease; thus it can be safely spared. The ability to perform a marginal mandibulectomy depends on the vertical height of the body of the mandible. Resorption of the mandible with age results in recession of the alveolar process, and the mandibular canal with the inferior alveolar nerve is at increased risk of involvement in these patients. In marginal resection in edentulous patients, the mandible is at risk of an iatrogenic fracture. Marginal mandibular resection is also best avoided in previously irradiated patients because of the more variable routes of tumor entry.

- It is also well recognized that metastasis to the cervical lymph nodes is the single most important prognostic factor in patients with head and neck cancer. The presence of a metastatic cervical node in a patient with oral cancer decreases the chance of a cure by 50% when compared with those with similar primary tumors without nodal metastases.

- In a patient with clinically negative neck nodes, the risk of metastasis to levels IV and V is very small and an SOHND is recommended. For similar patients with primary tumors of the tongue, inclusion of level IV in the dissection is indicated. In patients with palpable cervical nodes, levels I to IV are at highest risk. A comprehensive neck dissection is therefore recommended. This usually involves a type 1 modified radical neck dissection (RND) preserving the spinal accessory nerve. The classic RND is the gold standard against which the effectiveness of all other forms of neck dissection must be evaluated. When used alone, RND controls disease in the neck in more than 90% of N0 patients; however, as many as 60% of patients with bulky neck disease will have recurrence. The control rate for patients with clinically positive neck nodes improves to more than 80% if postoperative radiation therapy is added. For clinically N0 patients who are proven pathologically N0, failure rates of less than 10% have been reported. The 30% of patients who have pathologically proven occult metastases after SOHND develop neck recurrence 10% to 24% of the time, depending on the number of positive nodes and the presence of extracapsular extension. The addition of postoperative radiation therapy reduces the failure rate in these patients to 0% to 15%. The appropriate use of postoperative radiation therapy in combination with modified RND has resulted in control rates comparable with RND for similar patients. For lesions approaching or crossing the midline, bilateral neck dissections should be performed.

- Sentinel node biopsy can be done to identify patients who can be spared an elective neck dissection. The sentinel lymph node is defined as the first-echelon lymph node to which cancer spreads. Identification of the sentinel node requires the use of preoperative lymphoscintigraphy using radioactive technetium and then blue dye injection (toluidine blue) at the time of surgery. The sentinel node is identified with the use of a gamma probe and is confirmed with the injection of blue dye at the time of biopsy. Pathological examination of the sentinel node requires both hematoxylin and eosin staining and immunohistochemical analysis. The node requires serial sectioning at 150-micron sections for accurate analysis.

- Adjuvant radiation therapy is indicated for patients with positive or close surgical margins, lymphovascular invasion, perineural invasion, pathologically positive neck nodes, and extracapsular spreading. Postoperative doses of 60 Gy or more result in good locoregional control.

- Adjuvant chemoradiation therapy using cisplatin improves locoregional control in patients with extracapsular spreading, positive surgical margins, or both. In patients who cannot tolerate cisplatin, concurrent administration of cetuximab with radiation therapy has also shown improved locoregional control in locally advanced oral cavity cancer.

- Osteoradionecrosis is a complication of radiation to the mandible or maxilla. Diseased teeth within the radiation field are the prime initiator of osteoradionecrosis, and almost all bone necrosis occurs in patients who were dentulous before radiation therapy. Risk factors include the size and location of the lesion, the volume of the mandible within the radiation field, dosage of more than 65 Gy, and the health of the dentition. Patients may complain of severe pain. Early osteoradionecrosis may be treated with conservative measures such as the use of an oral irrigator (Waterpik), debridement, long-term antibiotics, and, very rarely, hyperbaric oxygen. There is no evidence that hyperbaric oxygen can reverse the effects of osteoradionecrosis. For more extensive necrosis, patients may benefit from aggressive surgical excision of the necrotic mandible and immediate microvascular reconstruction.

## SUGGESTED READING

Bernier J, Domenge C, Ozsahin M, Matuszewska K, Lefebvre JL, et al. Postoperative irradiation with or without concomitant chemotherapy for locally advanced head and neck cancer. N Engl J Med 2004;350(19):1945–52.

Byers R, Wolf P, Ballantyne A. Rationale for elective modified neck dissection. Head Neck Surg 1988;10(3):160–7.

Cooper JS, Pajak TF, Forastiere AA, Jacobs J, Campbell BH, et al. Postoperative concurrent radiotherapy and chemotherapy for high risk squamous cell carcinoma of the head and neck. N Engl J Med 2004;350(19):1937–44.

Ganly I, Patel S, Shah J. Early stage squamous cell cancer of the oral tongue—clinicopathologic features affecting outcome. Cancer 2012;118(1):101–11.

McGregor AD, MacDonald DG. Routes of entry of squamous cell carcinoma to the mandible. Head Neck Surg 1988;10(5):294–301.

McGregor AD, MacDonald DG. Patterns of spread of squamous cell carcinoma in the mandible. Head Neck 1989;11:457–61.

Morris LG, Patel SG, Shah JP, Ganly I. High rates of regional failure in squamous cell carcinoma of the hard palate and maxillary alveolus. Head Neck 2011;33(6):824–30.

Ross G, Shoaib T, Soutar DS, Camilleri IG, Gray HW, et al. The use of sentinel node biopsy to upstage the clinically N0 neck in head and neck cancer. Arch Otolaryngol Head Neck Surg 2002;128(11):1287–91.

Shah JP, Candela FC, Poddar AK. The patterns of cervical lymph node metastases from squamous carcinoma of the oral cavity. Cancer 1990;66(1):109–13.

Spiro RH, Huvos AG, Wong GY, Spiro JD, Gnecco CA, et al. Predictive value of tumor thickness in squamous carcinoma confined to the tongue and floor of the mouth. Am J Surg 1986;152(4):345–50.

Spiro RH, Koss LG, Hajdu SI, Strong EW. Tumors of minor salivary origin. A clinicopathologic study of 492 cases. Cancer 1973;31(1):117–29.

# 6 Pharynx and Esophagus

## Questions

### TRUE/FALSE

1. Malignant melanomas, minor salivary gland tumors, sarcomas, plasmacytomas, and lymphomas account for more than 20% of the malignant tumors of the oropharynx. (T/F)

2. The most common first-echelon nodal region for metastatic disease from the base of the tongue and tonsils is level II, although involvement of levels III and IV is also seen. (T/F)

3. Referred otalgia through cranial nerve (CN) IX and CN X could be one of the first symptoms of a patient with an oropharynx tumor. (T/F)

4. Human papillomavirus (HPV) type 16 is the cause of 90% of HPV-associated oropharyngeal cancers. (T/F)

5. E6 and E7 are the protooncogenes that play a role in the genetic alterations associated with HPV-related oropharynx squamous cell carcinoma (SCC). (T/F)

6. HPV-related tumors tend to be seen with a higher primary T stage and lower rate of nodal disease. (T/F)

7. Oral sex is associated with transmission of HPV. (T/F)

8. HPV types 11, 16, 18, and 33 are all associated with oropharyngeal carcinoma. (T/F)

9. Patients with HPV-associated oropharynx cancer have a worse prognosis than patients with non–HPV-associated oropharynx cancer. (T/F)

10. Patients with HPV-associated oropharynx cancer who are smokers have a worse prognosis than patients who have HPV-associated oropharynx cancer who are nonsmokers. (T/F)

11. Treatment options for stage I and II oropharynx cancer include definitive radiation therapy (RT) or primary surgical resection with or without neck dissection. (T/F)

12. The preferred interval between resection and postoperative RT is 6 weeks, and a prolonged delay is associated with increased locoregional failure and decreased survival times. (T/F)

13. Adjuvant contralateral neck treatment should be considered if the primary tumor approaches the midline because of the high probability of bilateral disease. (T/F)

14. Cervical metastasis from the soft palate may involve the retropharyngeal lymph nodes. (T/F)

15. Adenoid cystic carcinoma is the most commonly encountered minor salivary gland tumor. (T/F)

16. Nasopharyngeal tumors have a biological propensity for early lymphatic and distant metastatic spreading. (T/F)

17. Nasopharyngeal carcinoma (NPC) has a high propensity for nodal metastasis: reported rates are as high as 79%, and as many as 30% of patients have bilateral involvement. (T/F)

18. The nasopharynx is lined partly with pseudostratified columnar respiratory-type epithelium and partly with nonkeratinizing stratified squamous epithelium. (T/F)

19. The nerve supply to the nasopharyngeal mucosa is derived from the maxillary division of the trigeminal nerve, which arises in the pterygopalatine fossa. (T/F)

20. The majority of tumors in the nasopharynx arise in the region of the fossa of Rosenmüller or in the roof of the nasopharynx, followed by location in the posterior wall. (T/F)

21. Direct anterior extension of a nasopharyngeal tumor may lead to involvement of the posterior nasal cavity, or extension inferiorly along the pharyngeal wall may lead to involvement of the soft palate or the tonsils. (T/F)

22. Skull base involvement at presentation has rarely been reported. (T/F)

23. A strong association between NPC and Epstein-Barr virus has been reported. (T/F)

24. Parapharyngeal extension of NPCs, either as a direct extension of tumor or expansion of nodal disease, rarely occurs. (T/F)

25. The World Health Organization (WHO) has classified NPC as keratinizing SCC (type 1), non-keratinizing (differentiated) carcinoma (type 2), and undifferentiated carcinoma (type 3). (T/F)

26. The hypopharynx is divided into the right and left pyriform sinuses, the posterior and lateral wall, and the post cricoid region. (T/F)

27. The hypopharynx extends from the hyoid cartilage to the inferior border of the cricoid cartilage. (T/F)

28. The hypopharynx plays an important role in deglutition and protection of the airway from aspiration. (T/F)

29. As many as 60% of all hypopharyngeal SCCs arise from the piriform sinuses. (T/F)

30. The postcricoid area forms the anterior wall of the hypopharynx and connects the two piriform sinuses extending from the level of the arytenoid cartilages to the inferior border of the cricoid cartilage. (T/F)

31. Lymphatic drainage of the hypopharynx includes levels II and III, retropharyngeal lymph nodes, and the nodes of Rouvière. (T/F)

32. Carcinomas of the hypopharynx are usually found early when they are small and localized to the site of the primary lesion. (T/F)

33. Cancers involving the medial wall of the piriform sinus have a reported contralateral risk of metastasis as high as 20%. (T/F)

34. Both postcricoid and posterior pharyngeal wall tumors have a potential for bilateral metastasis. (T/F)

35. As many as two thirds of patients with hypopharyngeal cancers are initially found to have stage IV disease. (T/F)

36. Adenocarcinoma is the most common cancer of the cervical esophagus. (T/F)

37. Carcinoma involving the cervical esophagus is rare and often a direct extension from the hypopharynx. (T/F)

38. Cervical esophagus SCC has a poor prognosis with posttreatment 5-year survival rates as low as 20%. (T/F)

39. The primary treatment of cervical esophageal SCC has been surgical resection. (T/F)

40. The cervical esophagus extends from the cricopharyngeal sphincter to the thoracic inlet and is lined by a nonkeratinizing squamous epithelium. (T/F)

41. Primary adenocarcinoma of the cervical esophagus is rare but may arise from Barrett esophagus. (T/F)

42. The most common benign lesions reported in the cervical esophagus are pedunculated hyperplastic or fibrovascular polyps. (T/F)

43. T3 tumors of the cervical esophagus invade the muscularis propria. (T/F)

44. Hypopharyngeal and cervical esophageal cancers are predisposed to submucosal spreading that may be undetectable by clinical and endoscopic evaluation. (T/F)

45. A computed tomographic (CT) scan finding of more than 24 mm for the A-P diameter of the cervical esophagus should be considered abnormal. (T/F)

46. Two sensitive imaging criteria for the diagnosis of cervical esophageal cancer are thickening of the esophageal wall and effacement of the fat plane. (T/F)

47. The same staging criteria apply for SCC of the esophagus and adenocarcinoma of the esophagus. (T/F)

48. The current recommendation for SCC of the esophagus after R0 resection with or without positive nodes is observation. (T/F)

49. T1b tumors of the esophagus invade lamina propria or muscularis mucosae. (T/F)

50. The current treatment recommendation for T1b, N+ carcinoma of the cervical esophagus is chemoradiation therapy with salvage esophagectomy for persistent disease. (T/F)

## MULTIPLE CHOICE

51. What is the genetic signature associated with HPV-positive oropharyngeal cancer?
    i. Inactivation of p53
    ii. Downregulation of pRB
    iii. Increased p16
    iv. Decreased epidermal growth factor receptor (EGFR)
    v. Fewer p53 mutations
    vi. Downregulation of cyclin D1
    A. i, iv
    B. i, ii, iii
    C. i, ii, iii, iv
    D. All of the above

52. Surgical approaches to oropharynx tumors include
    i. Mandibulotomy.
    ii. Lateral pharyngotomy.
    iii. Suprahyoid pharyngotomy.
    iv. Transoral approaches.
    v. Median mandibuloglossotomy.
    vi. Pull through.
    A. i, iv
    B. i, ii, iii, iv, v, vi
    C. i, ii, iii, iv, v
    D. i, ii, iv

53. Postoperative adjuvant therapy should be considered in patients with
    i. Large primary tumors.
    ii. Close or positive margins.
    iii. Extracapsular extension.
    iv. Multiple positive nodes.
    v. Extensive vascular or perineural invasion.
    A. ii, iii
    B. i, ii, iii
    C. i, ii, iii, iv, v
    D. ii, iii, iv

54. Paramedian mandibulotomy is preferred compared with median and lateral mandibulotomy because
    i. Dental extraction is not required.
    ii. The inferior alveolar nerve is spared.
    iii. Division of genial muscles is not required.
    iv. The area lies outside the lateral radiation portals.
    A. ii
    B. i, iv
    C. i, ii
    D. All of the above

55. Current treatment options for N2 to 3 oropharyngeal cancer include
    i. Concurrent systemic therapy and RT.
    ii. Induction chemotherapy.
    iii. Surgery for the primary tumor and neck dissection.
    iv. Multimodality clinical trials.
    A. i, iii
    B. i, ii
    C. i, ii, iii
    D. All of the above

56. What is the paraneoplastic syndrome(s) associated with NPC?
    i. Hypertrophic osteoarthropathy
    ii. Pyrexia of unknown origin
    iii. Inappropriate antidiuretic hormone (ADH) secretion
    A. i
    B. iii
    C. i, ii
    D. i, ii, iii

57. Which of the following are surgical approaches to the nasopharynx?
    i. Transnasal/transantral
    ii. Le Fort I maxillotomy
    iii. Palatal split
    iv. Transpalatal flap
    v. Transcervicomandibulopalatal
    vi. Lateral infratemporal
    vii. Anterolateral maxillary swing
    A. iii, iv, vii
    B. i, iii, iv, v, vi, vii
    C. i, iii, iv, vii
    D. All of the above

58. Evidence suggesting a probable oncogenic role of Epstein-Barr virus (EBV) in the genesis of nasopharyngeal tumors includes
    i. Raised levels of antibodies against EBV.
    ii. Higher titers of IgA antibodies against EBV in patients with large tumor bulk.
    iii. Presence of EBV DNA or RNA in practically all tumor cells.
    iv. Presence of EBV in a clonal episomal form.
    v. Presence of EBV in the precursor lesion of NPC but not in the normal nasopharyngeal epithelium.
    A. i
    B. iii
    C. i, ii, iii

D. i, ii, iii, iv, v
E. i, iii, v

59. Which of the following are true about nasopharyngeal papillary adenocarcinoma?
    i. It is a low-grade adenocarcinoma.
    ii. It is characterized by an exophytic growth comprising papillary fronds and glandular structures.
    iii. The tumor most commonly involves the roof and lateral and posterior walls of the nasopharynx.
    iv. The tumor is usually confined within the nasopharynx.
    A. ii, iii
    B. i, ii
    C. i, ii, iii
    D. All of the above

60. Benign tumors that can arise from the nasopharynx include
    i. Angiofibroma.
    ii. Squamous papilloma.
    iii. Ectopic pituitary adenoma.
    iv. Craniopharyngioma.
    v. Salivary gland anlage tumor.
    A. i, ii
    B. i, ii, iii
    C. i, ii, iii, iv, v

61. Some of the treatment complications of NPC include
    i. Temporal lobe necrosis.
    ii. Encephalopathy.
    iii. Cranial nerve palsies.
    iv. Hypothalamic–pituitary dysfunction.
    v. Hearing impairment.
    A. i
    B. i, iii
    C. i, v
    D. i, ii, iii, iv, v
    E. i, ii, iii

62. Hypopharyngeal tumors have a poor prognosis compared with other head and neck cancer sites because of
    i. Vague early stage symptoms.
    ii. Locally advanced stage at presentation.
    iii. High rate of nodal metastasis.
    iv. High rate of distant metastasis.
    A. ii
    B. ii, iii
    C. i, ii, iii, iv
    D. ii, iv

63. Which of the following tumors arise from the hypopharynx?
    i. Sarcomas, including chondrosarcomas
    ii. Melanomas
    iii. Minor salivary gland tumors
    iv. Lymphomas
    v. Adenocarcinomas
    vi. SCCs
    A. iii, vi
    B. iii, v, vi

C. i, ii, iii, iv, v, vi
D. ii, iii, vi

64. Treatment options for T2-4a primary hypopharynx tumors or those with N+ disease include
    i. Induction chemotherapy.
    ii. Laryngopharyngectomy plus neck dissection including ± level VI.
    iii. Noncurrent chemotherapy and RT.
    iv. Multimodality clinical trials.
    v. Partial or conservation surgery plus neck dissection.
    A. i , ii, v
    B. i, ii, iii
    C. i, ii, iii, iv, v
    D. i, ii, iii, iv

65. Poor cure rates for cervical esophageal cancer are related to
    i. Advanced stage at diagnosis.
    ii. High incidence of submucosal spreading.
    iii. High rate of nodal metastasis.
    iv. High rate of second primary cancer of the esophagus.
    v. High incidence of long-term distant metastasis.
    A. i, iii
    B. i, iii, v
    C. i, ii, iii, iv, v
    D. i, ii
    E. i, ii, iii, iv

66. Reconstructive options for a laryngopharyngoesophagectomy include
    A. A gastric pull up.
    B. A free jejunal flap.
    C. A combination of free flap and regional flap.
    D. All of the above.

67. The most common site for carcinoma in the oropharynx is the
    A. Tonsil.
    B. Base of the tongue.
    C. Hard palate.
    D. Piriform fossa.

68. What structure has the highest risk of nodal metastases on presentation?
    A. Glottis
    B. Tonsil
    C. Maxillary sinus
    D. Anterior faucial pillar

69. The current recommended conventional dose of definitive RT for oropharyngeal cancer is
    A. 66 to 74 Gy in 2.0 Gy/fractions 5 days a week for 7 weeks.
    B. 56 to 66 Gy in 2.0 Gy/fractions 5 days a week for 7 weeks.
    C. 50 to 60 Gy in 2.0 Gy/fractions 5 days a week for 7 weeks.
    D. 70 to 75 Gy in 2.0 Gy/fractions 5 days a week for 7 weeks.

70. In nasopharyngeal cancer the most common site of metastases is the
    A. Bone.
    B. Liver.
    C. Lung.
    D. Brain.

71. The current treatment recommendation for T1 nasopharyngeal tumors includes
    A. Primary surgery and adjuvant RT.
    B. Definitive RT and elective neck irradiation.
    C. Irradiation to the nasopharynx alone.
    D. Whole-body irradiation.

72. Nasopharyngeal angiofibromas almost exclusively affect
    A. Adolescent girls.
    B. Boys and adolescent to young men with a peak in the second decade of life.
    C. Women in their second decade.
    D. Both sexes equally up to the age of 25 years.

73. NPC is highly sensitive to
    A. Doxorubicin (Adriamycin).
    B. Methotrexate.
    C. Cyclophosphamide.
    D. Platinum-based regimens.

74. The preferred imaging study for evaluating the intracranial or perineural extent of nasopharyngeal tumors is
    A. CT.
    B. Enhanced magnetic resonance imaging (MRI).
    C. Enhanced CT.
    D. Ultrasonography.

75. With reirradiation for recurrent or persistent nasopharyngeal cancer, temporal lobe necrosis rates are as high as
    A. 5%.
    B. 15%.
    C. 28%.
    D. 35%.

76. Primary piriform fossa tumors have a high incidence of nodal metastasis; reported rates are as high as
    A. 15%.
    B. 25%.
    C. 45%.
    D. 70%.

77. The primary lymphatic drainage of the oropharynx is to level
    A. I nodes.
    B. II nodes.
    C. III nodes.
    D. IV nodes.

78. The oropharynx extends from
    A. The level of the hard palate to the hyoid.
    B. The level of the superior border of the soft palate to the hyoid.
    C. The circumvallate papillae to the hyoid.
    D. The posterior border of the choanae to the hyoid.

79. The oropharynx includes the following, except the
    A. Tonsils.
    B. Epiglottis.
    C. Base of the tongue.
    D. Glossotonsillar sulcus.

80. The hypopharynx includes the following, except the
    A. Piriform sinus.
    B. Posterior tonsillar pillar.
    C. Epiglottis.
    D. Postcricoid region.

81. The nasopharynx extends
    A. Anteriorly from the posterior choana to the free border of the soft palate.
    B. Posteriorly from the choana to the tonsil.
    C. Anteriorly from the posterior choana to the upper plane of the tonsil.
    D. From the fossa of Rosenmüller to the base of the tongue.

82. The parapharyngeal space extends from the skull base to the
    A. Hyoid.
    B. Level of the epiglottis.
    C. Level of the angle of the mandible.
    D. Level of the postcricoid region.

83. The carotid (poststyloid) space contains the following, except
    A. CN IX.
    B. Internal carotid artery.
    C. External carotid artery.
    D. Internal jugular vein.

84. The masticator space includes the following muscles, except the
    A. Medial pterygoid.
    B. Lateral pterygoid.
    C. Posterior digastric.
    D. Temporalis.

85. An oropharyngeal tumor involving the medial pterygoid muscles is stage
    A. T3.
    B. T4a.
    C. T4b.
    D. T2.

86. An oropharyngeal tumor involving the lateral pterygoid muscle is stage
    A. T3.
    B. T4a.
    C. T4b.
    D. T2.

87. A 3.5-cm hypopharyngeal tumor with prevertebral fascia invasion is stage
    A. T2.
    B. T3.
    C. T4a.
    D. T4b.

88. In NPC, bilateral retropharyngeal lymph nodes smaller than 6 cm are
    A. N1.
    B. N2.

C. N3.
D. N3b.

89. In NPC, bilateral cervical lymph nodes smaller than 6 cm are
    A. N1.
    B. N2.
    C. N3.
    D. N3b.

90. In NPC, supraclavicular metastases smaller than 6 cm are
    A. N1.
    B. N2.
    C. N3.
    D. N3b.

91. The cervical esophagus begins
    A. 10 to 15 cm from the incisors.
    B. 15 to 20 cm from the incisors.
    C. 21 cm from the incisors.
    D. 25 cm from the incisors.

92. Which of the following is incorrect?
    A. The cervical esophagus lies in the neck.
    B. The upper thoracic esophagus is 15 to 25 cm from the incisors.
    C. The middle thoracic esophagus is 25 to 30 cm from the incisors.
    D. The lower thoracic esophagus is 30 to 40 cm from the incisors.

93. A nasopharyngeal primary SCC with parapharyngeal space extension is stage
    A. T1.
    B. T2.
    C. T3.
    D. T4.

94. A nasopharyngeal primary SCC with extension to the oropharynx without parapharyngeal space extension is stage
    A. T1.
    B. T2.
    C. T3.
    D. T4.

95. A nasopharyngeal primary SCC with extension into the nasal cavity without parapharyngeal space extension is stage
    A. T1.
    B. T2.
    C. T3.
    D. T4.

96. Overall 5-year survival rates for cancers of the hypopharynx and esophagus range from
    A. 10% to 30%.
    B. 20% to 40%.
    C. 30% to 50%.
    D. 50% to 80%.

97. What percent chance of occult metastases do T1 or 2 hypopharyngeal SCCs have?
    A. 10%
    B. 20%

C. 30%
D. 40%

98. Killian dehiscence is a triangular area
    A. Between the thyropharyngeus and the cricopharyngeus.
    B. Between the inferior and middle constrictor muscles.
    C. In the hypopharynx.
    D. Between the inferior constrictor and the upper esophagus.

99. A Zenker diverticulum is a
    A. True diverticulum.
    B. Pseudodiverticulum.
    C. False diverticulum.
    D. Partial diverticulum.

100. Esophageal webs are associated with the following, except
    A. Plummer-Vinson syndrome.
    B. Celiac disease.
    C. Gastroesophageal reflux disease (GERD).
    D. Bullous pemphigoid.

## Answers

| | | |
|---|---|---|
| 1. F | 27. T | 53. C |
| 2. T | 28. T | 54. D |
| 3. T | 29. T | 55. D |
| 4. T | 30. T | 56. D |
| 5. T | 31. T | 57. D |
| 6. F | 32. F | 58. D |
| 7. T | 33. T | 59. D |
| 8. F | 34. T | 60. C |
| 9. F | 35. T | 61. D |
| 10. T | 36. F | 62. C |
| 11. T | 37. T | 63. C |
| 12. T | 38. T | 64. D |
| 13. T | 39. T | 65. C |
| 14. T | 40. T | 66. D |
| 15. T | 41. T | 67. A |
| 16. T | 42. T | 68. B |
| 17. T | 43. F | 69. A |
| 18. T | 44. T | 70. A |
| 19. T | 45. T | 71. B |
| 20. T | 46. T | 72. B |
| 21. T | 47. F | 73. D |
| 22. F | 48. T | 74. B |
| 23. T | 49. F | 75. C |
| 24. F | 50. T | 76. D |
| 25. T | 51. D | 77. B |
| 26. T | 52. B | 78. B |

| | | |
|---|---|---|
| 79. B | 87. D | 95. A |
| 80. B | 88. A | 96. C |
| 81. A | 89. B | 97. D |
| 82. C | 90. D | 98. A |
| 83. C | 91. B | 99. C |
| 84. C | 92. B | 100. C |
| 85. B | 93. B | |
| 86. C | 94. A | |

## Core Knowledge

### HUMAN PAPILLOMAVIRUS

- The causative role of human papilloma virus (HPV) in cervical carcinogenesis was first noted in the 1970s. By the early 1980s, significant evidence had accumulated identifying HPV as the cause of benign neoplasms such as oral squamous papilloma, focal epithelial hyperplasia, and condyloma acuminatum. HPV is a small, circular, double-stranded DNA virus.

- In the head and neck, more than 90% of HPV-associated tumors appear to be caused by type 16. HPV is known to strike at anatomical areas of transition from one epithelial tissue to another (i.e., transition points) within the cervix or anus. In the head and neck, HPV concentrates within the reticulated epithelial tissue of the tonsillar crypts. The exact mechanism of carcinogenesis is still unknown; however, one interesting theory is the "hit and run" theory that HPV infection is an early and possibly initiating oncogenic event but perhaps not needed in the later steps of malignant progression. Two oncoproteins are recognized as having a pivotal role in carcinogenesis and maintenance of a malignant phenotype: E6 and E7. E6 leads to a decrease in p53, a key protein that prevents cell cycle progression in the presence of DNA damage. E7 also exerts its function on a key regulatory protein, pRb, by forming a complex with cullin 2 ubiquitin ligase. HPV plays a causative role in the development of oropharyngeal squamous cell carcinomas (SCCs) and confers a survival advantage as reported by the RTOG0129 study. The improved treatment response to chemoradiation therapy may be explained by the presence of wild-type p53 from HPV-positive tumor cells that possess intact apoptotic mechanisms in response to DNA damage caused by these treatment modalities. This has given rise to controversy over possible therapy deescalation for HPV-positive oropharyngeal cancers. Current research efforts are being directed at the development of therapeutic vaccines and at reducing the morbidity of treatment modalities against HPV-positive head and neck SCCs without compromising the survival advantage over HPV-negative tumors.

### OROPHARYNX

- Worldwide, the incidence of oropharyngeal cancers is increasing and the traditional "rules" of oncology are being tested as the implications of the HPV epidemic unfold.

- The oropharynx extends from the level of the superior surface of the soft palate above to the superior surface of the hyoid bone (or vallecula) below. It is further subdivided into four main anatomical subsites:
  - Anterior wall: glossoepiglottic area, base of tongue, vallecula (but not the lingual surface of the epiglottis).
  - Lateral wall: tonsil, tonsillar fossa and faucial pillars, glossotonsillar sulcus.
  - Posterior wall.
  - Superior wall: inferior surface of the soft palate, uvula.

- The primary lymphatic drainage of the oropharynx is to level II nodes; however, the tonsillar region, pharyngeal portion of the soft palate, lateral and posterior pharyngeal walls, and base of the tongue also drain to the retropharyngeal and parapharyngeal nodes. Tumors located near the midline have a higher propensity for bilateral metastasis.

- More than 90% of the tumors of the oropharynx are SCCs, the remainder of which are minor salivary gland tumors, sarcomas, plasmacytomas, lymphomas, and other rare tumors.

- The most common site for primary tumors of the oropharynx is the anterior tonsillar pillars and tonsils.

- Tonsillar tumors are seen in more advanced stages: as many as 75% of patients are seen with stage III or IV cancers, and as many as 11% are seen with contralateral nodal metastasis.

- Lymph node metastasis from the base of the tongue is common because of the rich lymphatic drainage. The most common first-echelon lymph nodes are level II, but involvement of levels III and IV is also seen, as shown by the fact that as many as 20% of patients are first diagnosed with bilateral metastasis.

- Referred otalgia can be one of the first symptoms of patients with oropharynx tumors.

- T staging for the tumors of the oropharynx:
  - T1 tumors are equal to 2 cm.
  - T2 tumors are greater than 2 cm but less than 4 cm.
  - T3 tumors are equal to 4 cm, or there is extension of disease to the lingual surface of the epiglottis.
  - T4a tumors show invasion of the larynx, deep/extrinsic muscles of the tongue, medial pterygoid, hard palate, or mandible.
  - T4b tumors show invasion of the lateral pterygoid muscle, pterygoid plates, or skull base or encasement of the carotid.

- N2 nodal metastasis from the oropharynx is divided into N2a (a single ipsilateral node with involvement that is greater than 3 cm but less than 6 cm), N2b (metastasis to multiple ipsilateral lymph nodes), and N2c (metastasis to bilateral or contralateral lymph nodes none of which are greater than 6 cm).

- The incidence of oropharynx SCC is increasing worldwide.

- The number of oral sex partners is associated with a higher risk of HPV transmission.

- HPV-associated oropharynx cancer usually affects younger men (in their 40s or 50s) and is mainly confined to the palatine tonsils and the base of tongue.

- Patients with HPV-associated oropharynx cancer have better prognoses and overall rates of survival compared with patients with HPV/P16-negative cancer.

- Patients with HPV-positive oropharynx cancer who are nonsmokers have better prognoses than patients with HPV-positive oropharynx cancer who are smokers.

- According to the current guidelines, treatment options for tumors of the oropharynx that are T1 to 2, N0 to 1 include definitive radiation therapy (RT) and surgical resection with ipsilateral or bilateral neck dissection; for T2N1 tumors, systemic therapy can be added to definitive RT.

- Advanced disease requires multidisciplinary discussion and therapy. The options include induction chemotherapy followed by RT (or chemoradiation therapy), surgery followed by RT (or chemoradiation therapy), or chemoradiation therapy alone.

- Observation is an option for the neck after organ-conserving treatment if posttreatment radiological studies such as positron emission tomography/computed tomography (PET/CT) scans show a complete response; however, close follow-up is recommended.

## NASOPHARYNX

- Nasopharyngeal carcinoma (NPC) is rare in the Western Hemisphere, showing its highest incidence in the Alaskan Eskimo and Mediterranean populations; however, it is endemic in southern China.

- The etiology of NPC is multifactorial and has viral, genetic, and environmental factors.

- Undifferentiated NPC is strongly associated with Epstein-Barr virus (EBV). EBV is also associated with earlier lesions such as carcinoma in situ.

- The nasopharynx extends anteriorly from the posterior choana to the free border of the soft palate. It comprises a vault, the lateral walls (including the fossa of Rosenmüller and mucosa covering the torus tubarius), a posterior wall, and the superior surface of the soft palate, which is the floor.

- The posterior lip of the opening of the eustachian tube is the torus tubarius, behind which is a mucosal fold called the fossa of Rosenmüller.

- The World Health Organization (WHO) classification for NPC encompasses keratinizing SCC, nonkeratinizing carcinomas, and basaloid squamous cell carcinoma.

- Keratinizing SCC is more common in North America and not associated with EBV, whereas nonkeratinizing carcinoma, undifferentiated type is highly associated with EBV.

- Nonkeratinizing carcinoma, undifferentiated type accounts for 60% of all NPCs in adults and is the most frequent type in the pediatric population.

- First-echelon lymphatic drainage of NPC includes the superior jugular, retropharyngeal, and posterior cervical chain nodes.

- Lymph node metastasis from NPC is common: as many as 90% of patients have evidence of unilateral nodal involvement, and as many as 50% have bilateral nodal involvement.

- T staging for NPC:
  - T1 tumors are confined to the nasopharynx or extend to the oropharynx and/or nasal cavity without parapharyngeal involvement.
  - T2 tumors have parapharyngeal involvement.
  - T3 tumors involve the bony structure of the skull base and/or paranasal sinuses.
  - T4 tumors have intracranial involvement and/or involvement of intracranial nerves, orbit, or hypopharynx or show extension to the infratemporal fossa/masticator space.

- N1 nodal disease involves unilateral cervical nodes(s) 6 cm or less above the supraclavicular fossa and/or unilateral or bilateral retropharyngeal nodes 6 cm or less. N2 is bilateral metastases in cervical nodes, ≤6 cm, above the supraclavicular fossa. N3 are nodes >6 cm or extending to the supraclavicular fossa.

- NPC is a highly radiosensitive cancer.

- Current National Comprehensive Cancer Network (NCCN) guidelines for the treatment of T1N0 disease is definitive RT to the nasopharynx and elective RT to the neck.

- Local control rates of 65% to 93% have been reported for T1 tumors of the nasopharynx with the use of conventional RT.

- Current treatment recommendation for larger nasopharyngeal primaries with or without nodal involvement is concurrent chemotherapy and RT or induction chemotherapy followed by concurrent chemoradiation therapy.

- The majority of the locoregional and distant failures occur within 2 years of treatment.

- When conventional doses of radiation are used, temporal lobe necrosis is reported to occur in about 1% of patients, and the latency interval is 4 years.

## HYPOPHARYNX AND ESOPHAGUS

- The overall survival rate for the cancers of hypopharynx and esophagus remains disappointing; the reported 5-year overall survival rates range from 30% to 50%.

- The poor survival rate is, in part, due to frequent multicentricity, submucosal spreading, and a high likelihood of advanced primary and nodal disease on presentation.

- The hypopharynx is divided into four subsites: the right and left pyriform sinuses, the posterior and lateral wall, and the post cricoid region.

- The Killian triangle is an area of relative anatomical weakness. It is a triangular region between the thyropharyngeus and the cricopharyngeus (both components of the inferior constrictor muscle). A Zenker diverticulum arising from this anatomical weakness is a false diverticulum. Endoscopic stapling is the surgical intervention of choice.

- Cervical esophageal cancers have a high incidence of positive results for cervical, mediastinal lymph nodes. As many as 80% of patients have incidences of paratracheal nodal involvement.

- T staging for hypopharyngeal tumors:
  - T1 tumors are limited to one subsite and are equal to 2 cm.
  - T2 tumors invade more than one subsite, measure more than 2 cm but are no greater than 4 cm, and do not show fixation of the hemilarynx.
  - T3 tumors are greater than 4 cm and show fixation of the hemilarynx.
  - T4a tumors invade thyroid/cricoid cartilage, hyoid bone, thyroid gland, esophagus, or central compartment soft tissue.
  - T4b tumors invade prevertebral fascia, the carotid artery, or mediastinal structures.

- Neck management for T1 and T2 hypopharyngeal tumors is indicated because patients with clinically N0 neck nodes have a high incidence of occult nodal metastasis (as high as 40%).

- T1 or T2 hypopharyngeal tumors can be managed with definitive RT or surgery (a partial laryngectomy, either open or endoscopic) with ipsilateral or bilateral neck dissection; larger tumors require multimodality therapy.

- The current treatment recommendation for T1 esophageal cancer without nodal disease is esophagectomy; if nodal disease is present, then chemotherapy and RT are recommended.

## SUGGESTED READING

Al-Sarraf M, LeBlanc M, Giri PG, Fu KK, Cooper J, et al. Chemoradiotherapy versus radiotherapy in patients with advanced nasopharyngeal cancer: phase III randomized Intergroup study 0099. J Clin Oncol 1998;16(4):1310–7.

Ang KK, Harris J, Wheeler R, Weber R, Rosenthal DI, et al. Human papillomavirus and survival of patients with oropharyngeal cancer. N Engl J Med 2010;363(1):24–35.

Baujat B, Audry H, Bourhis J, Chan AT, Onat H, et al. Chemotherapy in locally advanced nasopharyngeal carcinoma: an individual patient data meta-analysis of eight randomized trials and 1753 patients. Int J Radiat Oncol Biol Phys 2006;64(1):47–56.

Denis F, Garaud P, Bardet E, Alfonsi M, Sire C, et al. Final results of the 94-01 French Head and Neck Oncology and Radiotherapy Group randomized trial comparing radiotherapy alone with concomitant radiochemotherapy in advanced-stage oropharynx carcinoma. J Clin Oncol 2004;22(1):69–76.

Fakhry C, Westra WH, Li S, Cmelak A, Ridge JA, et al. Improved survival of patients with human papillomavirus-positive head and neck squamous cell carcinoma in a prospective clinical trial. J Natl Cancer Inst 2008;100(4):261–9.

Fischer CA, Zlobec I, Green E, Probst S, Storck C, et al. Is the improved prognosis of p16 positive oropharyngeal squamous cell carcinoma dependent of the treatment modality? Int J Cancer 2010;126(5):1256–62.

Lee AW, Tung SY, Chua DT, Ngan RK, Chappell R, et al. Randomized trial of radiotherapy plus concurrent-adjuvant chemotherapy vs radiotherapy alone for regionally advanced nasopharyngeal carcinoma. J Natl Cancer Inst 2010;102(15):1188–98.

Lefebvre JL, Chevalier D, Luboinski B, Kirkpatrick A, Collette L. Larynx preservation in pyriform sinus cancer: preliminary results of a European Organization for Research and Treatment of Cancer phase III trial. J Natl Cancer Inst 1996;88(13):890–9.

Setton J, Caria N, Romanyshyn J, Koutcher L, Wolden SL, et al. Intensity-modulated radiotherapy in the treatment of oropharyngeal cancer: an update of the Memorial Sloan-Kettering Cancer Center experience. Int J Radiat Oncol Biol Phys 2012;82(1):291–8.

# 7 Larynx and Trachea

## Questions

### TRUE/FALSE

1. The Broyle tendon is the anterior attachment of the true vocal cords (TVCs), which include the vocal ligament, conus elasticus, cricothyroid ligament, and inner perichondrium of the thyroid lamina. (T/F)

2. The Broyle tendon is a robust barrier to spreading of cancer from the glottis. (T/F)

3. The cricoid is the only circular structure of the larynx. (T/F)

4. The TVC is composed of respiratory epithelium. (T/F)

5. The vocalis muscle is part of the cricoarytenoid muscle. (T/F)

6. Subglottic tumors frequently spread to lymphatics. (T/F)

7. Glottic tumors frequently spread to regional lymphatics. (T/F)

8. Supraglottic tumors frequently spread to regional lymphatics. (T/F)

9. When supraglottic tumors spread to lymph nodes, bilateral lymph nodes are at risk. (T/F)

10. The thyrohyoid membrane is a barrier to anterior spreading from the preepiglottic space. (T/F)

11. Vocal cord paralysis suggests that the tumor has invaded the paraglottic space. (T/F)

12. Invasion into the preepiglottic space means that the stage of the tumor is T4. (T/F)

13. Cancers of the medial piriform sinus are associated with an elevated risk of contralateral metastasis. (T/F)

14. Voice outcomes of laser surgery are routinely better than radiation therapy alone for early T1 glottic tumors. (T/F)

### Case 7-1

*Case 7-1 pertains to Questions 15 through 20.*

A 65-year-old smoker presents with a new lesion of the larynx. The tumor is squamous cell carcinoma (SCC) and involves the infrahyoid epiglottis and left aryepiglottic

fold and extends to the false vocal cord without vocal cord fixation. No lymphadenopathy is present.

15. Poor pulmonary function would be a contraindication to conservation laryngeal surgery in Case 7-1. (T/F)

16. In Case 7-1, transoral laser resection would be appropriate treatment for the primary tumor. (T/F)

17. Bilateral neck dissections are indicated in Case 7-1. (T/F)

18. Vocal cord fixation of one arytenoid is a contraindication to surgery in Case 7-1. (T/F)

19. Radiation therapy alone would be appropriate management of the patient in Case 7-1. (T/F)

20. If no disease is present in the neck, surgery alone would be appropriate treatment of the patient described in Case 7-1. (T/F)

21. Tracheoesophageal puncture (TEP) and esophageal speech are the only options for postlaryngectomy voice rehabilitation. (T/F)

22. Long-term durable control of larynx cancer with chemotherapy alone, without surgery or radiation therapy, has been reported. (T/F)

23. Human papilloma virus (HPV) is commonly found in larynx cancer specimens. (T/F)

24. HPV-18 is the most common virus found in larynx cancer specimens. (T/F)

25. Data are still inconclusive, but HPV is likely to be a contributing cause to laryngeal cancer oncogenesis. (T/F)

26. A small but measurable survival benefit has been observed in HPV-positive laryngeal cancer patients compared with age- and stage-matched control subjects. (T/F)

27. HPV-associated laryngeal disease is more common in supraglottic than glottic tumors. (T/F)

### MULTIPLE CHOICE

28. What is responsible for sensation above the vocal cords?
    A. Recurrent laryngeal nerve
    B. External branch of the superior laryngeal nerve

C. Internal branch of the superior laryngeal nerve
D. Glossopharyngeal nerve (cranial nerve [CN] IX)

29. What accompanies the superior laryngeal artery?
    A. Recurrent laryngeal nerve
    B. External branch of the superior laryngeal nerve
    C. Internal branch of the superior laryngeal nerve
    D. Glossopharyngeal nerve (CN IX)

30. What innervates the posterior cricoarytenoid muscle?
    A. Recurrent laryngeal nerve
    B. External branch of the superior laryngeal nerve
    C. Internal branch of the superior laryngeal nerve
    D. Glossopharyngeal nerve (CN IX)

31. What innervates the thyroarytenoid muscle?
    A. Recurrent laryngeal nerve
    B. External branch of the superior laryngeal nerve
    C. Internal branch of the superior laryngeal nerve
    D. Glossopharyngeal nerve (CN IX)

32. What innervates the cricothyroid muscle?
    A. Recurrent laryngeal nerve
    B. External branch of the superior laryngeal nerve
    C. Internal branch of the superior laryngeal nerve
    D. Glossopharyngeal nerve (CN IX)

33. What innervates the interarytenoid muscle?
    A. Recurrent laryngeal nerve
    B. External branch of the superior laryngeal nerve
    C. Internal branch of the superior laryngeal nerve
    D. Glossopharyngeal nerve (CN IX)

34. What innervates the cricopharyngeus muscle?
    A. Recurrent laryngeal nerve
    B. External branch of the superior laryngeal nerve
    C. Internal branch of the superior laryngeal nerve
    D. Glossopharyngeal nerve (CN IX)

35. What is responsible for sensation below the vocal cords?
    A. Recurrent laryngeal nerve
    B. External branch of the superior laryngeal nerve
    C. Internal branch of the superior laryngeal nerve
    D. Glossopharyngeal nerve (CN IX)

36. What enters the larynx through the thyrohyoid membrane?
    A. Recurrent laryngeal nerve
    B. External branch of the superior laryngeal nerve
    C. Internal branch of the superior laryngeal nerve
    D. Glossopharyngeal nerve (CN IX)

*For Questions 37 through 41, match the feature of larynx cancer to its stage.*

37. Cancer erodes part of the thyroid lamina but does not penetrate it.
    A. T1a
    B. T1b
    C. T2
    D. T3
    E. T4a

38. Cancer is limited to the TVC unilaterally, and there is complete movement.
    A. T1a
    B. T1b

C. T2
D. T3
E. T4a

39. Cancer is limited to the TVC, but paralysis is present.
    A. T1a
    B. T1b
    C. T2
    D. T3
    E. T4a

40. Cancer is noted in the preepiglottic space.
    A. T1a
    B. T1b
    C. T2
    D. T3
    E. T4a

41. Cancer is limited to both TVCs, and movement is intact.
    A. T1a
    B. T1b
    C. T2
    D. T3
    E. T4a

42. The layer most responsible for maintaining the mucosal wave is the
    A. Epithelial layer.
    B. Superficial lamina propria.
    C. Deep lamina propria.
    D. Vocalis tendon.

43. Vocal cord fixation is most likely due to invasion of the
    A. Conus elasticus.
    B. Quadrangular membrane.
    C. Paraglottic space.
    D. Broyle tendon.

44. Which of the following is not a subsite of the hypopharynx?
    A. Posterior pharyngeal wall
    B. Piriform sinus
    C. Postcricoid area
    D. Interarytenoid space

*For Questions 45 through 52, indicate the level(s) of tissues addressed in the given cordectomy type, as defined by the European Laryngological Society.*

    i. Epithelium
    ii. Superficial lamina propria
    iii. Reinke space
    iv. Vocal ligament
    v. Thyroarytenoid muscle
    vi. Perichondrium of cartilage
    vii. Unilateral cord
    viii. Contralateral cord
    ix. Anterior commissure
    x. Ipsilateral arytenoid
    xi. False vocal cord
    xii. Subglottis to 1 cm

45. Type I cordectomy
    A. i, ii, iii
    B. ii, iii, vi

C. i, ii, vii
D. iii, vii, xi

46. Type II cordectomy
    A. i, ii, iii, iv, v
    B. ii, iii, vi
    C. i, ii, iii, iv, vii
    D. ii, vii, x, xi, xii

47. Type III cordectomy
    A. i, ii, iii, iv, v, vi
    B. i, ii, iii, iv, v, vii
    C. i, ii, vii, x
    D. iii, vii, xi

48. Type IV cordectomy
    A. i, ii, iii, iv, v, vi, vii
    B. i, ii, iii, iv, v, vii
    C. i, ii, vii, x, xi, xii
    D. ii, iii, vii, ix, xi

49. Type Va cordectomy
    A. i, ii, iii, iv, v
    B. ii, iii, vi, vii, viii, x
    C. i, ii, vii, ix, x, xi, xii
    D. i, ii, iii, iv, v, vi, vii, viii

50. Type Vb cordectomy
    A. i, ii, iii, iv, v, vi
    B. ii, iii, vi, vii, viii, x
    C. i, ii, vii, ix, x, xi, xii
    D. i, ii, iii, iv, v, vi, vii, viii

51. Type Vc cordectomy
    A. i, ii, iii, iv, v, vi
    B. i, ii, iii, iv, v, vi, x
    C. i, ii, vii, ix, x, xi, xii
    D. i, ii, iii, iv, v, vi, xi

52. Type Vd cordectomy
    A. i, ii, iii, iv, v, vi
    B. i, ii, iii, iv, v, vi, x
    C. i, ii, vii, ix, x, xi, xii
    D. i, ii, iii, iv, v, vi, xi

*For Questions 53 through 61, match the following features of larynx cancer with the stage.*

    A. T1
    B. T1a
    C. T1b
    D. T2
    E. T3
    F. T4a
    G. T4b
    H. Not enough information

53. A 1-cm sessile tumor of the epiglottis tip

54. An exophytic 3-cm tumor anchored at the epiglottis tip only

55. Tumor limited to the mobile unilateral vocal cord with extension into the subglottis

56. Tumor limited to the mobile unilateral vocal cord with extension into the ventricle

57. Tumor extending through the cricothyroid membrane anteriorly

58. Tumor eroding through the thyroid lamina into the soft tissue

59. Tumor encasing the carotid artery 270 degrees

60. Tumor involving the false vocal cord, infrahyoid epiglottis, and ipsilateral aryepiglottic fold with no fixation of the vocal cord

61. Tumor centered at the left arytenoid but causing bilateral vocal cord paralysis, without extralaryngeal extension

62. Which of the following statements are true about the VA Larynx Trial?
    i. The VA Larynx Trial was a randomized trial.
    ii. Concomitant chemotherapy with radiation therapy was one of the trial arms.
    iii. Surgery with adjuvant radiation therapy was one of the trial arms.
    iv. Cisplatin and 5-fluorouracil (5FU) were the chemotherapy agents used in the trial.
    A. ii, iii, iv
    B. i, iii, iv
    C. ii, iii
    D. i, ii, iv
    E. ii, iv
    F. i, ii, iii, iv

63. Which of the following statements are true about the VA Larynx Trial?
    i. Patients who had a partial response to induction chemotherapy went on to definitive chemoradiation therapy.
    ii. Patients who had no response to induction chemotherapy went on to receive total laryngectomy with adjuvant therapy.
    iii. Patients who had a complete response to induction chemotherapy went on to receive radiation therapy.
    iv. Patients in the surgery arm also received adjuvant chemotherapy.
    A. i, ii, iii, iv
    B. i, iii, iv
    C. i, iv
    D. ii, iii
    E. iii, iv
    F. ii, iii, iv

64. Which of the following statements are true about the VA Larynx Trial?
    i. The trial included only advanced stage III and stage IV tumors.
    ii. T1N1 tumors were excluded from the trial.
    iii. Patients with N0 nodes made up more than half of all patients in the study (both arms).
    iv. Patients with T4 tumors made up more than half of all patients in the study (both arms).
    A. i, ii, iii, iv
    B. i, iii, iv
    C. i, iv
    D. i, ii, iii
    E. iii, iv
    F. ii, iii, iv

65. Which of the following statements are true about the VA Larynx Trial?
    i. Patients randomly assigned to surgery with adjuvant therapy did better than those assigned to chemotherapy.
    ii. Patients randomly assigned to chemotherapy had a better overall survival rate than did those assigned to surgery with adjuvant therapy.
    iii. More than one third of chemotherapy arm patients went on to have a total laryngectomy.
    A. i
    B. i, ii
    C. ii
    D. iii
    E. ii, iii

66. Which of the following statements about the RTOG 91-11 trial are true?
    i. One arm was induction chemotherapy followed by radiation therapy alone.
    ii. One arm was concurrent cisplatin with radiation therapy.
    iii. One arm was surgery followed by total laryngectomy.
    A. i
    B. i, ii
    C. ii
    D. iii
    E. ii, iii

67. Which of the following statements about the RTOG 91-11 trial are true?
    i. Induction chemotherapy was with cisplatin and 5FU.
    ii. The addition of chemotherapy, whether concurrent or induction, increased treatment toxicity.
    iii. The rate of concurrent chemoradiation mucositis was significantly higher than that in the other two treatment arms.
    A. i
    B. i, ii, iii
    C. ii
    D. iii
    E. ii, iii

68. Which of the following statements about the RTOG 91-11 trial are true?
    i. Concurrent chemoradiation therapy improved locoregional control.
    ii. Concurrent chemoradiation therapy had equivalent toxicity to radiation therapy alone.
    iii. Concurrent chemoradiation therapy was associated with the highest rate of larynx preservation.
    iv. Concurrent chemoradiation therapy was associated with improved overall survival rates compared with the other arms.
    A. i, ii, iii, iv
    B. ii, iii, iv

C. i, iv
D. i, ii, iii
E. iii, iv
F. i, iii

69. Which of the following statements are true regarding advanced larynx cancer?
    i. Regarding locoregional control, concurrent chemoradiation therapy is superior to radiation therapy alone.
    ii. Surgery with adjuvant therapy has been compared with concurrent chemoradiation therapy for treatment in a phase III randomized controlled trial.
    iii. Concurrent chemoradiation therapy has shown improved overall survival rates compared with surgery with adjuvant therapy.
    A. i
    B. i, ii, iii
    C. ii
    D. iii
    E. ii, iii

70. Which of the following suggests only superficial invasion (lamina propria only) of an early glottic cancer?
    i. Retention of the mucosal wave on videostroboscopy
    ii. Impairment but no fixation of TVC mobility
    iii. Complete elevation of the lesion with fluid injection into Reinke space
    iv. Vocal cord fixation but retention of arytenoid mobility
    A. i
    B. ii, iii, iv
    C. i, iv
    D. i, ii, iii
    E. iii, iv
    F. i, iii

71. After total laryngectomy, a patient undergoes an air-insufflation test to determine candidacy for a TEP. There is no production of voice. Which of the following tests would help identify the cause?
    A. Advancing the air-insufflation catheter further into the esophagus
    B. Having the patient swallow while insufflating
    C. Injection of lidocaine into the cricopharyngeal muscle
    D. Having the patient press harder around the tracheostoma during insufflation

72. In the patient described in Question 71, what intraoperative maneuver may have resulted in a better candidate for TEP placement?
    A. Cricopharyngeal myotomy at the time of total laryngectomy
    B. Primary TEP placement rather than delayed TEP placement
    C. Performing a vertical line rather than T-closure of the pharyngeal mucosa during total laryngectomy
    D. Beveling the trachea during tracheostoma formation

## Case 7-2

A 65-year-old man presents with 6 months of occasional hoarseness. A complete head and neck examination is performed and shows no lymphadenopathy. Flexible laryngoscopy shows a fullness of the subglottis that is incompletely visualized. Normal vocal cord movement is noted. A computed tomographic (CT) scan is displayed in Figure 7-1.

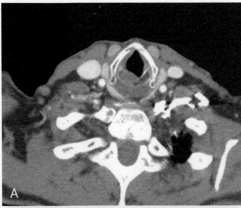
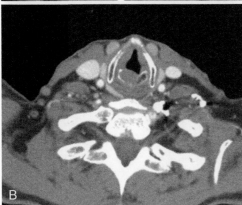

**Figure 7-1**

73. The next best step in the management of Case 7-2 should be
    A. Positron emission tomography (PET)/CT.
    B. Magnetic resonance imaging (MRI).
    C. Direct laryngoscopy with biopsy.
    D. Videostroboscopy.

74. Which of the following is the least likely diagnosis of the patient in Case 7-2?
    A. Chondrosarcoma
    B. Chondroma
    C. SCC
    D. Benign cricoid cyst

75. Biopsy of this lesion in Case 7-2 demonstrates cartilage elements, but the pathologist is unable to confirm chondroma versus chondrosarcoma. Further metastatic evaluation results are negative. The next step in management should be
    A. Endoscopic cricoidectomy with or without tracheostomy.
    B. Total laryngectomy.

C. Open partial cricoidectomy with appropriate reconstruction.
D. Observation with serial CT scans.

76. Biopsy of the lesion in Case 7-2 confirms chondrosarcoma. Which of the following surgical options is best for this patient?
    A. Endoscopic cricoidectomy with or without tracheostomy
    B. Total laryngectomy
    C. Open partial cricoidectomy with appropriate reconstruction

77. Biopsy of this lesion in Case 7-2 shows SCC in the subglottis, with no vocal cord impairment. Regional and distant metastatic workup results are negative. The next appropriate treatment is
    A. Total laryngectomy with adjuvant radiation therapy.
    B. Partial or endoscopic cricoidectomy with adjuvant radiation therapy.
    C. Primary radiation therapy.
    D. Concomitant chemoradiation therapy with cisplatin.

78. Biopsy of this lesion in Case 7-2 shows adenoid cystic carcinoma. Regional and distant metastatic workup results are negative. The next appropriate treatment is
    A. Total laryngectomy with adjuvant radiation therapy.
    B. Partial or endoscopic cricoidectomy with adjuvant radiation therapy.
    C. Primary radiation therapy.
    D. Concomitant chemoradiation therapy with cisplatin.

79. Biopsy of this lesion in Case 7-2 shows small cell neuroendocrine carcinoma. Regional and distant metastatic workup results are negative. The next appropriate treatment is
    A. Total laryngectomy with adjuvant radiation therapy.
    B. Partial or endoscopic cricoidectomy with adjuvant radiation therapy.
    C. Primary radiation therapy.
    D. Concomitant chemoradiation therapy with possible additional chemotherapy.

## Case 7-3

A 70-year-old man with a history of long-term smoking, as well as chronic obstructive pulmonary disease, presents with 1 year of hoarseness. Neck examination shows right level II lymphadenopathy with a 1.5-cm lymph node. Flexible fiberoptic laryngoscopy shows a right transglottic lesion with right vocal cord fixation. The disease extends to the left aryepiglottic fold. There is no impairment or involvement of the left vocal cord. PET/CT shows no distant metastasis, fluorodeoxyglucose (FDG)-avid lymphadenopathy as previously described, and an FDG-avid primary lesion of the larynx. The CT scan is shown in Figure 7-2.

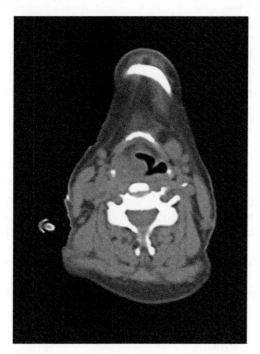

**Figure 7-2**

shows impaired movement without fixation. Regional and distant workup results are negative. Direct laryngoscopy shows an exophytic lesion confined to the vibratory surface of the TVC only; the lesion does not involve either arytenoid. The neuroradiology department states that no obvious erosion of the thyroid cartilage is present on the CT scan (see Figure 7-3), only age-related changes.

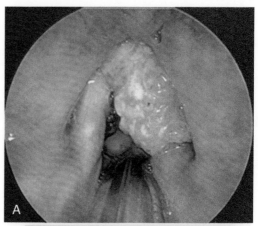

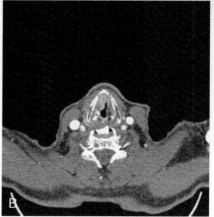

**Figure 7-3**

80. What is the next appropriate step in management of Case 7-3?
    A. Direct laryngoscopy with biopsy
    B. Referral to medical oncology
    C. Needle biopsy of an enlarged FDG-avid lymph node
    D. Tracheostomy

81. Tissue biopsy of the lesion in Case 7-3 confirms SCC. The patient desires surgery. What is the best surgical treatment for this patient?
    A. Total laryngectomy with bilateral neck dissection
    B. Total laryngectomy with dissection of the left side of the neck
    C. Transoral endoscopic laser partial laryngectomy with bilateral neck dissection
    D. Transoral endoscopic laser partial laryngectomy with dissection of the left side of the neck
    E. Vertical partial laryngectomy, reconstruction with strap musculature, and bilateral neck dissection
    F. Vertical partial laryngectomy, reconstruction with strap musculature, and dissection of the left side of the neck

82. What adjuvant therapy will likely be indicated for the tumor described in Case 7-3?
    A. Radiation therapy to the laryngeal bed and left side of the neck
    B. Radiation therapy to the laryngeal bed and both sides of the neck
    C. Chemoradiation therapy to the laryngeal bed and left side of the neck
    D. Chemoradiation therapy to the laryngeal bed and both sides of the neck

**Case 7-4**

A 69-year-old man presents with the lesion pictured in Figure 7-3. The left TVC is mobile, but the right TVC

83. Which of the following is the most appropriate T stage for the glottis tumor described in Case 7-4?
    A. T1a
    B. T1b
    C. T2
    D. T3

84. Which of the following is the most appropriate nonsurgical treatment for the patient in Case 7-4?
    A. Primary radiation therapy alone to the larynx
    B. Primary radiation therapy to the larynx and bilateral neck
    C. Concomitant chemoradiation therapy
    D. Induction chemotherapy with cisplatin, followed by radiation therapy alone

85. Which of the following is appropriate surgical management of the disease described in Case 7-4?
    i. Transoral laser endoscopic resection only with type III cordectomy
    ii. Transoral laser endoscopic resection with neck dissection

iii. Open anterolateral partial laryngectomy only

iv. Open anterolateral partial laryngectomy with neck dissection

A. i
B. ii, iii, iv
C. i, iv
D. i, ii, iii
E. iii, iv
F. i, iii

## Case 7-5

A 55-year-old man with good pulmonary function presents with the lesion in Figure 7-4. The lesion is confined to the laryngeal surface, and no disease is seen on the lingual surface of the epiglottis. The true vocal folds are mobile and are free of disease. The lesion extends to the false vocal fold only. On a CT scan, no lymphadenopathy is seen and the preepiglottic space is not involved.

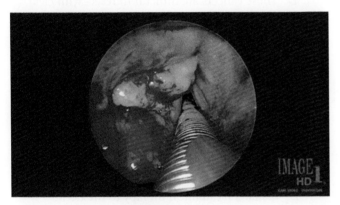

**Figure 7-4**

86. Which of the following is the most appropriate T stage for the supraglottic tumor described in Case 7-5?
A. T1
B. T2
C. T3
D. T4a
E. T4b

87. Which of the following is the most appropriate nonsurgical treatment for the patient in Case 7-5?
A. Primary radiation therapy alone to the larynx
B. Primary radiation therapy to the larynx and bilateral neck
C. Concomitant chemoradiation therapy
D. Induction chemotherapy with cisplatin, followed by radiation therapy alone

88. Which of the following is the most appropriate surgical management of the disease described in Case 7-5?
A. Transoral laser endoscopic resection
B. Open supraglottic partial laryngectomy
C. Open supracricoid laryngectomy
D. Total laryngectomy

89. Which of the following is appropriate management of the neck after surgical management of the primary lesion described in Case 7-5?
A. No neck dissection; observation only
B. No neck dissection; radiation therapy only
C. Unilateral neck dissection
D. Bilateral neck dissection

*For Questions 90 through 94, select the most appropriate airway management for each of the following scenarios.*

90. A 50-year-old man has a bulky T3 glottic tumor with vocal cord fixation. The airway is easily visible on fiberoptic laryngoscopy.
A. Routine anesthesia induction, direct laryngoscopy, and intubation
B. Routine anesthesia induction and flexible fiberoptic transoral asleep intubation
C. Awake transnasal fiberoptic intubation
D. Awake tracheostomy with local anesthesia

91. A 50-year-old man with a bulky transglottic tumor presents to the emergency department with stridor and is unable to breathe. No visible airway is seen on fiberoptic laryngoscopy.
A. Routine anesthesia induction, direct laryngoscopy, and intubation
B. Routine anesthesia induction, and flexible fiberoptic transoral asleep intubation
C. Awake transnasal fiberoptic intubation
D. Awake tracheostomy with local anesthesia

92. A 50-year-old male presents with a bulky supraglottic tumor partially obscuring the view of the glottis. After manipulation of the flexible scope, the TVCs are completely visualized and uninvolved.
A. Routine anesthesia induction, direct laryngoscopy, and intubation
B. Routine anesthesia induction and flexible fiberoptic transoral asleep intubation
C. Awake transnasal fiberoptic intubation
D. Awake tracheostomy with local anesthesia.

93. A patient has a pedunculated lesion of the TVC that is acting like a ball valve in the glottic opening.
A. Routine anesthesia induction, direct laryngoscopy, and intubation
B. Routine anesthesia induction and flexible fiberoptic transoral asleep intubation
C. Awake transnasal fiberoptic intubation
D. Awake tracheostomy with local anesthesia

94. A 50-year-old man has bulky supraglottic and glottic disease. The larynx cannot be visualized on laryngoscopy. The patient is comfortable and has no stridor or distress.
A. Routine anesthesia induction, direct laryngoscopy, and intubation
B. Routine anesthesia induction and flexible fiberoptic transoral asleep intubation
C. Awake transnasal fiberoptic intubation
D. Awake tracheostomy with local anesthesia.

## Case 7-6

A 65-year-old man presents with the lesion pictured in Figure 7-5. He has bilateral bulky 3-cm cervical lymphadenopathy but no distant metastasis.

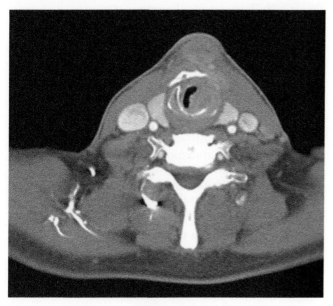

**Figure 7-5**

95. Which of the following is the most appropriate T stage for this tumor based on data presented in Case 7-6?
    A. T1
    B. T2
    C. T3
    D. T4a
    E. T4b

96. What is the preferred method of treatment for the patient in Case 7-6?
    A. Radiation therapy alone
    B. Concomitant chemoradiation therapy with cisplatin
    C. Total laryngectomy with bilateral neck dissection
    D. Induction chemotherapy with cisplatin, followed by concomitant chemoradiation therapy

97. Under what circumstances, supported by published data, is chemotherapy recommended in addition to radiation therapy for postoperative adjuvant therapy?
    i. Negative margins were achieved on resection of the primary tumor, but the resection extended into the base of the tongue.
    ii. Lymph nodes in the neck show extracapsular extension.
    iii. The tumor has perineural invasion on pathological examination.
    iv. A free flap or pectoralis flap is used for closure rather than primary closure.
    v. A positive margin is found at the base of the tongue and is unable to be surgically cleared.
    A. i, ii, iii
    B. i, ii, iv, v

C. ii, v
D. v

98. Which of the following would not be recommended as part of the treatment for a T1 piriform sinus hypopharynx tumor?
    A. Transoral laser resection of the primary tumor with negative margins
    B. Radiation therapy alone
    C. Transcervical lateral pharyngectomy
    D. Bilateral neck dissection after surgery for the primary tumor
    E. Concomitant chemoradiation therapy

99. Why is the hypopharynx SCC survival rate consistently worse than that of other head and neck cancers?
    A. These cancers are routinely more aggressive than other head and neck cancers.
    B. These cancers are HPV-related.
    C. These cancers tend to be seen at more advanced stages.
    D. These cancers are difficult to resect with clear margins.
    E. These cancers tend to be chemotherapy and radiation therapy resistant.

100. A 75-year-old woman presents with an incidentally found T1 hypopharynx tumor of the medial piriform sinus. CT and PET findings are negative for cervical disease. She undergoes surgical resection of the primary lesion. Which of the following is the best next step in treatment of the neck?
    A. No neck dissection necessary
    B. Ipsilateral neck dissection only
    C. Bilateral neck dissection
    D. Ipsilateral radiation therapy to the neck
    E. Bilateral radiation therapy to the neck

## Answers

| | | |
|---|---|---|
| 1. F | 17. T | 33. A |
| 2. T | 18. F | 34. B |
| 3. T | 19. T | 35. A |
| 4. F | 20. T | 36. C |
| 5. F | 21. F | 37. D |
| 6. T | 22. T | 38. A |
| 7. F | 23. T | 39. D |
| 8. T | 24. F | 40. D |
| 9. T | 25. T | 41. B |
| 10. T | 26. F | 42. B |
| 11. T | 27. F | 43. C |
| 12. F | 28. C | 44. D |
| 13. T | 29. C | 45. C |
| 14. F | 30. A | 46. C |
| 15. T | 31. A | 47. B |
| 16. T | 32. B | 48. A |

| 49. D | 67. B | 85. F |
|-------|-------|-------|
| 50. A | 68. F | 86. B |
| 51. D | 69. A | 87. B |
| 52. C | 70. F | 88. A |
| 53. A | 71. C | 89. D |
| 54. A | 72. A | 90. A |
| 55. D | 73. C | 91. D |
| 56. D | 74. D | 92. C |
| 57. F | 75. D | 93. A |
| 58. F | 76. B | 94. D |
| 59. G | 77. C | 95. D |
| 60. D | 78. A | 96. C |
| 61. E | 79. D | 97. C |
| 62. B | 80. A | 98. E |
| 63. D | 81. A | 99. C |
| 64. D | 82. B | 100. C |
| 65. D | 83. C | |
| 66. B | 84. A | |

## Core Knowledge

### ANATOMY AND PATTERNS OF SPREADING

- The larynx is a unique organ. It has many functions, including generating noise for speech, directing food, liquids, and saliva into the esophagus, and directing air into the trachea.
- It is divided into three areas: the subglottis, glottis, and supraglottis. The three main types of cartilage are the cricoid, hyoid, and thyroid.
- Studies using injections into cadaveric larynges showed that the larynx is compartmentalized.
- The Broyle tendon is the anterior attachment of the vocal ligament to the inner perichondrium of the thyroid. It consists of the vocal ligament, conus elasticus, thyroarytenoid ligament, and thyroid perichondrium. It is very tough, and injections of the true vocal cord (TVC) show it to be an anterior barrier to tumor spreading.
- Prior studies have shown that anterior commissure lesions routinely extend supraglottically or subglottically to cross to the contralateral cord.
- The TVC is made of stratified squamous epithelium, not respiratory epithelium.
- Lymphatic drainage is highly variable to different parts of the larynx. In general, the supraglottic and subglottic structures are rich in lymphatics; therefore bilateral lymph nodes are at risk from tumors in this area.
- Glottic lymphatic drainage is minimal. Hence, regional lymphatics are not routinely addressed in early glottic cancer.

- There are multiple barriers in the larynx to cancer spreading, including the conus elasticus, quadrangular membrane, and the Broyle tendon.
- Vocal cord fixation is usually a sign of paraglottic space invasion or arytenoid involvement.
- All muscles of the intrinsic larynx are innervated by the recurrent laryngeal nerve except one muscle.
- The cricothyroid is innervated by the external branch of the superior laryngeal nerve. This nerve also innervates the cricopharyngeus, which is part of the inferior constrictor, not the larynx.
- The internal branch of the superior laryngeal nerve is responsible for sensation above the vocal cords. Sensation of the vocal cords and below is related to the recurrent laryngeal nerve.
- The internal branch of the superior laryngeal nerve enters the larynx with the superior laryngeal artery, which is a branch of the superior thyroid artery, at the thyrohyoid membrane.
- The recurrent laryngeal nerve is also known as the inferior laryngeal nerve.
- The posterior cricoarytenoid muscle is the only abductor of the vocal cords.
- The TVC is a complex organ with multiple layers. Superficial to deep the layers are as follows:
  - Epithelial layer, composed of stratified squamous epithelium
  - Superficial lamina propria (SLP)
  - Deep lamina propria
  - Vocalis tendon (the vocalis is the medial part of the thyroarytenoid muscle)
  - Vocalis muscle
- The SLP is responsible for the elasticity that allows TVC vibration and phonation. It allows the mucosal wave to occur.
- Injection of the SLP can differentiate between superficial and deep lesions. Superficial lesions will separate from the vocalis tendon, while deeper lesions will remain tethered with injection.

### STAGING AND TREATMENT

- Please see the American Joint Committee on Cancer (AJCC) manual for the most up-to-date staging.
- Please see National Comprehensive Cancer Network (NCCN) guidelines for consensus recommendations on larynx cancer management by stage.

### EARLY GLOTTIC CANCER

- These are defined as T1 or T2 tumors of the glottis with N0 neck nodes.
- Single modality treatment with surgery or irradiation alone is appropriate.
- Regional lymphatics are not routinely addressed in management because of a low risk of metastasis.

- Tumor control is largely independent of the treatment modality. Both surgery and primary irradiation have similar local control rates.
- Voice outcomes have not favored one treatment modality over another.

## ADVANCED LARYNGEAL CANCER AND TRIALS

- Multimodality therapy is the preferred method of treatment.
- The options for partial laryngectomy techniques, either open or endoscopic, versus total laryngectomy are dependent on many factors. These include tumor-related factors such as location of the tumor, patient-related factors such as lung status, and surgeon-related factors such as comfort and expertise in minimally invasive techniques.
- The VA Larynx Trial was a randomized controlled trial of advanced larynx cancer that examined two arms: either total laryngectomy with irradiation or induction chemotherapy followed by definitive radiation therapy. Patients who had either no response to chemotherapy or a biopsy-proven tumor after induction chemotherapy and radiation therapy underwent total laryngectomy.
  - There was no use of concomitant chemotherapy in this trial.
  - Stage III tumors were the most common tumor stage represented.
  - The overall survival rate was the same for all conditions.
  - More than one third of chemotherapy patients still had to undergo total laryngectomy.
- The RTOG 91-11 was a randomized controlled trial of treatment of advanced larynx cancer. The three arms were induction chemotherapy followed by radiation therapy, radiation therapy alone, or concomitant chemoradiation therapy.
  - There was no surgical arm in the study.
  - Larynx preservation was the primary study endpoint.
  - The addition of chemotherapy increased treatment toxicity, primarily mucositis.
  - Concurrent chemoradiation therapy had the highest locoregional control rate.
  - The overall survival rate was the same in all three arms.
  - Ten-year data are now available for this study.

## VOICE REHABILITATION AFTER TOTAL LARYNGECTOMY

- Three major approaches to voice rehabilitation are possible after total laryngectomy: esophageal speech, electrolarynx usage, and tracheoesophageal puncture (TEP).
- The air-insufflation test is used to evaluate candidacy for TEP. It is a functional test that evaluates neopharyngeal function to determine whether TEP placement will be successful. It involves connecting

a conduit, in the form of a catheter, from the tracheostoma, through the nose, and into the neopharynx/esophagus. The goal is to insufflate the neopharynx/esophagus at the level of TEP placement to determine whether phonation can occur.
- The results are affected by many factors, including type of closure (primary versus flap), residual pharyngeal function, and whether a cricopharyngeal myotomy has been performed at the time of surgery. Unsuccessful production of voice is usually due to a cricopharyngeal spasm. If lidocaine injection into the cricopharyngeus is successful at generating a voice, then a cricopharyngeal spasm is usually confirmed as the cause.

## PARTIAL LARYNGEAL SURGERY

- A variety of laryngeal procedures aim to retain portions of the larynx while still maintaining its necessary function in lieu of a total laryngectomy.
- Open procedures include supraglottic laryngectomy, supracricoid laryngectomy, vertical partial laryngectomy, horizontal laryngectomy, and any other variation of open partial laryngectomy.
- Reconstruction of open procedures commonly uses the strap musculature. Therefore open partial laryngectomy is a poor choice for tumors that extend through the cartilage because the strap muscles usually need to be resected to achieve a clear margin.
- Transoral endoscopic or transoral laser microsurgery has also been used as an "inside out" approach for removal of tumors.
- Whatever the surgical strategy, a few key elements are common among all approaches:
  - Surgery affects the major functions of the larynx: speech, breathing, and swallowing or control of saliva and food into the esophagus.
  - Maintenance of at least one cricoarytenoid unit is critical in retaining laryngeal function.
  - Patients with poor pulmonary status may not be good candidates for surgery because of the risk of aspiration with these procedures.

## OTHER LARYNGEAL PATHOLOGIES

- In the vast majority of larynx cancer cases, the focus is on management and treatment of squamous cell carcinoma (SCC).
- Meta-analysis has suggested that up to 20% of SCCs in the larynx may be human papillomavirus (HPV)-associated.
- HPV-associated larynx cancer has not been linked with a poor prognosis or outcome, which is dramatically different than that seen for oropharynx cancer.
- Cartilage tumors are rarely seen in the larynx. Pathological differentiation of chondroma versus chondrosarcoma on biopsy can be difficult. Appropriate treatment should weigh the morbidity of resection,

sometimes requiring total laryngectomy, against the risk of observation.

- For more details about chondrosarcoma behavior, see Chapter 12 on soft tissue tumors.

- Primary lesions of the cricoid can have a broad differential diagnosis, from SCCs, to salivary gland tumors, to sarcomas. In general, it is difficult to resect these lesions and maintain the larynx. Single institutions have noted some success with select patients. Total laryngectomy is the conservative management when cricoid resection is necessary.

- Minor salivary gland tumors such as adenoid cystic carcinoma and mucoepidermoid carcinoma are occasionally seen in the larynx. Resection with negative margins is the recommended approach, and adjuvant radiation therapy should be used when appropriate.

- Small cell neuroendocrine carcinoma is a rare and distinct tumor of the larynx. Total laryngectomy has not usually been successful at control, even with complete resection. Concomitant chemoradiation therapy is the recommended modality for treatment.

## SUGGESTED READING

Ang KK, Harris J, Wheeler R, Weber R, Rosenthal DI, et al. Human papillomavirus and survival of patients with oropharyngeal cancer. N Engl J Med 2010;363(1):24–35.

Bernier J, Cooper JS. Chemoradiation after surgery for high-risk head and neck cancer patients: how strong is the evidence? Oncologist 2005;10(3):215–24.

Ferlito A, Rinaldo A. Primary and secondary small cell neuroendocrine carcinoma of the larynx: a review. Head Neck 2008;30(4):518–24.

Forastiere AA, Goepfert H, Maor M, Pajak TF, Weber R, et al. Concurrent chemotherapy and radiotherapy for organ preservation in advanced laryngeal cancer. N Engl J Med 2003;349 (22):2091–8.

Forastiere AA, Zhang Q, Weber RS, Maor MH, Goepfert H, et al. Long-term results of RTOG 91-11: a comparison of three nonsurgical treatment strategies to preserve the larynx in patients with locally advanced larynx cancer. J Clin Oncol 2013;31(7): 845–52.

Induction chemotherapy plus radiation compared with surgery plus radiation in patients with advanced laryngeal cancer. The Department of Veterans Affairs Laryngeal Cancer Study Group. N Engl J Med 1991;324(24):1685–90.

Johnson JT, Bacon GW, Myers EN, Wagner RL. Medial vs lateral wall pyriform sinus carcinoma: implications for management of regional lymphatics. Head Neck 1994;16(5):401–5.

Kirchner JA, Carter D. Intralaryngeal barriers to the spread of cancer. Acta Otolaryngol 1987;103(5-6):503–13.

Li X, Gao L, Li H, Gao J, Yang Y, et al. Human papillomavirus infection and laryngeal cancer risk: a systematic review and meta-analysis. J Infect Dis 2013;207(3):479–88.

Peretti G, Piazza C, Bolzoni A. Endoscopic treatment for early glottic cancer: indications and oncologic outcome. Otolaryngol Clin North Am 2006;39(1):173–89.

Spielmann PM, Majumdar S, Morton RP. Quality of life and functional outcomes in the management of early glottic carcinoma: a systematic review of studies comparing radiotherapy and transoral laser microsurgery. Clin Otolaryngol 2010;35(5):373–82.

Zeitels SM, Burns JA, Wain JC, Wright CD, Rosenberg AE. Function preservation surgery in patients with chondrosarcoma of the cricoid cartilage. Ann Otol Rhinol Laryngol 2011;120(9):603–7.

# 8 Cervical Lymph Nodes

## Questions

### TRUE /FALSE

1. A modified radical neck dissection (MRND) implies preservation of one or more of the following: sternomastoid muscle, internal jugular vein, or accessory nerve. (T/F)

2. The demarcation between levels III and IV is the upper belly of the omohyoid muscle. (T/F)

3. The demarcation between levels I and II is the posterior belly of the digastric muscle. (T/F)

4. In a patient with a 2-cm squamous cell carcinoma (SCC) confined to the nasopharynx and multiple metastatic lymph nodes in unilateral level II, of which the largest measures 4.5 cm, the staging is T1N2b. (T/F)

5. In a 62-year-old patient with a 4.5-cm Hurthle cell carcinoma of the thyroid with a single 4-cm metastatic lymph node in level III, the staging is T3N1. (T/F)

6. Upregulation of matrix metalloproteinases is an important step in development of lymph node metastases. (T/F)

7. SCC is usually characterized by simultaneous tumor growth in the lymph node's subcapsular sinus and juxtacapsular lymphatics. (T/F)

8. Distant metastases are rare in non–human papillomavirus (HPV)-related oropharyngeal SCCs in the absence of lymph node metastases. (T/F)

9. Tumor classification is a more significant prognostic indicator than nodal classification in HPV-related oropharyngeal cancer. (T/F)

10. Previous neck surgery can lead to diversion of lymphatic flow to the contralateral side of the neck with increased risk of contralateral lymph node metastases in a patient with a lateral tongue SCC. (T/F)

11. Ultrasound (US) alone has a lower sensitivity than computed tomography (CT) for detection of metastatic disease in the clinically negative neck. (T/F)

12. Ultrasound-guided fine-needle aspiration (US-FNA) cytology is less sensitive than positron emission tomography fused with CT (PET-CT) for the detection of metastatic disease in the clinically negative neck. (T/F)

13. Round shape, mobility, and lack of central necrosis are features that do not indicate malignancy in the case of a 1-cm lymph node in level I in a patient with floor of the mouth SCC. (T/F)

14. The main value of PET-CT performed 3 months after completion of chemoradiation therapy is its very high positive predictive value for detection of persistent viable tumor in cervical nodes. (T/F)

15. The negative predictive value of CT of the neck for restaging after chemoradiation therapy is similar to that of PET-CT performed 3 months after completion of treatment. (T/F)

16. In patients with oral cavity cancers clinically staged T2-4N0, elective neck dissection should be performed because of its proven survival benefit. (T/F)

17. An MRND incorporating levels II through V should be performed on patients with laryngeal SCC with established cervical metastases in level II or III because of the 10% to 20% risk of microscopic metastases in level V. (T/F)

18. A 61-year-old patient with T1N2b tonsil cancer is treated with chemoradiation therapy and initially achieves a complete response in both the primary site and neck but 1 year later develops a recurrent level II neck mass that is confirmed to be SCC by FNA. In this scenario, a highly selective (level IIA/III) neck dissection offers the same control rate as an MRND. (T/F)

19. A 56-year-old patient with supraglottic cancer, initially staged T2N0 and treated with radiation therapy, now has recurrence at the primary site but no evidence on neck CT of nodal metastases. The patient is scheduled for salvage laryngectomy. A concomitant bilateral neck dissection should be performed because of the 20% to 30% risk of cervical metastatic disease. (T/F)

20. In patients undergoing transoral robotic or laser resection of supraglottic cancers, bilateral neck dissection should always be deferred for 1 to 2 weeks after the primary procedure because of the risk of laryngeal edema and the need for a tracheostomy. (T/F)

21. During level V neck dissection, the surgeon should avoid trying to identify the accessory nerve at the posterior limit, around the trapezius muscle, because of the deep location and possibility of branching. (T/F)

22. In the case of metastatic SCC in which the surgeon finds metastatic nodes adherent to the accessory nerve but able to be dissected from the nerve without leaving gross tumor behind, the nerve sacrifice should be avoided on the basis that residual microscopic disease can be treated with radiation therapy. (T/F)

23. The common carotid artery does not have any branches before the carotid bifurcation. (T/F)

24. Care should be taken to avoid unnecessary damage to cervical plexus nerves because of their motor innervation of the levator scapulae muscle and risk of aggravating shoulder dysfunction if damaged. (T/F)

25. The glossopharyngeal nerve courses between the internal and external carotid arteries with the styloid muscles. (T/F)

26. Unilateral damage to the phrenic nerve during neck dissection is usually asymptomatic for the patient. (T/F)

27. If a large hole is inadvertently made in the internal jugular vein during dissection and heavy bleeding occurs, the anesthesiologist should be instructed to position the patient head down (Trendelenburg position). (T/F)

28. Chyle leakage in the lower neck can be avoided by keeping the plane of dissection superficial to that of the transverse cervical vessels. (T/F)

29. In selective (level II/III) neck dissections, disturbance to accessory nerve function is rare. (T/F)

30. Blindness after neck dissection is a very rare complication that has usually been associated with carotid artery ligation. (T/F)

31. A complete clinical response to chemoradiation therapy or radiation treatment of cervical neck disease is reduction of the tumor size by at least 50% in all dimensions within 3 months. (T/F)

32. In cases of advanced metastatic neck disease treated primarily with chemoradiation therapy that show only a partial response, the incidence of finding viable tumor within the neck at neck dissection is around 40%. (T/F)

33. In cases of neck dissection in which pathological examination shows a single metastatic node less than 3 cm without extranodal extension, postoperative radiotherapy improves regional control but not survival rates. (T/F)

34. In the case of patients with multiple positive nodes at neck dissection, no extracapsular spreading, and negative resection margins of the primary tumor, a significant survival advantage for postoperative chemoradiation therapy over postoperative radiation therapy alone has not been shown. (T/F)

35. For the clinically N0 neck undergoing treatment with elective neck irradiation, the dose required to give a regional control rate of approximately 95% is 45 Gy to 50 Gy. (T/F)

36. The risk of major neurological morbidity due to resection of the carotid artery without reconstruction is on the order of 30% to 50%. (T/F)

37. Division of the accessory nerve will result in drooping and posterior rotation of the scapula, with consequent shoulder deformity and weakness. (T/F)

38. If chyle leakage is suspected, then suction drains should be avoided in the postoperative period. (T/F)

39. In cases of bilateral internal jugular vein invasion, staged neck dissections performed 6 weeks apart can be performed safely without undue risk of cerebral edema. (T/F)

40. Unilateral right-sided hypoglossal nerve injury will cause impairment in the patient's ability to protrude the tongue to the left. (T/F)

41. The treatment of choice for primary atypical mycobacterial infection in cervical nodes is antibacterial chemotherapy. (T/F)

42. Granulomatous lymphadenitis may be associated with primary toxoplasma infection. (T/F)

43. Avoidance of contact sports for 3 months in patients with infectious mononucleosis is advisable because of the risk of splenic rupture. (T/F)

44. Castleman disease is characterized by progressive lymph node enlargement, iron-deficiency anemia, and risk of progression to non-Hodgkin lymphoma. (T/F)

45. Bartonella lymphadenitis is most commonly seen in farmers or abattoir workers. (T/F)

46. In a 35-year-old patient with a 2-cm papillary thyroid carcinoma, the risk of micrometastatic disease in levels II through V is approximately 40% to 50%. (T/F)

47. The first echelon of drainage of cancer of the maxillary sinus is into the jugulodigastric node at level II. (T/F)

48. Adenoid cystic carcinoma of the parotid gland has a low risk of cervical metastases; thus elective neck dissection is not considered necessary. (T/F)

49. Patients with primary parotid cancers that involve the overlying skin but who have clinically negative necks have a 25% to 35% risk of harboring metastases in level V; thus these patients should all undergo MRND including level V. (T/F)

50. Patients with established cervical metastases from non–oral cavity primary tumors have a low risk of harboring metastases in level I; thus level I may be omitted in patients undergoing MRND. (T/F)

## SINGLE-BEST ANSWER

51. Which of the following are established adverse prognostic factors?
    i. Lymph node metastases in level IV

ii. Minimal extranodal extension in oral cavity cancer

iii. High nodal ratio (the number of positive metastatic lymph nodes divided by the number of lymph nodes removed at neck dissection)

iv. Presence of level V lymph nodes in low-risk papillary thyroid cancer

v. Persistent positive node 3 months after completion of chemoradiation therapy

vi. Poorly differentiated histological type in primary larynx cancer

vii. Poorly differentiated histological type in primary oropharynx cancer

A. i, iii, iv
B. i, iii, vi
C. v, vi, vii
D. ii, iii, iv
E. iv, vi, vii

52. Dissection of level IV is indicated in which of the following cases?

i. A 62-year-old patient with a 3-cm epiglottic SCC and a radiologically negative neck undergoing transoral robotic surgery

ii. A 51-year-old patient with initial N2b neck disease with a residual 1.5-cm node in level II detected by a PET/CT scan 12 weeks after completion of chemoradiation therapy

iii. A 69-year-old patient with a large base-of-the-tongue SCC and a 3-cm metastatic node in level II

iv. A 37-year-old patient with a 2-cm unilateral medullary thyroid carcinoma and a radiologically negative neck

v. A 67-year-old patient with a 4.5-cm papillary thyroid carcinoma and a radiologically negative neck

vi. An 81-year-old patient with 3-cm cystic SCC metastasis from an unknown primary in level II

A. i, ii, vi
B. i, iii, vi
C. iv, v, vi
D. iii, iv, v, vi
E. iii, iv

53. Which of the following primary sites may drain initially to lymph nodes located above the lower border of the mandible (facial nodes)?

i. Floor of the mouth
ii. Buccal mucosa
iii. Anterior nasal cavity
iv. Tip of the tongue
v. Lateral border of the tongue
vi. Lower eyelid
vii. Soft palate

A. i, ii, iii, iv
B. i, ii, iv
C. ii, iii, vi
D. i, iii, vii
E. i, ii, iv, v

54. Arrange the following scenarios according to the likelihood of harboring occult cervical metastases in the radiologically negative neck, giving the most likely first.

i. T1N0 SCC of the lateral border of the oral tongue
ii. T1N0 SCC of the soft palate
iii. T1N0 SCC of the upper alveolus
iv. T1N0 SCC of the epiglottis
v. T1N0 acinic cell carcinoma of the parotid gland
vi. T1N0 medullary carcinoma of the thyroid gland
vii. T1N0 Hurthle cell carcinoma of the thyroid gland
viii. T3N0 transglottic SCC

A. vi, iv, i, viii
B. iv, iii, i, viii
C. vi, vii, i, ii
D. i, v, ii, iii
E. i, ii, iii, iv

55. Arrange the following risk factors in order of importance in predicting cervical metastases in a patient with oral cavity cancer and a clinically negative neck, giving the highest risk factor first.

i. T stage
ii. Tumor thickness
iii. Subsite within the oral cavity
iv. Age of the patient
v. HPV status
vi. Smoking status
vii. Histological pattern of invasion (pushing versus invasive)

A. i, ii, iii
B. v, ii, iii
C. vii, i, ii
D. ii, vi, iv
E. ii, i, iii

56. Arrange the following in order of likelihood of obtaining regional control, from greatest likelihood to least.

i. Observation alone of a clinically negative neck in a patient with T2N0 oral cavity SCC

ii. Neck dissection alone for management of the neck in a patient with T1N1 oral cavity cancer and a single ipsilateral 2.5-cm metastatic level II node

iii. Neck dissection alone for management of the neck in a patient with T1N1 tonsil cancer and a single ipsilateral 2.5-cm metastatic level II node

iv. Radiation therapy alone for management of the clinically negative neck in a patient with T2N0 oral cavity SCC

v. Therapeutic neck dissection in a patient with an initial diagnosis of T2N0 oral cavity cancer who develops neck "metastases" in level I 6 months after surgery to the primary tumor and observation of the neck

vi. Therapeutic neck dissection in a patient with an initial diagnosis of T1N1 tonsil cancer who develops "metastases" on the contralateral (previously untreated) side of the neck, 1 year after undergoing tonsillectomy plus neck dissection plus postoperative radiation therapy

vii. Salvage neck dissection in a patient with an initial diagnosis of T1N1 tonsil cancer who develops a recurrent metastatic cervical mass on the ipsilateral (previously treated) side of the neck, 1 year after undergoing tonsillectomy plus neck dissection plus postoperative radiation therapy

viii. Neck dissection plus postoperative radiation therapy for management of the neck in a patient with T1N2b oral cavity cancer, with three metastatic nodes in levels II and III, the largest of which is 3 cm, without extracapsular spreading

A. i, ii, vi, vii
B. i, viii, vi, v
C. iv, iii, vi, v
D. viii, ii, v, vi
E. viii, vi, vii, i

57. Which of the following statements regarding functional outcomes of neck dissection are true?

i. Despite preservation of the accessory nerve during MRND with dissection of the accessory nerve through level V, a large proportion of patients will have long-term functional shoulder impairment.

ii. Resection of the sternomastoid muscle in MRND exacerbates postoperative functional shoulder impairment.

iii. Despite preservation of the greater auricular nerve, most patients will have numbness of the neck.

iv. The risk of postoperative lower lip weakness is increased when dissection of level I is performed.

v. Shoulder dysfunction is rare after selective neck dissection.

A. i, iv, v
B. i, ii, v
C. i, ii, iii
D. ii, iv, v
E. i, iii, iv

58. Which of the following statements are true regarding treatment of the neck with chemoradiation therapy for established metastatic disease?

i. The presence of N3 neck disease is considered a contraindication for nonsurgical treatment.

ii. In cases of complete clinical response, the incidence of developing recurrence in the neck in patients who do not undergo neck dissection is approximately 5%.

iii. Neck dissection performed within 6 weeks of completion of treatment may show a higher incidence of residual cancer in lymph nodes than neck dissection performed beyond 12 weeks after completion of treatment.

iv. If the primary tumor does not recur, the development of distant metastases is usually preceded by regional recurrence.

v. Large-volume neck disease has a lower likelihood of response to chemoradiation therapy than does small-volume neck disease.

vi. In cases in which a fluorodeoxyglucose (FDG)-avid node persists for 3 months after completion of radiation therapy, the likelihood of residual cancer is 75% to 80%.

A. ii, iii, v
B. i, ii, iii
C. i, iii, iv
D. ii, iii, iv
E. ii, v, vi

59. Which of the following statements regarding metastatic cervical cancers of unknown primary site are true?

i. Most level II unknown primary SCCs have an occult primary site within the tonsil.

ii. The use of PET/CT to detect the primary site has a high false-positive rate because of nonspecific inflammation within the Waldeyer ring, leading to increased FDG-avidity.

iii. Epstein–Barr virus (EBV) serological type may be helpful in discovering the primary site.

iv. A metastatic adenocarcinoma in level II is more likely to have originated from an infraclavicular primary site than from a head and neck primary site.

v. In cases in which the histological type is uncertain, immunohistochemical analysis with S100 should be performed to exclude lymphoma.

vi. Metastatic SCC from an unknown primary site carries a worse prognosis than metastatic SCC from a known primary site, when the burden of neck disease is taken into account.

A. i, ii, v
B. i, ii, iii
C. ii, iii, vi
D. i, ii, vi
E. i, ii, iv

60. Which of the following statements are true?

i. The hypoglossal nerve is always located deep to the facial vein.

ii. The phrenic nerve can be distinguished from branches of the cervical plexus by its direction (lateral to medial).

iii. Bilateral neck dissection at the same time as total laryngectomy has been associated with an increased rate of salivary fistula.

iv. N stage is less important than T stage as a prognosticator for overall survival in patients with supraglottic SCC.

v. The outcomes of primary chemoradiation therapy for metastatic adenocarcinoma of the neck are similar to those observed for SCC in cases of similar N stage.

vi. The greater cornu of hyoid bone overlies the superior laryngeal nerve.
A. i, ii, iv
B. ii, iii, iv
C. ii, iii, vi
D. i, ii, iii

## MULTIPLE CHOICE

61. The phrenic nerve
A. Runs from lateral to medial, over the scalenus anterior muscle, deep to the transverse cervical vessels.
B. Runs from medial to lateral, over the scalenus anterior muscle, deep to the transverse cervical vessels.
C. Runs from medial to lateral, over the scalenus anterior muscle, superficial to the transverse cervical vessels.
D. Runs from lateral to medial, over the scalenus anterior muscle, and has a variable relationship with the transverse cervical vessels.

62. A 60-year-old patient with cT1N2b oropharyngeal SCC is initially treated with radiation therapy and achieves a complete response at the primary site and in the neck at 3 months after completion of treatment. She subsequently develops a recurrent level II nodal mass. This will be most appropriately treated by
A. "Super-selective" level IIA/upper level III neck dissection, with removal of lymph node–bearing tissue between the posterior belly of digastric muscle, accessory nerve, omohyoid muscle, internal jugular vein, and cervical plexus rootlets.
B. Selective neck dissection including levels II, III, and IV, with sparing of the accessory nerve, sternomastoid muscle, and internal jugular vein.
C. Modified radical or radical neck dissection, with sacrifice of the sternomastoid muscle and accessory nerve or internal jugular vein, if these structures are involved.
D. Induction chemotherapy with the choice of further surgical treatment depending on the response.

63. Postoperative radiation therapy for patients with pN1 disease
A. Has been shown to offer a clear survival benefit in all patients with head and neck SCC.
B. Has been shown to offer a clear survival benefit in patients with non–HPV-related SCC but not in patients with HPV-related SCC.
C. Improves regional control but without a clearly demonstrated survival benefit.
D. Improves the likelihood of regional control in patients who have undergone selective neck dissection but has not been clearly shown to improve regional control in patients who have undergone MRND.

64. During the course of a neck dissection, the surgeon inadvertently punctures the lower end of the internal jugular vein, causing profuse bleeding. The most appropriate immediate management is to
A. Raise the head of the bed, identify the tear, and repair it with polypropylene sutures (5-0 Prolene).
B. Raise the head of the bed, identify the tear, and repair it with a patch graft from a saphenous vein.
C. Lower the head of the bed, use two suctions, identify the tear, and repair it with polypropylene sutures.
D. Pack the lower part of the wound with moist gauze and request a thoracic surgery consultation, leaving the pack in place until a partial upper sternotomy is performed.

65. During the course of a selective neck dissection for SCC, gross cancer is found to be densely adherent to the accessory nerve. The correct management is to
A. Sacrifice the accessory nerve.
B. Sharply dissect the cancer from the accessory nerve, with the aim of removing all macroscopic disease; nerve sacrifice should be reserved for cases of nerve encasement or inability to separate all grossly visible disease from the nerve.
C. Perform sharp dissection with the aim of separating as much cancer as possible from the accessory nerve, then treat the patient with postoperative chemoradiation therapy.
D. Convert to a radical neck dissection, levels I through V, with sacrifice of the accessory nerve, sternomastoid muscle, and internal jugular vein.

66. Which of the following is the most appropriate rule of thumb for when lateral selective neck dissection should be performed for patients with papillary thyroid carcinoma?
A. Only in cases of FNA-proven metastatic disease in the lateral neck
B. In patients of Japanese or Korean extraction
C. For grossly invasive primary thyroid cancers greater than 4 cm
D. For patients with grossly enlarged metastatic central compartment lymph nodes

67. The most appropriate neck surgery for patients with supraglottic SCCs and clinically negative necks who are undergoing laser or robotic resection of the primary tumor is
A. Ipsilateral level IIA and III neck dissection.
B. Ipsilateral level IIA, III, and IV neck dissection.
C. Ipsilateral level IIA, IIB, III, and IV neck dissection.
D. Bilateral level IIA and III neck dissection.

68. For which of the following cancers does the presence of metastatic neck disease portend the worst prognosis in terms of overall survival?
A. Oral tongue SCC
B. HPV-related tonsil SCC
C. Maxillary sinus SCC
D. Papillary thyroid SCC in a patient older than 45 years whose primary tumor is greater than 4 cm

69. A patient undergoing concurrent chemoradiation therapy as primary treatment for metastatic neck disease achieves a reduction in cervical node volume of 40% to 50% as assessed by a posttreatment CT scan. This is considered to be
    A. A complete clinical response.
    B. A partial clinical response.
    C. Stable disease.
    D. Progressive disease.

70. A patient with a primary SCC of the vallecula staged T2N2b is treated with primary chemoradiation therapy and achieves a complete response at the primary site and a partial response in the neck. The likelihood of viable tumor in cervical lymph nodes being found at neck dissection is
    A. 10%.
    B. 20% to 30%.
    C. 40% to 50%.
    D. 70% to 80%.

71. Which of the following patients whose necks are managed with observation is most at risk of developing a recurrence in the neck?
    A. An 80-year-old with T4N0 glottic SCC, treated with total laryngectomy without neck dissection and without postoperative radiation therapy
    B. A 65-year-old with a 1.8-cm (diameter) × 10-mm (thickness) lateral tongue SCC who undergoes wide resection of the tongue cancer with negative margins and observation of the neck
    C. A 54-year-old patient with a 3-cm SCC of the tonsil with a 4-cm metastatic node who undergoes primary chemoradiation therapy and shows a complete response at the primary site and a residual 1-cm neck node, as measured by CT 3 months after completion of treatment
    D. A 59-year-old patient undergoing salvage laryngectomy without neck dissection for a rT4N0 SCC of the supraglottis, initially staged T3N2c and treated with chemoradiation therapy

72. Which of the following salivary cancers arising in the parotid gland is most likely to metastasize to cervical nodes?
    A. Adenoid cystic carcinoma
    B. Low-grade mucoepidermoid carcinoma
    C. Epithelial–myoepithelial carcinoma
    D. Carcinoma ex pleomorphic adenoma

73. A 32-year-old woman with a 1.5-mm thick malignant melanoma undergoes sentinel node mapping and excision at the same time as wide local excision, and metastases are confirmed by histopathological analysis of the sentinel node. The incidence of finding further metastatic nodes with completion neck dissection is
    A. 10%.
    B. 20% to 30%.
    C. 40% to 50%.
    D. 70% to 80%.

74. The surgical demarcation between level III and level IV in the neck is
    A. The upper border of the omohyoid muscle.
    B. The lower border of the omohyoid muscle.
    C. A horizontal line along the inferior border of the cricoid cartilage.
    D. The transverse cervical vessels.

75. The radiological demarcation between level I and level II in the neck is:
    A. A vertical line through the posterior border of the submandibular gland.
    B. The posterior belly of the digastric muscle.
    C. The mylohyoid muscle.
    D. A vertical line through the tip of the greater cornu of the hyoid bone.

76. Which of the following is not required to make a diagnosis of primary branchiogenic SCC (SCC arising primarily in a branchial cyst)?
    A. Not HPV-positive
    B. Tumor seen on histological examination to be clearly arising from the wall of the branchial cyst
    C. No clinical evidence of primary aerodigestive tract SCC
    D. No radiation therapy given at a 5-year follow-up

77. Which of the following is most accurate at staging the neck in patients with SCC of the larynx who have not received any previous treatment?
    A. Clinical palpation
    B. MRI
    C. PET-CT
    D. US-FNA

78. In metastatic SCC of the neck from an unknown primary, which of the following blood tests is likely to be most useful at pinpointing a primary site?
    A. HPV-16 DNA
    B. Anti-VCA EBV IgA antibodies
    C. Anti-p16 antibodies
    D. Prostate-specific antigen (PSA)

79. The treatment of choice for lymphadenopathy caused by atypical mycobacteria in children is
    A. Rifampicin-based antimicrobial chemotherapy.
    B. Sulfa-based antimicrobial chemotherapy.
    C. Complete surgical excision without antimicrobials.
    D. Surgical curettage and debulking followed by antimicrobial therapy.

80. The accessory nerve
    A. Supplies the sternomastoid, levator scapulae, and trapezius muscle, aiding in elevation and rotation of the scapula.
    B. Supplies the upper and middle fibers of the trapezius, but not the lower fibers, such that injury leads to unopposed depression and "winging" of the scapula.
    C. Supplies the lower fibers of the trapezius, which is responsible for rotation of the scapula.

D. Supplies the sternomastoid muscle, which assists in elevating the clavicle and turning the head to the ipsilateral side.

81. The cervical plexus
   A. Provides a contribution to the accessory nerve, which is responsible for proprioceptive function of the trapezius muscle.
   B. Provides a solely sensory function.
   C. Arises from the anterior rami of the first seven cervical nerves.
   D. Gives rise to the phrenic nerve, which is the sole motor supply to the diaphragm.

82. A 48-year-old patient with bulky bilateral cervical metastatic disease involving both internal jugular veins is to undergo surgical treatment. Which of the following statements is true?
   A. Simultaneous bilateral internal jugular vein ligation will lead to a 30% to 40% risk of serious neurological sequelae.
   B. Simultaneous bilateral internal jugular vein ligation will have minimal adverse sequelae, provided both external jugular veins are preserved.
   C. At least one internal jugular vein should be preserved, and low-volume residual disease should be treated with postoperative chemoradiation therapy.
   D. Bilateral internal jugular vein ligation will have minimal adverse sequelae provided that dissection of the other side of the neck is performed 6 weeks after the first.

83. A 59-year-old patient has bulky metastatic disease invading the carotid artery. Which of the following statements is true?
   A. Resection of the internal carotid artery without reconstruction is associated with a 70% to 90% rate of serious neuromorbidity.
   B. Resection of the external carotid artery without reconstruction is associated with a 10% to 25% rate of serious neuromorbidity.
   C. As long as encasement of the carotid artery is less than 180 degrees, surgery should be considered as first-line treatment because metastatic disease involving the carotid artery is unlikely to respond to primary chemoradiation therapy.
   D. Even with resection of the involved carotid artery and reconstruction with a saphenous vein graft, more than 80% of patients will die of their cancer.

84. Which of the following is most likely to give rise to isolated metastasis at level IV?
   A. SCC in the body of the tongue
   B. SCC of the supraglottic larynx
   C. SCC of the subglottic larynx
   D. Papillary thyroid carcinoma

85. What dose of radiation therapy is required to control the clinically negative neck in a patient with cT3N0 oral tongue SCC?
   A. 45 to 50 Gy
   B. 60 Gy

C. 66 Gy
   D. 66 to 70 Gy combined with chemotherapy

86. The neck staging of a patient with poorly differentiated thyroid cancer with a 4-cm metastatic node in the supraclavicular fossa on the right side and a 2-cm metastatic node on the left side at level II is
   A. N1a.
   B. N1b.
   C. N2c.
   D. N3.

87. The neck staging of a patient with nasopharyngeal SCC with a 4-cm metastatic node in the supraclavicular fossa on the right side and a 2-cm metastatic node on the left side at level II is
   A. N1a.
   B. N1b.
   C. N2c.
   D. N3.

88. Which of the following is least likely to metastasize to cervical nodes?
   A. Osteosarcoma of the mandible
   B. Adenoid cystic carcinoma of the floor of the mouth
   C. Neuroendocrine carcinoma of the supraglottic larynx
   D. Adenocarcinoma of the parotid gland, not otherwise specified (NOS)

89. Sacrifice of which of the following structures constitutes an extended MRND?
   A. Accessory nerve, hypoglossal nerve, internal jugular vein
   B. Sternomastoid muscle, omohyoid muscle, and internal jugular vein
   C. Accessory nerve, sternomastoid muscle, and internal jugular vein
   D. Accessory nerve, internal jugular vein, and submandibular gland

90. The brachial plexus
   A. Lies on the scalenus anterior muscle, tethered by deep cervical fascia.
   B. Enters into the neck from deep to the internal jugular vein and leaves by going deep to the trapezius.
   C. Enters the neck from deep to the posterior belly of the digastric and leaves by going deep to the trapezius.
   D. Enters the neck between the scalenus anterior and medius muscles, tethered by deep cervical fascia.

91. The most likely consequence of injury to the brachial plexus during neck dissection is
   A. Weakness of the shoulder.
   B. Weakness of intrinsic muscles of the hand.
   C. Numbness of the entire arm.
   D. Raised hemidiaphragm.

92. Which of the following tumors is most at risk of giving rise to distant metastases without any evidence of cervical metastases?
   A. T4N0 SCC of the hypopharynx
   B. T3N0 medullary thyroid cancer

C. T3N0 adenoid cystic carcinoma of the parotid
D. T4N0 SCC of the nasopharynx

93. The major benefit of PET-CT scanning in restaging the neck in the postradiation therapy setting is
   A. High negative predictive value.
   B. High positive predictive value.
   C. High sensitivity.
   D. High specificity.

94. The optimal timing for performing PET-CT to restage the neck in a patient with initial T3N2b SCC of the oropharynx treated with primary chemoradiation therapy
   A. Is within 2 weeks of completion of treatment.
   B. Is 6 to 8 weeks after completion of treatment.
   C. Is 3 to 4 months after completion of treatment.
   D. Is 6 months after completion of treatment.

95. Which of the following statements regarding bilateral neck dissection is true?
   A. Most patients undergoing bilateral neck dissection should also undergo tracheostomy.
   B. Bilateral neck dissection should not be performed simultaneously with transoral laser or robotic resection of large supraglottic cancers.
   C. Bilateral blindness is a rarely reported complication.
   D. Bilateral neck dissection should only be performed in cases of FNA-proven metastases or grossly abnormal nodes on both sides of the neck.

96. Which of the following statements regarding second arch branchial cysts is true?
   A. The peak age of presentation is in the teenage years.
   B. Most cases will have a rudimentary tract extending deeply to the tonsillar fossa.
   C. Approximately 10% to 30% are bilateral.
   D. These cysts may become inflamed in patients with acute tonsillitis because of lymphoid tissue in the wall.

97. Which of the following best describes the course of a second arch branchial fistula?
   A. A second arch branchial fistula goes from the skin of the lower neck, deep to the posterior belly of the digastric muscle, between the carotid arteries, superior to the hypoglossal nerve, and into the tonsillar fossa.
   B. A second arch branchial fistula goes from the skin of the lower neck, deep to the posterior belly of the digastric muscle, between the superior laryngeal nerve and hypoglossal nerves, and into the tonsillar fossa.
   C. A second arch branchial fistula goes from the skin of the neck around the level of the hyoid bone, over the posterior belly of the digastric muscle, and into the tonsillar fossa.
   D. A second arch branchial fistula goes from the skin of the neck around the level of the hyoid bone, through the parotid gland, has a variable relationship with the facial nerve, then

courses parallel to the external auditory canal and ultimately into the external auditory canal at the junction of the bony and cartilaginous sections.

98. The concept of MRND with preservation of certain structures based on the rationale that "lymph nodes of the neck do not form part of the adventitia of veins nor are located with muscular aponeuroses" was chiefly espoused by
   A. Suarez
   B. Bocca
   C. Crile
   D. Shah

99. Elective neck dissection in patients with clinically negative necks is most strongly recommended in the case of which of the following patients who are undergoing surgery for treatment of the primary tumor?
   A. A 42-year-old with a 5-mm thick malignant melanoma of the cheek
   B. A 78-year-old man with a 4.5-cm medullary thyroid carcinoma with preoperative vocal palsy
   C. A 68-year-old nonsmoker with a 3-cm adenoid cystic carcinoma of the hard palate
   D. A 42-year-old smoker with a 1.5-cm adenosquamous carcinoma of the soft palate

100. A 39-year-old woman initially presents with cT1N0 SCC of the tongue and undergoes partial glossectomy and elective neck dissection (levels I, II, and III). Pathological examination shows no metastases in the neck, so the patient does not undergo postoperative radiation therapy. She presents 6 months later with a level I mass on the same side. FNA confirms SCC. Which of the following would be the recommended next treatment at this point?
   A. Radiation therapy
   B. Chemoradiation therapy
   C. Further surgery
   D. Palliative treatment

## Answers

| | | |
|---|---|---|
| 1. T | 13. F | 25. T |
| 2. F | 14. F | 26. T |
| 3. F | 15. T | 27. T |
| 4. F | 16. F | 28. F |
| 5. T | 17. F | 29. F |
| 6. T | 18. F | 30. F |
| 7. F | 19. F | 31. F |
| 8. T | 20. F | 32. T |
| 9. T | 21. F | 33. T |
| 10. T | 22. F | 34. T |
| 11. F | 23. T | 35. T |
| 12. F | 24. T | 36. T |

| | | |
|---|---|---|
| 37. F | 59. B | 81. D |
| 38. F | 60. D | 82. D |
| 39. T | 61. A | 83. D |
| 40. T | 62. C | 84. D |
| 41. F | 63. C | 85. A |
| 42. T | 64. C | 86. B |
| 43. T | 65. A | 87. D |
| 44. T | 66. A | 88. A |
| 45. F | 67. D | 89. A |
| 46. T | 68. C | 90. D |
| 47. F | 69. C | 91. A |
| 48. T | 70. C | 92. C |
| 49. F | 71. B | 93. A |
| 50. T | 72. D | 94. C |
| 51. B | 73. A | 95. C |
| 52. E | 74. C | 96. D |
| 53. C | 75. A | 97. A |
| 54. A | 76. A | 98. A |
| 55. E | 77. D | 99. D |
| 56. C | 78. B | 100. C |
| 57. E | 79. C | |
| 58. A | 80. C | |

## Core Knowledge

- The presence of cervical nodal metastases is a very significant adverse prognosticator in nearly all types of head and neck cancer. Further important prognostic indicators are the number of positive nodes, the presence of bilateral metastatic nodes, metastatic involvement of lower neck levels (level IV), and the presence of extranodal tumor extension. The nodal ratio and the presence of matted nodes have also been shown to have prognostic significance. Nodal status is the most important prognostic indicator in squamous cell carcinoma (SCC) of the oral cavity, hypopharynx, and larynx; however, it would appear to be less important than T stage in the case of human papillomavirus (HPV)-related oropharyngeal cancer. Papillary thyroid carcinoma in young patients is unique among cancers in that nodal metastases do not appear to have any significant adverse effect on survival.

- Nodal status is incorporated into the American Joint Committee on Cancer (AJCC)/International Union Against Cancer (UICC) TNM staging for head and neck cancer. Note that the N staging for nasopharynx and thyroid cancer differs from that for other mucosal sites.

- The risk of nodal metastases varies with the primary site. Primary sites within the pharynx (i.e., nasopharynx, oropharynx, and hypopharynx) and supraglottic larynx are particularly high risk. The oral cavity has an intermediate risk, whereas the glottic larynx, nasal cavity, and paranasal sinuses are low risk. Other predictors of risk of metastases are higher T stage and thickness (in case of oral cavity cancers).

- For cancers at high-risk primary sites, the neck must always be addressed in the treatment plan, regardless of whether clinical nodal enlargement is present. Elective treatment of the neck is usually not required in glottic or sinonasal carcinomas unless nodes clinically suggestive of cancer are present. The management of the clinically negative neck in oral cavity SCC is discussed further on.

- The clinical status of the neck (cN0 or cN+) is determined on the basis of clinical examination and imaging. Ultrasound (US) is highly sensitive and offers the advantage of combination with fine-needle aspiration (FNA) for definitive diagnosis of metastatic disease. Computed tomography (CT) and/or magnetic resonance imaging (MRI) should be performed in cases of clinically enlarged nodes for assessment of the extent and invasion of adjacent structures. Positron emission tomography (PET)/CT lacks sensitivity for the cN0 neck but is particularly useful in monitoring the response of cervical metastases to nonsurgical treatment.

- Cervical lymph nodes are categorized into six nodal levels, and additional subcategorization divides levels 1, 2, and 5 into sublevels A and B. For most head and neck cancers, metastatic involvement of cervical lymph nodes tends to occur in an orderly and predictable fashion; each primary site usually drains to a particular neck level. Thus in the case of the clinically negative neck or neck with limited metastatic involvement, treatment can be directed at those nodes at greatest risk of harboring metastases without compromising regional control or survival.

- Elective treatment of the clinically negative neck involves either surgery or radiation therapy. Both offer approximately 95% regional control rates. In most cases, the same modality being used to treat the primary site will also be used to treat the neck.

- Surgical treatment of the clinically negative neck usually comprises elective selective neck dissection (SND), wherein only those nodes at greatest risk of harboring metastases are removed. This significantly reduces morbidity to the shoulder compared with modified radical neck dissection (MRND) because of less extensive dissection of the accessory nerve.

- Management of the clinically negative neck in oral cavity cancer is controversial. Elective neck dissection (END) offers superior regional control over observation but has not been conclusively shown to provide survival benefit because many patients who convert from observation to treatment will undergo successful salvage surgery with delayed therapeutic neck dissection. Most authors prefer a policy of END on the basis that (1) the success of salvage neck dissection in many surgeons' hands is low because of more advanced stage neck disease by the time of conversion and difficulty in practice in detecting the earliest conversion of the neck from cN0 to cN+; (2) morbidity of SND is low; and (3) pathological information obtained from the END specimen may identify patients with high-risk adverse pathological indicators who may benefit from adjuvant radiation therapy.

- Adjuvant radiation therapy is usually indicated in patients whose neck dissection pathological analysis shows multiple positive nodes, involvement of a node greater than 3 cm, or extranodal spreading. An improved survival rate with postoperative chemoradiation therapy has been shown for patients with extranodal spreading, although at a cost of increased toxic effects. The management of a single positive node less than 3 cm (pN1) is controversial. Adjuvant radiation therapy in this setting has been shown to improve regional control but not the survival rate.

- The clinically positive neck is usually best treated by combined treatment, either surgery with postoperative irradiation or primary chemoradiation therapy.

- Surgical treatment of the clinically positive neck usually consists of MRND or radical neck dissection (RND). Recently, modified SND has gained acceptance for the treatment of cases with early, low-volume metastatic disease.

- Patients undergoing primary chemoradiation therapy to the N+ neck should undergo restaging scans 3 months after completion of treatment. A complete clinical response (CCR) is defined as complete disappearance of detectable disease. The success of chemoradiation therapy in achieving a CCR is related to the N stage of the neck and also appears to be higher in patients with HPV-related cancers.

- Patients achieving a CCR have no more than a 5% to 10% risk of developing neck recurrence without surgery, so they can be safely observed. In patients with less than a CCR, it is generally recommended that they undergo neck dissection; however, select patients with low-volume residual disease may be safely observed with repeated scans in 3-month intervals.

- In patients who have undergone chemoradiation therapy but who still have residual cervical disease that is confined to a single level on imaging, highly selective neck dissection appears to offer regional control similar to that after MRND or RND. The incidence of finding viable metastatic cancer on histological examination in these cases is around 40%. In contrast, patients with multilevel neck disease, a poor response to chemoradiation therapy, or with recurrent metastatic disease in the neck after previously having achieved a CCR should undergo MRND or RND.

## SUGGESTED READING

Ambrosch P, Kron M, Pradier O, Steiner W. Efficacy of selective neck dissection: a review of 503 cases of elective and therapeutic treatment of the neck in squamous cell carcinoma of the upper aerodigestive tract. Otolaryngol Head Neck Surg 2001;124(2):180–7.

Andersen PE, Cambronero E, Shaha AR, Shah JP. The extent of neck disease after regional failure during observation of the N0 neck. Am J Surg 1996;172(6):689–91.

Basheeth N, O'Leary G, Sheahan P. Elective neck dissection for N0 neck during salvage total laryngectomy. JAMA Otolaryngol Head Neck Surg 2013;139(8):790–6.

Goenka A, Morris LG, Rao SS, Wolden SL, Wong RJ, et al. Long-term regional control in the observed neck following definitive chemoradiation for node-positive oropharyngeal squamous cell cancer. Int J Cancer 2013;133(5):1214–21.

Kligerman J, Lima RA, Soares JR, Prado L, Dias FL, et al. Supraomohyoid neck dissection in the treatment of T1/T2 squamous cell carcinoma of oral cavity. Am J Surg 1994;168(5):391–4.

Ong SC, Schöder H, Lee NY, Patel SG, Carlson D, et al. Clinical utility of 18F-FDG PET/CT in assessing the neck after concurrent chemoradiotherapy for locoregional advanced head and neck cancer. J Nucl Med 2008;49(4):532–40.

Shah JP. Patterns of cervical lymph node metastasis from squamous carcinomas of the upper aerodigestive tract. Am J Surg 1990;160(4):405–9.

Sheahan P, O'Keane C, Sheahan JN, O'Dwyer TP. Effect of tumour thickness and other factors on the risk of regional disease and treatment of the N0 neck in early oral squamous carcinoma. Clin Otolaryngol Allied Sci 2003;28(5):461–71.

Watkins JP, Williams GB, Mascioli AA, Wan JY, Samant S. Shoulder function in patients undergoing selective neck dissection with or without radiation and chemotherapy. Head Neck 2011;33(5):615–9.

Yuen AP, Ho CM, Chow TL, Yuen AP, Ho CM, et al. Prospective randomized study of selective neck dissection versus observation for N0 neck of early tongue carcinoma. Head Neck 2009;31(6):765–72.

# 9  Thyroid and Parathyroid

## Questions

### TRUE/FALSE

1. Thyroid nodules are uncommon in the general population.  (T/F)

2. The majority of thyroid nodules are malignant.  (T/F)

3. Thyroid nodules at the extremes of age are higher risk for malignancy.  (T/F)

4. Open biopsy should be routine in diagnosis of thyroid nodules.  (T/F)

5. Ultrasound scanning is the initial diagnostic imaging technique used in the workup of thyroid nodules.  (T/F)

6. The most common thyroid malignancy of follicular cell origin is follicular carcinoma.  (T/F)

7. Multiple recurrent differentiated cancers of follicular cell origin may degenerate to undifferentiated histological types.  (T/F)

8. The peak age at presentation of thyroid cancers of follicular cell origin is 50 to 59 years.  (T/F)

9. Up to 30% of thyroid cancers of follicular cell origin are inherited.  (T/F)

10. Mutations in the RET protooncogene are associated with cancers of follicular cell origin.  (T/F)

11. The blood supply of the thyroid gland is from the superior, middle, and inferior thyroid arteries.  (T/F)

12. The external branch of the superior laryngeal nerve runs posteromedial to the superior thyroid artery.  (T/F)

13. Normally, the recurrent laryngeal nerve is encountered posterior to the inferior thyroid artery.  (T/F)

14. The normal weight of a parathyroid gland is approximately 100 mg.  (T/F)

15. The superior parathyroid glands tend to lie more ventrally than the inferior parathyroid glands.  (T/F)

16. For select patients with disease limited to one lobe of the thyroid, thyroid lobectomy gives oncological results equal to total thyroidectomy.  (T/F)

17. If malignancy has been proven in one lobe of a multinodular gland, total thyroidectomy is the procedure of choice.  (T/F)

18. The presence of luminal airway involvement from thyroid cancer is a contraindication to surgery.  (T/F)

19. In the presence of malignancy, subtotal thyroidectomy to protect the recurrent laryngeal nerve should be performed.  (T/F)

20. Computed tomographic (CT) scanning with iodine contrast is contraindicated in the workup of thyroid cancer.  (T/F)

21. Elective lateral neck dissection should be offered in high-risk cases.  (T/F)

22. Because of a significant rate of metastasis, level I should routinely be included in a lateral neck dissection for differentiated thyroid cancer.  (T/F)

23. Elective central neck dissection improves survival rates in low-risk cases.  (T/F)

24. Parathyroid glands immediately on the capsule of the gland can be preserved during surgery for proven malignancy.  (T/F)

25. Before resection of a functioning recurrent laryngeal nerve that is encased by cancer, contralateral lobe dissection is sound policy so that the integrity of the contralateral nerve is ensured.  (T/F)

26. The major aim of surgery is to control disease in the central compartment.  (T/F)

27. Thyroid lobectomy is appropriate for unilateral disease.  (T/F)

28. Metastasectomy for isolated distant metastases should be considered in select cases.  (T/F)

29. During disease progression, metastases tend to become increasingly radioiodine avid.  (T/F)

30. Distant metastasis is an absolute contraindication to resection of airway structures to control the primary lesion.  (T/F)

31. A rapidly growing thyroid cancer with obvious extrathyroidal extension should be considered to be anaplastic thyroid cancer and managed without the need for biopsy.  (T/F)

32. Anaplastic cancers develop de novo or from dedifferentiation of other thyroid cancers. (T/F)

33. Surgery for anaplastic cancers should not be considered other than for biopsy. (T/F)

34. Development of chemoradiation protocols offers the chance of a cure to patients with anaplastic cancers. (T/F)

35. Patients with anaplastic cancer that is resectable in the head and neck should be considered candidates for major resection. (T/F)

36. The majority of medullary thyroid cancers are familial. (T/F)

37. Genetic screening for medullary thyroid cancer involves testing for the RAS protooncogene. (T/F)

38. Patients with preoperatively identified disease in the lateral part of the neck are generally cured with total thyroidectomy and neck dissection. (T/F)

39. Thyroid and neck surgery should not be considered in the setting of distant metastatic disease. (T/F)

40. Vascular endothelial growth factor receptor inhibitor therapy has received U.S. Food and Drug Administration approval for use in patients with advanced medullary thyroid cancer. (T/F)

41. Preoperative localization of parathyroid glands offers little in surgical planning. (T/F)

42. In primary hyperparathyroidism, a drop in intraoperative parathyroid hormone levels to less than 50% of the highest preexcisional levels predicts a 97% cure rate. (T/F)

43. All four glands should routinely be explored in primary hyperparathyroidism. (T/F)

44. All four glands should routinely be explored in multiple endocrine neoplasia syndromes. (T/F)

45. A lateral approach to the posterior aspect of the thyroid may facilitate access in revision parathyroid surgery. (T/F)

46. The diagnosis of parathyroid carcinoma is primarily histological. (T/F)

47. Mutations in the *HRPT2* gene have been implicated in parathyroid carcinoma. (T/F)

48. The presence of hypercalcemia and a palpable neck mass are suggestive of parathyroid carcinoma. (T/F)

49. During surgery parathyroid carcinoma should be carefully dissected from the ipsilateral thyroid lobe. (T/F)

50. Recurrent or persistent parathyroid carcinoma is rapidly progressive. (T/F)

## MULTIPLE CHOICE

51. Based on Figure 9-1, the operating surgeon should expect to encounter which of the following?

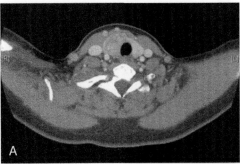
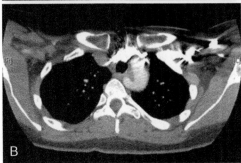

**Figure 9-1** (Courtesy of Memorial Sloan Kettering Cancer Center, New York.)

A. Invasion of the airway
B. Bulky nodal disease
C. The nonrecurrent inferior laryngeal nerve
D. Encasement of the carotid artery
E. Tracheomalacia

52. Select the correct AJCC stage for the following patients based on TNM.
    i. Stage I
    ii. Stage II
    iii. Stage III
    iv. Stage IV
    (a) A 16-year-old boy has a 5-cm papillary thyroid carcinoma and evidence of nodal disease in the lateral side of the neck but no evidence of distant metastatic disease.
    (b) A 50-year-old woman has a 3-cm papillary thyroid carcinoma and evidence of involvement of the strap muscles. There is evidence of distant disease, but biopsy-positive nodes are present in the central part of the neck.
    (c) A 75-year-old woman has a 1.5-cm follicular carcinoma of the thyroid without evidence of extrathyroidal extension, nodal metastases, or distant metastases.
    (d) A 60-year-old man has a 3-cm tumor limited to the thyroid and disease in the central part of the neck but no distant metastases.
    (e) A 33-year-old woman has a 3-cm follicular carcinoma and evidence of pulmonary metastases.

53. In Figure 9-2, which of the following features are identifiable:

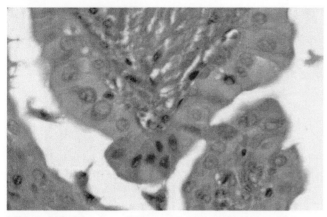

**Figure 9-2** (Courtesy of Memorial Sloan Kettering Cancer Center, New York.)

 i. Vascular invasion.
 ii. Nuclear clearing.
 iii. Extracapsular extension.
 iv. Nuclear pseudoinclusions.
 v. Tall cell features.
A. i, iii
B. ii, iv, v
C. ii, iv
D. i, v
E. i, iii, v

54. Select from the list below the initial surgical therapy most appropriate for the following patients.
 i. Thyroid lobectomy
 ii. Total thyroidectomy
 iii. Total thyroidectomy with bilateral central neck dissection
 iv. Total thyroidectomy with central and lateral neck dissection
 v. Total thyroidectomy, laryngectomy, and central neck dissection
 vi. Open biopsy
(a) A 10-year-old child has a confirmed RET mutation and a family history of medullary thyroid carcinoma.
(b) A 35-year-old patient has a uninodular follicular lesion on fine-needle aspiration biopsy of the left thyroid.
(c) A 72-year-old patient has a rapidly enlarging thyroid gland, which is hard on examination and is causing respiratory distress.
(d) A 66-year-old patient has progressive hoarseness and hemoptysis related to locally aggressive, poorly differentiated thyroid carcinoma with pulmonary metastases stable in size over 5 years.
(e) A 49-year-old patient has biopsy-proven papillary microcarcinoma in the setting of a multinodular thyroid gland.

55. From the following imaging techniques, select the most appropriate initial investigation(s) for localization of a hyperfunctioning parathyroid gland.

 i. Ultrasound
 ii. Magnetic resonance imaging (MRI)
 iii. CT
 iv. Sestamibi scan
 v. Positron emission tomography (PET)-CT
A. i, iv
B. ii, iv
C. v
D. i, iii
E. ii, iii

56. From Figure 9-3, identify the possible data described by lines A and B.

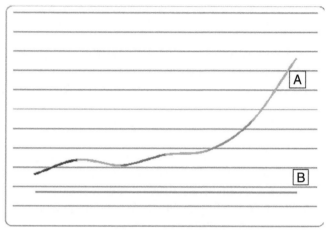

**Figure 9-3** (Courtesy of Memorial Sloan Kettering Cancer Center, New York.)

A. *A* is the percentage of thyroid surgeries that are lobectomy; *B* is the incidence.
B. *A* is the incidence; *B* is the percentage of patients receiving radioactive iodine.
C. *A* is the percentage of thyroid cancers that are follicular carcinoma; *B* is the mortality from thyroid cancer.
D. *A* is the mortality from thyroid cancer; *B* is thyroid cancer incidence.
E. *A* is the incidence of thyroid cancer; *B* is the mortality from thyroid cancer.

57. From the following options, identify those features that are an indication for sternotomy when resection of a substernal goiter is planned.
 i. Kyphosis
 ii. Malignancy with extrathyroidal extension
 iii. Multinodular disease
 iv. Extension of disease below the great vessels
 v. Tumor size greater than the diameter of the thoracic inlet
 vi. Revision surgery
 vii. Nonpapillary histological type
A. i, iv, vii
B. ii, iv, v, vi
C. iii, v, vi, vii
D. i, iii, v
E. None of the above

58. The following responses relate to the anatomy and embryology of the thyroid and parathyroid glands.

Select the response or responses that are true in relation to the statements below.

 i. Dorsal to the recurrent laryngeal nerve
 ii. Foramen cecum
 iii. Foramen rotundum
 iv. Fourth and fifth pharyngeal pouches
 v. Hyoid bone
 vi. Levator muscle of the thyroid gland
 vii. Pyramidal lobe
 viii. Third and fourth pharyngeal pouches
 ix. Thyroid cartilage
 x. Ventral to the recurrent laryngeal nerve

(a) This is the point of origin of the thyroid in the embryo.
(b) This is traversed by the thyroid during its migration to the adult position.
(c) This is a remnant of the thyroglossal duct.
(d) This is the origin of the parathyroid glands.
(e) This is the usual anatomical position of the superior parathyroid glands.

*For Questions 59 through 63, select the correct thyroidectomy surgical technique(s) from the following list.*

 i. Intubation with an endotracheal tube with inbuilt electromyographic (EMG) monitoring of the larynx
 ii. Infiltration of lidocaine with epinephrine into the skin incision
 iii. Identification of the recurrent laryngeal nerve
 iv. Thyroid lobectomy
 v. Subtotal thyroidectomy
 vi. Extracapsular total thyroidectomy
 vii. Elective central neck dissection
 viii. Elective lateral neck dissection
 ix. Insertion of cellulose hemostatic agent
 x. Use of a suction drainage

59. Which technique(s) have been associated with reduced rates of recurrent nerve injury?
 A. iii, vi
 B. iii, iv, v
 C. i, viii, ix
 D. vi, vii
 E. ii, ix, x
 F. x

60. Which technique(s) are oncologically sound management of the thyroid gland in the cancer setting?
 A. v, vi
 B. iii, iv, v
 C. i, viii, ix
 D. vi, vii
 E. ii, ix, x
 F. x

61. Which technique(s) have been associated with increased rates of recurrent nerve injury?
 A. iii, vi
 B. iii, iv, v
 C. i, viii, ix
 D. vi, vii

 E. ii, ix, x
 F. x

62. Which technique(s) have been shown not to reduce postoperative hematoma rates?
 A. iii, vi
 B. iii, iv, v
 C. i, viii, ix
 D. vi, vii
 E. ii, ix, x
 F. x

63. Which technique(s) have been associated with increased rates of hypocalcemia?
 A. iii, vi
 B. iii, iv, v
 C. i, viii, ix
 D. vi, vii
 E. ii, ix, x
 F. x

64. Which of the following clinical scenarios should be expected when the intraoperative finding displayed in Figure 9-4 is encountered?

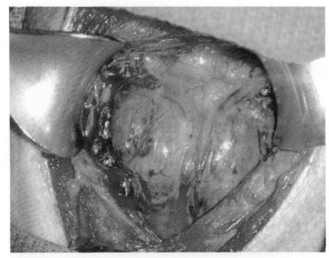

**Figure 9-4** (Courtesy of Memorial Sloan Kettering Cancer Center, New York.)

 i. Metastatic melanoma
 ii. Anaplastic thyroid carcinoma
 iii. Fibrosarcoma
 iv. Angiosarcoma
 v. Treatment of acne
 vi. Recent chemotherapy
 vii. Previous radiation therapy to the neck
 viii. Recent radioiodine therapy

 A. i, vi
 B. v
 C. viii
 D. iii, iv
 E. ii, vii

65. Locally advanced, differentiated thyroid cancer without distant metastases
 A. Should be excised with preservation of the laryngeal framework and treated with postoperative external beam radiation therapy.

B. Should be excised with preservation of the laryngeal framework and treated with postoperative radioactive iodine.
C. Should be managed with complete resection with negative margins so that uncontrolled disease in the central part of the neck is avoided.
D. Should be treated with preoperative induction chemotherapy.

66. Lateral nodal disease in papillary thyroid cancer
A. Predicts improved survival rates for young patients.
B. Predicts lower recurrence rates in young patients.
C. Predicts worse survival rates for older patients.
D. Predicts local recurrence in older patients.

67. Children at risk of medullary thyroid cancer on genetic screening
A. Should undergo total thyroidectomy as soon as possible after birth.
B. Should undergo total thyroidectomy before the age of 1 year.
C. Should remain under observation until nodular disease is identified in the thyroid gland.
D. Should undergo risk assessment depending on the genetic mutation detected.

68. Patients with medullary thyroid cancer that is unresectable or distantly metastatic *and* who have evidence of disease progression
A. Should be considered for wide-field external beam radiation therapy.
B. Should be considered for platinum-based chemotherapy.
C. Should be considered for targeted therapies.
D. Should be considered for best supportive therapy.

69. The prognosis of patients with unresectable medullary cancer is best assessed with the use of
A. Calcitonin doubling time.
B. Serial cross-sectional imaging.
C. Serial PET scans.
D. Serum calcium monitoring.

70. The patient most likely to benefit from postoperative radioiodine is
A. A 74-year-old with T3N1bM0 papillary thyroid cancer.
B. A 55-year-old with T1N0M0 papillary thyroid cancer.
C. A 30-year-old with T2N1aM0 medullary thyroid cancer.
D. A 13-year-old with T1N1aM1 papillary thyroid cancer.

71. In patients with differentiated thyroid cancer that presents with lateral neck node metastases, the levels that should routinely be included in a therapeutic lateral neck dissection are
A. I through V.
B. IIa through Vb.
C. IIb through Va.
D. II through IV.

72. Subtotal thyroidectomy may be indicated in which clinical situation?
A. Unifocal T2 lateralized well-differentiated thyroid cancer, in order to protect the contralateral nerve
B. Bilateral nodular goiter causing compressive symptoms
C. In regions of the world where there is little access to thyroid hormone replacement
D. In no clinical situation

73. In patients with differentiated thyroid cancer metastatic to the lateral side of the neck, which preoperative investigation should be considered routine?
A. Ultrasound examination
B. PET scan
C. Contrast-enhanced CT of the neck
D. Diagnostic radioiodine scan

74. Which of the following side effects is associated with the administration of radioactive iodine?
A. Dysphagia
B. Xerostomia
C. Secondary malignancy
D. All of the above

75. Which size of thyroid tumor is increasing most rapidly in incidence?
A. Greater than 4 cm
B. 2 to 4 cm
C. 1 to 2 cm
D. Less than 1 cm

76. What is the rate of incidental malignancy in multinodular goiters?
A. Less than 5%
B. 5% to 10%
C. 10% to 30%
D. 30% to 50%

77. The ideal incision for a thyroidectomy and neck dissection should run
A. In a skin crease at the level of the cricoid cartilage.
B. From the mastoid tip, parallel with the trapezius, to the inferior part of the neck, then within a skin crease at the level of the cricoid cartilage.
C. From the mastoid tip to the cricoid cartilage with a "lazy S" extension to the clavicle.
D. In two parallel skin creases two fingerbreadths below the mandible and two fingerbreadths above the clavicle.

78. Access to level V during a therapeutic neck dissection for thyroid cancer without overt nodal disease in the posterior triangle
A. Cannot be achieved through a single horizontal incision.
B. Is obtained by extending the incision to the anterior border of the trapezius laterally.
C. Is obtained by dissecting posterolaterally under the sternomastoid muscle and retracting the nodal tissue from behind the muscle.
D. Is not required because this level is rarely involved.
E. Requires division of the accessory nerve to ensure a comprehensive nodal dissection.

79. In patients with papillary thyroid cancer and without evidence of central neck metastases at presentation, management of the neck with observation rather than elective central neck dissection results in what percentage of cases requiring further central neck surgery in the subsequent 10 years?
    A. 50%
    B. 30%
    C. 15%
    D. Less than 5%

80. When treatment options are considered in patients with T4 differentiated thyroid cancer with distant metastases, what percentage will still be alive after 5 years if adequate surgical resection of the primary tumor is performed?
    A. 0%
    B. 25%
    C. 33%
    D. 50%

81. Elective central neck dissection in differentiated thyroid cancers has been shown to result in
    A. Lower recurrence rates.
    B. Improved survival rates.
    C. Lower postoperative thyroglobulin levels.
    D. No improvement in outcomes.

82. Fatality from differentiated thyroid cancer is predominantly due to
    A. Complications of pulmonary metastases.
    B. Uncontrolled disease in the central part of the neck.
    C. Uncontrolled disease in the lateral part of the neck.
    D. Complications of therapy.

83. The disease that presents most commonly to surgeons as metastatic disease *to* the thyroid is
    A. Malignant melanoma.
    B. Bronchial carcinoma.
    C. Renal cell carcinoma.
    D. Prostatic adenocarcinoma.

84. Extrathyroidal extension that is not evident in the operating room but that is identified microscopically on histopathological examination
    A. Has not been shown to affect survival.
    B. Is an indication for adjuvant radioiodine.
    C. Is an indication for completion thyroidectomy after initial lobectomy.
    D. Results in high rates of local recurrence.

85. Multicentricity in papillary thyroid cancer
    A. Is an indication for elective neck surgery.
    B. Justifies total thyroidectomy for all patients.
    C. Predicts worse survival rates.
    D. Has no impact on outcomes.

86. Which statement about radioactive iodine avidity in thyroid cancers of follicular cell origin is true?
    A. It is proportional to fluorodeoxyglucose-PET avidity.

B. It is inversely related to the risk of death from thyroid cancer.
    C. It is homogeneous throughout primary lesions.
    D. It is more common in older patients.

87. Which of the following areas is a common site for nodal metastases from thyroid cancers?
    A. The perifacial lymph nodes
    B. Level IV posterior to the great vessels
    C. Level II superior to the accessory nerve
    D. The parapharyngeal space

88. Papillary thyroid metastasis to the Delphian nodes has been shown to be associated with
    A. Low survival rates.
    B. High rates of recurrence.
    C. Extrathyroidal extension.
    D. Reduced rates of lateral neck metastases.

89. Genomic analysis of Hurthle cell carcinoma suggests
    A. Significant similarities to papillary carcinoma.
    B. Significant similarities to follicular cancers.
    C. Significant differences from both papillary and follicular cancers.
    D. Significant similarities to medullary cancers.

90. National database studies of outcomes related to differentiated thyroid cancer
    A. Are reliable; treatment decisions may be based on them.
    B. Suggest that survival rates for differentiated cancers are improving.
    C. Show trends toward less aggressive therapies in the United States.
    D. Lack sufficient detail to allow analysis of the impact of treatment on outcome.

91. After routine total thyroidectomy, suction drains
    A. Reduce postoperative hematoma rates.
    B. Reduce postoperative seroma rates.
    C. Improve cosmetic outcomes.
    D. Should not be used.

92. Factors that have been shown to predict the risk of postthyroidectomy hematoma include the
    A. Size of the thyroid tumor.
    B. Experience of the surgeon.
    C. Use of an electrosurgical device.
    D. Duration of surgery.

93. During follow-up of low-risk differentiated thyroid cancers, serial thyroglobulin monitoring
    A. Reduces recurrence rates.
    B. Is of unproven benefit.
    C. Improves survival rates.
    D. Prevents unnecessary surgery.

94. Which treatment modality is most effective for managing recurrent nodal disease in differentiated thyroid cancer?
    A. Surgery
    B. Radioiodine
    C. External beam radiation therapy
    D. Alcohol ablation

95. Children who are seen with papillary thyroid cancer are at high risk of
    A. Locally advanced primary tumors.
    B. Bony metastases.
    C. Pulmonary metastases.
    D. Local recurrence.

96. Which of the following factors is not an independent predictor of survival in differentiated thyroid cancer?
    A. Age
    B. Extrathyroidal extension
    C. Multicentric disease
    D. Completeness of resection

97. Which of the following features is suggestive of malignancy in a parathyroid lesion?
    A. Palpable neck mass
    B. Normocalcemia
    C. Prior history of thyroid malignancy
    D. Increased thyroglobulin level

98. The next step in managing a patient with normal clinical examination results and a rising thyroglobulin level after surgery for thyroid cancer is
    A. Elective neck dissection.
    B. Ultrasound imaging.
    C. Therapeutic radioiodine.
    D. Tyrosine kinase inhibitor therapy.

99. Which of the following statements about targeted therapy in medullary thyroid cancers is true?
    A. Side effects are uncommon.
    B. Survival rates are improved.
    C. Dose reduction is required in a significant number of patients.
    D. The duration of therapy is 6 weeks.

100. The most important differential diagnosis in patients with suspected anaplastic thyroid cancer is
    A. Poorly differentiated thyroid cancer.
    B. Lymphoma.
    C. Sarcoma.
    D. Metastatic melanoma.

## Answers

| | | |
|---|---|---|
| 1. F | 13. T | 25. T |
| 2. F | 14. F | 26. T |
| 3. T | 15. F | 27. F |
| 4. F | 16. T | 28. T |
| 5. T | 17. T | 29. F |
| 6. F | 18. F | 30. F |
| 7. T | 19. F | 31. F |
| 8. F | 20. F | 32. T |
| 9. F | 21. F | 33. F |
| 10. F | 22. F | 34. F |
| 11. F | 23. F | 35. T |
| 12. T | 24. T | 36. F |

| | | |
|---|---|---|
| 37. F | 57. B | 78. B |
| 38. T | 58. (a) ii (b) v (c) vii (d) viii (e) i | 79. D |
| 39. F | | 80. D |
| 40. T | | 81. D |
| 41. F | 59. B | 82. A |
| 42. T | 60. A | 83. C |
| 43. F | 61. D | 84. A |
| 44. T | 62. F | 85. D |
| 45. T | 63. D | 86. B |
| 46. F | 64. B | 87. B |
| 47. T | 65. C | 88. C |
| 48. T | 66. C | 89. C |
| 49. F | 67. D | 90. D |
| 50. F | 68. C | 91. D |
| 51. C | 69. A | 92. A |
| 52. (a) i (b) iii (c) i (d) ii (e) ii | 70. D | 93. B |
| | 71. B | 94. A |
| | 72. C | 95. C |
| 53. C | 73. A | 96. C |
| 54. (a) ii (b) i (c) vi (d) v (e) ii | 74. D | 97. A |
| | 75. D | 98. B |
| 55. A | 76. C | 99. C |
| 56. E | 77. A | 100. B |

## Core Knowledge

- The incidence of thyroid cancer is rising in the United States and around the world.

- Most of the increase can be explained by the increasing detection of microscopic disease.

- This has led to a change in the histological distribution of disease: papillary carcinoma now constitutes more than 90% of cases.

- In tandem with the increase in microcarcinomas, an increase has also been seen in larger volume disease, which has not yet been explained.

- All patients with nodules and lymph nodes suggestive of thyroid cancer should undergo ultrasound assessment with fine-needle aspiration biopsy.

- Cross-sectional imaging should be considered in patients with bulky local disease or in those with possible extrathyroidal extension, particularly into the laryngotracheal axis.

- Although contrast administration may delay the provision of radioactive iodine (RAI) treatment, it should not deter the surgeon when information gained will allow more accurate surgical planning—it is the surgery that will cure the patient rather than the iodine.

- All patients should undergo risk assessment before surgical management.

- Risk assessment strategies exist for predicting survival (grade, age, metastases, extension, size [GAMES]) and recurrence (American Thyroid Association).

- For differentiated thyroid carcinoma (i.e., follicular, Hurthle cell, and papillary), the only procedures that should be performed are thyroid isthmusectomy, lobectomy, or total thyroidectomy.

- For low-risk cases, more extensive surgery has never been shown to improve outcomes; lobectomy has provided equivalent results to total thyroidectomy in terms of survival and recurrence.

- In high-risk cases, total thyroidectomy is generally preferred because it facilitates adjuvant RAI treatment.

- No group has convincingly shown improved outcomes for elective lateral neck dissection.

- There is evidence that elective central neck dissection allows identification of occult disease in up to 50% of cases; however, this has not translated into improved outcomes.

- Central neck dissection, particularly outside of centers of excellence, is associated with significant morbidity in terms of nerve injury and hypocalcemia.

- The role of RAI is far from clear. In low-risk patients, there is no proven benefit.

- In high-risk patients, particularly in those with distant metastases, RAI appears to have a role; its use in high-risk patients is generally considered routine.

- In the large group of patients who are at intermediate risk, RAI should be used selectively, with the understanding that benefits are probably minimal and that risks do exist but are small.

- As differentiated thyroid cancer undergoes dedifferentiation, it becomes more aggressive and shows less avidity for RAI and more avidity for fluorodeoxyglucose used in positron emission tomography (PET). As such, RAI becomes less useful, and adjuvant therapy for extrathyroidal extension or residual disease should involve external beam radiation.

- For patients who are seen with distant metastases, a thyroidectomy will allow concentration of iodine in the distant metastases in addition to providing control of disease in the central area of the neck.

- In the setting of locally advanced tumors with distant metastatic disease, an attempt to quantify the progression of distant disease should be made. In the event of stable distant disease and progressive local disease, aggressive surgery in the central area of the neck may prevent complications such as asphyxia and provide meaningful quality of life.

- Medullary thyroid cancer is more aggressive and difficult to cure.

- In the absence of regional disease, a total thyroidectomy and central neck dissection should be performed.

- If tumor spreading is present in the neck (particularly the lateral part of the neck), the rate of biochemical cure is low. Disease in the central part of the neck should be approached with central neck dissection and a low threshold for lateral neck dissection if lymphadenopathy suggestive of cancer is encountered.

- If the disease is advanced at presentation, central neck surgery may be performed to prevent complications. However, if the disease is incurable, a tradeoff must be made between preventing complications from disease and causing complications with surgery.

- Genetic screening should be arranged for all patients with medullary thyroid cancer because up to 25% will have a heritable genetic defect.

- In families with RET mutations, specific codon analysis will provide detailed information regarding the level of risk and therefore the timing of prophylactic thyroidectomy.

- In patients with advanced or inoperable disease, tyrosine kinase inhibitors play a role in slowing disease progression. The only agent currently licensed for use in the United States is vandetanib.

- Anaplastic thyroid cancer is rapidly progressive and almost universally fatal.

- On occasion, patients may be seen while they are still able to undergo surgery. In those very select cases, significant resections will be possible; however, in most settings, a biopsy to rule out lymphoma will be followed by best supportive or palliative care.

- In select patients, radiation therapy, chemotherapy, or both may provide some additional quality of life.

- The finding of black thyroid has been associated with administration of minocycline, commonly prescribed for acne vulgaris.

- Parathyroid surgery should be performed by surgeons with extensive experience in thyroid surgery.

- Careful preoperative assessment including biochemical analysis, parathyroid hormone (PTH) levels, and imaging are essential.

- Ultrasound with sestamibi scanning allows identification of the majority of adenomas; however, local practice will vary.

- A minimally invasive parathyroidectomy after identification of an adenoma on a preoperative workup is reasonable, if it can be assumed that intraoperative PTH levels will drop below 50% after removal of the adenoma.

- Parathyroid carcinoma is rare but should be considered when a parathyroid mass is palpable, when calcium levels are extremely high, or when metastases are present.

- The diagnosis of malignancy often cannot be made on histological analysis; therefore clinical suspicion is important.

- Parathyroid cells are extremely liable to implantation; therefore when such surgery is performed, the capsule of the gland must remain intact.

- In the setting of parathyroid malignancy, ipsilateral thyroid lobectomy will allow en bloc resection of disease.

## SUGGESTED READING

American Thyroid Association Guidelines Task Force, Kloos RT, Eng C, Evans DB, Francis GL, Gagel RF, et al. Medullary thyroid cancer: management guidelines of the American Thyroid Association. Thyroid 2009;19(6):565–612.

American Thyroid Association (ATA) Guidelines Taskforce on Thyroid Nodules and Differentiated Thyroid Cancer, Cooper DS, Doherty GM, Haugen BR, Kloos RT, Lee SL, et al. Revised American Thyroid Association management guidelines for patients with thyroid nodules and differentiated thyroid cancer. Thyroid 2009;19(11):1167–214.

Barney BM, Hitchcock YJ, Sharma P, Shrieve DC, Tward JD. Overall and cause-specific survival for patients undergoing lobectomy, near-total, or total thyroidectomy for differentiated thyroid cancer. Head Neck 2011;33(5):645–9.

Hay ID, Thompson GB, Grant CS, Bergstralh EJ, Dvorak CE, Gorman CA, et al. Papillary thyroid carcinoma managed at the Mayo Clinic during six decades (1940-1999): temporal trends in initial therapy and long-term outcome in 2444 consecutively treated patients. World J Surg 2002;26(8):879–85.

Hodin R, Angelos P, Carty S, Chen H, Clark O, Doherty G, et al. No need to abandon unilateral parathyroid surgery. J Am Coll Surg 2012;215(2):297 ; author reply 297–300.

Nixon IJ, Ganly I, Patel SG, Palmer FL, Whitcher MM, Tuttle RM, et al. Thyroid lobectomy for treatment of well differentiated intrathyroid malignancy. Surgery 2012;151(4):571–9.

Norman J, Lopez J, Politz D. Abandoning unilateral parathyroidectomy: why we reversed our position after 15,000 parathyroid operations. J Am Coll Surg 2012;214(3):260–9.

Patel KN, Shaha AR. Poorly differentiated and anaplastic thyroid cancer. Cancer Control 2006;13(2):119–28.

Shah JP, Patel SG, Singh B. Jatin Shah's head and neck surgery and oncology. 4th ed. Philadelphia: Mosby; 2012. p. 471–525.

Wells Jr SA, Robinson BG, Gagel RF, Dralle H, Fagin JA, Santoro M, et al. Vandetanib in patients with locally advanced or metastatic medullary thyroid cancer: a randomized, double-blind phase III trial. J Clin Oncol 2012;30(2):134–41.

# 10 Salivary Glands

## Questions

### TRUE/FALSE

1. The parotid gland is the first major salivary gland to develop. (T/F)

2. Immunoglobulin G is the primary immunoglobulin found in saliva. (T/F)

3. Salivary immunoglobulins are primarily produced in plasma cells in the parenchyma of the gland. (T/F)

4. Saliva tonicity is similar to that of intracellular fluid. (T/F)

5. An increase in parasympathetic tone will lead to increased salivary flow. (T/F)

6. The major salivary glands are endodermal in origin. (T/F)

7. Sjögren syndrome (SjS) can be ruled out by negative results for anti-SSA (Ro) and SSB (La) antibodies. (T/F)

8. Salivary stones are most commonly found in the Wharton duct. (T/F)

9. Parotid stones tend to be radiopaque, whereas submandibular stones are more radiolucent. (T/F)

10. Gustatory sweating is the most common postoperative complication of parotid surgery. (T/F)

11. The incidence of gustatory sweating is less with a total parotidectomy. (T/F)

12. Preservation of the great auricular nerve is correlated with an improved quality of life. (T/F)

13. Electromyographic (EMG) monitoring of the facial nerve has been shown to decrease temporary and permanent facial paralysis after parotid surgery. (T/F)

14. Pleomorphic adenoma is the most common benign tumor of the minor salivary glands. (T/F)

15. Pleomorphic adenoma may demonstrate calcifications on imaging. (T/F)

16. Pleomorphic adenoma is not more likely to recur with enucleation. (T/F)

17. Pleomorphic adenomas are thought to originate from excretory duct cells. (T/F)

18. Malignant degeneration is reported in 35% to 40% of pleomorphic adenomas. (T/F)

19. Mucoepidermoid carcinoma is the most common malignancy of the submandibular gland. (T/F)

20. The majority of primary submandibular neoplasms are malignant. (T/F)

21. Adenoid cystic carcinoma is the most common minor salivary gland neoplasm. (T/F)

22. Pediatric parotid neoplasms are more likely to be malignant. (T/F)

23. Mucoepidermoid carcinoma is the most common pediatric parotid malignancy. (T/F)

24. Identification of both pseudocysts and true glandular lumina is required for a diagnosis of adenoid cystic carcinoma. (T/F)

25. Adenoid cystic carcinoma was formerly known as a cylindroma. (T/F)

26. Adenoid cystic carcinoma is considered a slow-growing highly malignant tumor. (T/F)

27. The typical pattern of adenoid cystic carcinoma is described as *cribriform*. (T/F)

28. Combined patterns of growth (tubular and solid) are common in adenoid cystic carcinoma. (T/F)

29. Combined patterns of growth are only seen in the original tumor of adenoid cystic carcinoma. (T/F)

30. Combined patterns of growth are commonly seen in original tumors and in recurrences of adenoid cystic carcinomas. (T/F)

31. The prognosis of adenoid cystic carcinoma is not influenced by the pattern of growth. (T/F)

32. The cribriform growth pattern of adenoid cystic carcinoma is associated with a higher incidence of metastases. (T/F)

33. The solid growth pattern of adenoid cystic carcinoma is associated with a higher incidence of metastases. (T/F)

34. Metastases to the lungs are usually asymptomatic or "silent" in adenoid cystic carcinoma. (T/F)

35. Lymph node metastases are common findings on neck dissections for adenoid cystic carcinoma. (T/F)

36. High-grade variants of mucoepidermoid carcinoma have a more solid infiltrative pattern of growth. (T/F)

37. Nuclear atypia, frequent mitoses, and extensive necrosis are classic features of high-grade mucoepidermoid carcinomas. (T/F)

38. There is a marked difference in prognosis for mucoepidermoid carcinoma depending on the grade of the tumor. (T/F)

39. High-grade mucoepidermoid carcinomas closely resemble squamous cell carcinomas. (T/F)

40. The t11;19 Q21;P13 chromosomal translocation is present in up to 80% of mucoepidermoid carcinomas and is a good prognostic indicator. (T/F)

41. On computed tomography (CT), a small benign mixed tumor of the parotid is a smoothly marginated, homogenously enhancing ovoid mass. (T/F)

42. On T2 magnetic resonance imaging (MRI), a benign mixed tumor (BMT) is a sharply marginated mass with uniform hypointensity. (T/F)

43. A BMT is a hypoechoic hypervascular mass on ultrasound. (T/F)

44. Angiography may assist in distinguishing a deep lobe BMT from a glomus tumor. (T/F)

45. A $^{99m}$Tc-pertechnetate result for a BMT is similar to that for a Warthin tumor. (T/F)

46. Saliva contains muramidase. (T/F)

47. Saliva stimulated by sympathetic innervation is thicker. (T/F)

48. Saliva stimulated parasympathetically is more watery. (T/F)

49. Everyday human saliva secretion amounts to 2.0 to 2.5 L. (T/F)

50. The submandibular gland contributes approximately 75% of saliva secretion. (T/F)

## MULTIPLE CHOICE

51. Dry eyes, lobular atrophy, and dental caries are characteristic findings in which disease?
    A. Mikulicz disease
    B. Sarcoidosis
    C. SjS
    D. Atypical tuberculosis

52. Dry eyes, hilar lymphadenopathy, and dental caries are characteristic of which disease?
    A. Mikulicz disease
    B. Sarcoidosis
    C. SjS
    D. Atypical tuberculosis

53. A patient with SjS and an enlarging parotid gland should be suspected of having
    A. Chronic sialadenitis.
    B. Warthin tumor.
    C. Mucoepidermoid carcinoma.
    D. Mucosa-associated lymphoid tissue (MALT) lymphoma.

54. Gustatory sweating after parotidectomy is caused by
    A. Stimulation of sweat glands by parasympathetic fibers from the auriculotemporal branch of the trigeminal nerve.
    B. Stimulation of sweat glands by sympathetic fibers from the auriculotemporal branch of the trigeminal nerve.
    C. Stimulation of sweat glands by preganglionic fibers via the glossopharyngeal nerve.
    D. Stimulation of sweat glands originating in the superior salivatory ganglion.
    E. A and C.
    F. A and D.
    G. B and C.

55. The most reliable landmark for the facial nerve is the
    A. Tragal pointer.
    B. Posterior belly of the digastric.
    C. Tympanomastoid suture line.
    D. Bony cartilaginous ear canal.

56. Characteristic MRI findings for pleomorphic adenoma include
    A. Hyperintensity on T1.
    B. Hyperintensity on T2.
    C. Enhancement with gadolinium.
    D. A and B.
    E. A and C.
    F. B and C.

57. The potential cells of origin for pleomorphic adenomas include
    A. Myoepithelial cells.
    B. Intercalated duct cells.
    C. Excretory duct cells.
    D. A and B.
    E. A and C.
    F. B and C.

58. All of the following are found within the parapharyngeal space, except the
    A. Hypoglossal nerve.
    B. Spine of the sphenoid.
    C. Nerve to the tensor veli palatini.
    D. Foramen ovale.

59. Which of the following is the correct sequence for increasing risk of malignancy in a salivary neoplasm?
    A. Parotid < submandibular < minor
    B. Minor < submandibular < parotid
    C. Submandibular < parotid < minor
    D. Parotid < minor < submandibular

60. List the following adult malignancies in order from most frequent to least frequent.
    A. Mucoepidermoid > adenoid cystic > acinic cell > malignant mixed tumor
    B. Mucoepidermoid > adenoid cystic > malignant mixed tumor > adenocarcinoma
    C. Mucoepidermoid > adenoid cystic > adenocarcinoma > acinic cell carcinoma
    D. Mucoepidermoid > adenocarcinoma > adenoid cystic > acinic cell carcinoma

61. List the following pediatric parotid neoplasms in order from most frequent to least frequent.
    A. Pleomorphic adenoma > acinic cell > mucoepidermoid > adenoid cystic
    B. Pleomorphic adenoma > mucoepidermoid > acinic cell > adenoid cystic
    C. Pleomorphic adenoma > adenoid cystic > mucoepidermoid > acinic cell
    D. Mucoepidermoid > pleomorphic adenoma > acinic cell > adenoid cystic

62. Which of the following statements about saliva is correct?
    A. In humans, the submandibular gland contributes about 85% of secretions, the parotid gland secretes about 15%, and small amounts are secreted from the other salivary glands.
    B. In humans, the submandibular gland contributes about 20% to 25% of secretions, the parotid gland secretes about 70% to 75%, and small amounts are secreted from the other salivary glands.
    C. In humans, the submandibular gland contributes about 35% to 45% of secretions, the parotid gland secretes about 35% to 40%, and small amounts are secreted from the other salivary glands.
    D. In humans, the submandibular gland contributes about 70% to 75% of secretions, the parotid gland secretes about 20% to 25%, and small amounts are secreted from the other salivary glands.

63. Which of the following statements is correct?
    A. Sympathetic stimulation of saliva facilitates digestion, whereas parasympathetic stimulation facilitates respiration.
    B. Sympathetic stimulation of saliva facilitates respiration, whereas parasympathetic stimulation facilitates digestion.
    C. Sympathetic stimulation of saliva facilitates respiration and digestion, whereas parasympathetic stimulation facilitates digestion.
    D. Sympathetic stimulation of saliva facilitates respiration, whereas parasympathetic stimulation facilitates digestion and respiration.

64. Which of the following statements is correct?
    A. Human saliva is 85% water, whereas the other 15% consists of electrolytes, mucus, glycoproteins, enzymes, and antibacterial compounds such as secretory immunoglobulin A (IgA) and lysozyme.
    B. Human saliva is 95.0% water, whereas the other 5% consists of electrolytes, mucus, glycoproteins, enzymes, and antibacterial compounds such as secretory IgA and lysozyme.
    C. Human saliva is 99.5% water, whereas the other 0.5% consists of electrolytes, mucus, glycoproteins, enzymes, and antibacterial compounds such as secretory IgA and lysozyme.

D. Human saliva is 92.5% water, whereas the other 7.5% consists of electrolytes, mucus, glycoproteins, enzymes, and antibacterial compounds such as secretory IgA and lysozyme.

65. Which of the following statements is correct?
    A. Parotid glands produce a serous type of saliva, whereas sublingual glands secrete a predominantly mucous type of saliva.
    B. Parotid glands produce a mucous type of saliva, whereas sublingual glands secrete a predominantly serous type of saliva.
    C. Parotid glands produce a serous type of saliva, whereas sublingual glands secrete saliva that is equally serous and mucous.
    D. Parotid glands produce equally serous and mucous saliva, whereas sublingual glands secrete a predominantly mucous type of saliva.

66. Minor salivary glands secrete
    A. Mucous saliva.
    B. Serous saliva.
    C. Predominantly serous saliva.
    D. Equally serous and mucous saliva.

67. Which of the following statements is correct?
    A. Overall, 50% of salivary gland cancers arise in the parotid gland, 25% arise in the minor salivary glands, and 25% arise in the submandibular gland.
    B. Overall, 65% of salivary gland cancers arise in the parotid gland, 27% arise in the minor salivary glands, and 8% arise in the submandibular gland.
    C. Overall, 25% of salivary gland cancers arise in the parotid gland, 50% arise in the minor salivary glands, and 25% arise in the submandibular gland.
    D. Overall, 85% of salivary gland cancers arise in the parotid gland, 10% arise in the minor salivary glands, and 5% arise in the submandibular gland.

68. Which of the following statements is correct?
    A. There is no distinct staging system for tumors arising in minor salivary glands; hence there is no uniformity for the staging of salivary gland tumors.
    B. Minor salivary gland tumors less than 4 cm are staged T3.
    C. The American Joint Committee on Cancer (AJCC) staging system for tumors arising in minor salivary glands is the same as for major salivary glands.
    D. Minor salivary gland carcinomas with extracapsular extension are staged T3.

69. Which of the following statements is correct?
    A. Staging of minor salivary gland tumors is an independent AJCC staging system.
    B. Staging of minor salivary gland tumors is based on that of major salivary glands.

C. Staging of minor salivary gland tumors is based on the site of origin.

D. Staging of minor salivary gland tumors is based on the depth of invasion.

70. Which of the following statements about salivary gland cancer is correct?
    A. Adjuvant radiation therapy to the primary site maximizes the potential for locoregional control and adds a considerable survival advantage in high-staged cancers.
    B. Adjuvant radiation therapy to the primary site maximizes the potential for locoregional control only in early stage tumors.
    C. Adjuvant radiation therapy to the primary site has little impact on locoregional control but reduces the risk of distant metastases.
    D. Adjuvant radiation therapy is largely ineffective.

71. Which of the following statements about salivary gland cancer is most accurate?
    A. Patients with an early T stage, high-grade tumor, and positive surgical margins should receive postoperative radiation therapy.
    B. Patients with an advanced T stage tumor should receive postoperative radiation therapy.
    C. Patients with positive surgical margins, perineural invasion, and lymph node metastasis should receive postoperative radiation therapy.
    D. Patients with an advanced T stage, high-grade tumor, positive surgical margins, perineural invasion, and lymph node metastasis should receive postoperative radiation therapy.

72. Which of the following statements about recurrent minor salivary gland cancer is correct?
    A. Local recurrences require chemoradiation therapy.
    B. Local recurrences indicate a palliative course.
    C. Local recurrences do not necessarily portend a decreased chance of survival.
    D. Surgical intervention is not a therapeutic option for local recurrences.

73. Which of the following statements about the facial nerve in salivary gland cancer is correct?
    A. Sacrifice of a functional facial nerve is not appropriate.
    B. Sacrifice of a functional facial nerve is appropriate for facilitation of a monobloc resection.
    C. Sacrifice of the facial nerve is necessary within 1 cm of malignant disease so that clearance is facilitated.
    D. Sacrifice of a functional facial nerve is justified if the tumor directly invades the nerve or when resection facilitates a monobloc excision.

74. Which of the following statements about parotid gland cancer margins is correct?
    A. Microscopically positive margins on the facial nerve are unacceptable.
    B. Close or microscopically positive margins on the facial nerve are acceptable because adjuvant radiation therapy offers acceptable local control rates.

C. Microscopically positive margins on the facial nerve do not necessitate radiation therapy.

D. Close margins warrant revision surgery and adjuvant radiation therapy for improved local control.

75. Which of the following statements is correct?
    A. Nearly 80% of the parotid gland is lateral to the facial nerve, and the 20% medial is considered the "deep lobe."
    B. Nearly 20% of the parotid gland is lateral to the facial nerve, and the 80% medial is considered the "deep lobe."
    C. Nearly 40% of the parotid gland is lateral to the facial nerve, and the 60% medial is considered the "deep lobe."
    D. Nearly 50% of the parotid gland is lateral to the facial nerve, and the 50% medial is considered the "deep lobe."

76. Which of the following statements about sialadenitis is correct?
    A. Persistent reduction in salivary flow from the parotid gland occurs at a total dose of 50 to 60 Gy.
    B. Persistent reduction in salivary flow from the parotid gland occurs at a total dose of 10 to 20 Gy.
    C. Persistent reduction in salivary flow from the parotid gland occurs at a total dose of 30 to 40 Gy.
    D. Persistent reduction in salivary flow from the parotid gland occurs at a total dose of 70 to 80 Gy.

77. Which of the following statements about sialadenitis is correct?
    A. The submandibular gland is considerably more radiation-sensitive than the parotid gland.
    B. The parotid gland is considerably more radiation-sensitive than the submandibular gland.
    C. The parotid gland and the submandibular gland have equal radiosensitivity.
    D. The parotid gland is highly radioinsensitive.

78. Which of the following statements about sialadenitis is correct?
    A. Dry skin is the most frequent complication of $^{131}I$ therapy for thyroid cancer.
    B. Headaches are the most frequent complication of $^{131}I$ therapy for thyroid cancer.
    C. Sialadenitis is the most frequent complication of $^{131}I$ therapy for thyroid cancer.
    D. Gastrointestinal upset is the most frequent complication of $^{131}I$ therapy for thyroid cancer.

79. Which of the following statements about the marginal mandibular nerve is correct?
    A. Surface marking is the tragal pointer.
    B. Surface marking is the masseter muscle.
    C. Surface marking is the angle of the mandible.
    D. Surface marking is the posterior belly of the digastric muscle.

80. The most consistent anatomical landmark of the facial nerve is the
    A. Anterior border of the posterior belly of the digastric muscle.
    B. Posterior border of the posterior belly of the digastric muscle.
    C. Superior border of the posterior belly of the digastric muscle.
    D. Inferior border of the posterior belly of the digastric muscle.

81. The facial nerve exits
    A. Medial to the stylomastoid foramen.
    B. Superior to the stylomastoid foramen.
    C. Posterior to the stylomastoid foramen.
    D. Lateral to the stylomastoid foramen.

82. The buccal branch of the facial nerve, as shown in Figure 10-1,

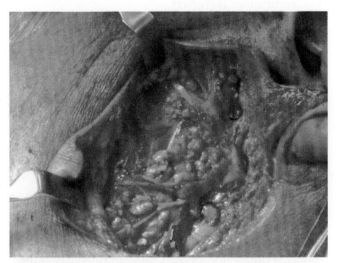

**Figure 10-1** (Courtesy of Memorial Sloan Kettering Cancer Center, New York.)

    A. Extends along the path of the Stensen duct.
    B. Extends between the tragus and the lateral canthus of the eye.
    C. Extends along the path of the marginal mandibular nerve.
    D. Extends superior to the zygomatic branch.

83. Which of the following statements about the deep lobe of the parotid is correct?
    A. Most tumors within the deep lobe are benign.
    B. Most tumors within the deep lobe are malignant.
    C. Most tumors within the deep lobe are sarcomas.
    D. Most tumors within the deep lobe are neurofibromas.

84. Which of the following statements about the deep lobe of the parotid, as shown in Figure 10-2, is correct?
    A. Most tumors present in the retromandibular location.
    B. Most tumors present in the parapharyngeal space.

C. Most tumors present in the retromandibular and parapharyngeal space.
D. Most tumors present in the retromandibular and retropharyngeal space.

85. A Warthin tumor is also known as a
    A. Benign mixed tumor.
    B. Papillary cystadenoma.
    C. Papillary cystadenoma sarcomatosum.
    D. Papillary cystadenoma lymphomatosum.

86. Which of the following statements about a Warthin tumor is correct?
    A. 90% of tumors are unilateral.
    B. 10% of tumors are unilateral.
    C. 50% of tumors are bilateral.
    D. 40% of tumors are bilateral.

87. Which of the following statements about salivary gland cancer is correct?
    A. Parotid carcinomas overall have the worst prognosis.
    B. Submandibular carcinomas have the best prognosis overall.
    C. Parotid carcinomas overall have the best prognosis.
    D. Sublingual carcinomas overall have the best prognosis.

88. The most reliable prognostic indicators of salivary gland cancer are the
    A. Stage of disease and radiological findings.
    B. Stage of disease and histological grade.
    C. Histological grade and radiological findings.
    D. Stage of disease and facial nerve paralysis.

89. The most favorable histological type for salivary gland cancer is
    A. Acinic cell and low-grade mucoepidermoid carcinoma.
    B. Squamous cell and low-grade mucoepidermoid carcinoma.

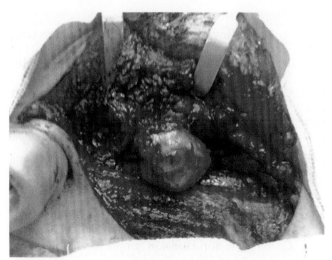

**Figure 10-2** (Courtesy of Memorial Sloan Kettering Cancer Center, New York.)

C. Squamous cell and anaplastic carcinoma.

D. Fibromyxoid sarcoma and low-grade mucoepidermoid carcinoma.

90. Which of the following statements about metastatic disease to the parotid gland is correct?

A. The skin of the face, external ear, and scalp account for 90% of primary tumor locations.

B. The skin of the face, external ear, and scalp account for 50% of primary tumor locations.

C. The skin of the face, external ear, and scalp account for 75% of primary tumor locations.

D. The skin of the face, external ear, and scalp account for 40% of primary tumor locations.

91. Which of the following statements about the salivary glands is correct?

A. A normal parotid has no intraparotid nodes.

B. All intraparotid lymph nodes are pathological.

C. The normal parotid has 2 to 32 intraglandular nodes.

D. All salivary glands have intraglandular lymph nodes.

92. Which of the following descriptions is true about lymphoma (Figure 10-3)?

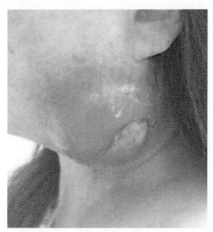

**Figure 10-3** (Courtesy of Memorial Sloan Kettering Cancer Center, New York.)

A. Parotid involvement most commonly seen with diffuse large A-cell lymphoma

B. Parotid involvement most commonly seen with diffuse large B-cell lymphoma

C. Parotid involvement most commonly seen with diffuse large C-cell lymphoma

D. Parotid involvement most commonly seen with diffuse large D-cell lymphoma

93. Which of the following statements about lymphoma is correct?

A. Systemic non-Hodgkin lymphoma involves the parotid in 1% to 8% cases.

B. Systemic non-Hodgkin lymphoma involves the parotid in 8% to 16% cases.

C. Systemic non-Hodgkin lymphoma involves the parotid in 1% to 2% cases.

D. Systemic non-Hodgkin lymphoma involves the parotid in 10% to 20% cases.

94. Which of the following statements about metastases to the parotid is correct?

A. Metastases to the parotid most commonly result from squamous cell carcinoma of the skin.

B. Metastases to the parotid most commonly result from melanoma.

C. Metastases to the parotid most commonly result from lymphoma.

D. Metastases to the parotid most commonly result from sarcoma.

95. Which of the following are immunohistochemical features of melanoma within parotid nodes?

A. S-100 and HMV-45 positive

B. S-200 and HMD-45 positive

C. S-100 and HMB-45 positive

D. S-500 and HMB-45 positive

96. Which of the following statements about parotid embryology is correct?

A. "Early" encapsulation explains lymph node incorporation within its capsule.

B. "Late" encapsulation explains lymph node incorporation within its capsule.

C. "Delayed" encapsulation explains lymph node incorporation within its capsule.

D. "Failed" encapsulation explains lymph node incorporation within its capsule.

97. Which of the following statements about Sjögren syndrome (SjS) is correct?

A. Collagen vascular disease is not part of primary SjS.

B. Collagen vascular disease is a feature of primary SjS.

C. Rheumatoid arthritis is a common feature of primary SjS.

D. Primary SjS develops into secondary SjS in the elderly.

98. What is the best imaging modality for diagnosis of SjS?

A. MRI with MR sialography

B. Ultrasound

C. Radionucleotide study

D. CT

99. Each of the following is a differential diagnosis for SjS, except

A. Human immunodeficiency virus (HIV)-associated benign lymphoepithelial lesions (BLLs)

B. Non-Hodgkin lymphoma

C. Epstein–Barr viral infection

D. Sarcoidosis

100. Which of the following statements about BLL-HIV infection is correct?

A. 25% of HIV-positive patients develop BLLs of the parotid.

B. 5% of HIV-positive patients develop BLLs of the parotid.

C. 75% of HIV-positive patients develop BLLs of the parotid.

D. 90% of HIV-positive patients develop BLLs of the parotid.

## Answers

| | | |
|---|---|---|
| 1. T | 35. F | 69. C |
| 2. F | 36. T | 70. A |
| 3. T | 37. F | 71. D |
| 4. T | 38. T | 72. C |
| 5. T | 39. T | 73. D |
| 6. F | 40. T | 74. B |
| 7. F | 41. T | 75. A |
| 8. T | 42. F | 76. A |
| 9. F | 43. F | 77. B |
| 10. T | 44. T | 78. C |
| 11. F | 45. F | 79. C |
| 12. T | 46. T | 80. C |
| 13. F | 47. T | 81. D |
| 14. T | 48. T | 82. A |
| 15. T | 49. F | 83. A |
| 16. F | 50. T | 84. C |
| 17. F | 51. C | 85. D |
| 18. F | 52. B | 86. A |
| 19. F | 53. D | 87. C |
| 20. F | 54. E | 88. B |
| 21. T | 55. C | 89. A |
| 22. T | 56. F | 90. C |
| 23. T | 57. A | 91. C |
| 24. T | 58. D | 92. B |
| 25. T | 59. A | 93. A |
| 26. T | 60. C | 94. A |
| 27. T | 61. B | 95. C |
| 28. T | 62. D | 96. B |
| 29. F | 63. B | 97. A |
| 30. T | 64. C | 98. A |
| 31. F | 65. A | 99. C |
| 32. F | 66. A | 100. B |
| 33. T | 67. B | |
| 34. T | 68. A | |

## Core Knowledge

- Salivary gland neoplasms are thought to arise either from pleuripotent stem cells of the salivary duct system in the reserve cell theory or from differentiated cells along the salivary gland unit in the multicellular theory. Because of the heterogeneity of tumors, the etiology of salivary neoplasms is unclear. Ionizing radiation, Epstein–Barr virus, nickel exposure, and employment in the rubber industry have been associated with salivary malignancies. Current smoking and heavy alcohol use have been demonstrated to cause increased risk of malignancy in men, but this risk has not been seen in women.

- There are five main histopathological categories: malignant epithelial tumors (e.g., mucoepidermoid, adenoid cystic, and acinic cell), benign epithelial tumors (e.g., pleomorphic adenoma and papillary cystadenoma lymphomatosum), lymphomatous tumors (Hodgkin lymphoma), soft tissue tumors, and metastatic tumors. The epidemiology of these tumors is not well documented; however, the global annual incidence of salivary gland tumors is estimated at 0.4 to 13.5 per 100,000 people.

- The incidence of malignancy in the parotid, submandibular, and minor salivary glands is 25%, 50%, and 80%, respectively. Overall, 65% of salivary gland cancers arise in the parotid gland, 27% arise in the minor salivary glands, and 8% arise in the submandibular gland. Approximately 3% to 5% of all head and neck neoplasms arise in the salivary glands.

- Mucoepidermoid carcinoma is the most frequently encountered parotid malignancy, comprising 12% to 29% of malignant salivary gland tumors. Adenoid cystic cancers are characterized by high metastatic potential, perineural invasion, and late local recurrence, sometimes up to a decade after initial surgery. Acinic cell carcinoma represents 7% to 17.5% of salivary malignancies.

- Pediatric salivary lesions are more likely to be inflammatory than those found in adults and are associated with a preponderance of congenital lesions such as vascular malformations and remnants of the branchial apparatus. Neoplastic salivary lesions in the pediatric population tend to have a similar pathological distribution to that seen in adults but are more likely to be malignant. Approximately 35% of parotid neoplasms in children are malignant.

- The majority of salivary tumors in general and parotid tumors in particular are seen as palpable masses. Although clinical signs of local invasion (such as fixation to skin, reduced mobility, and facial paralysis) or nodal metastases may suggest malignancy, these are often not present.

- Five major indications have been suggested for salivary gland fine-needle aspiration cytology (FNAC) of the parotid gland. FNAC can be used to rule out inflammatory lesions, identify systemic diseases such as reticuloendothelial tumors, rule out direct invasion of the gland or metastases, evaluate unresectable lesions and tumors in patients who are considered to be poor surgical candidates, and evaluate lesions when the probability of a neoplasm is low, such as in children. The argument against routine performance of an FNAC test in benign disease is that it does not affect the indication for or the extent of surgery for well-demarcated tumors confined to the parotid gland. Overall, the extent of surgery should not be based on FNAC results alone; however, it is a valuable surgical adjunct and an accurate method of determining histological type.

- The literature reflects high sensitivity and specificity values for FNAC of benign lesions, but these values decrease for malignant variants. Pleomorphic adenoma is the most frequently reported benign tumor, histologically confirmed in 95% of cases. Cytological accuracy of more than 90% is also achieved for papillary cystadenoma lymphomatosum (Warthin tumor).

- The fundamental principle for parotid tumor surgery is gross total excision of the tumor with preservation of the functioning facial nerve as long as it is not directly involved by the tumor.

- Facial nerve identification: the posterior belly of the digastric, mastoid tip, tragal pointer, and the tympanomastoid suture line are key anatomical landmarks. The nerve lies 2 to 4 mm inferior to the tympanomastoid suture line. The most consistent intraoperative landmark is the superior aspect of the posterior belly of the digastric.

- Computed tomography (CT) with and without contrast is a commonly used preoperative imaging modality offering excellent information with regard to salivary calculi, neoplasms, tumor size, surrounding structural anatomy (particularly bony information), and regional lymph node involvement. Magnetic resonance imaging (MRI) is the optimal imaging modality for salivary gland disease, offering the added advantage of assessment of perineural spreading. Perineural tumor spreading, in particular, the spreading of parotid cancers along the course of the facial nerve into the mastoid segment of the temporal bone, has to be ruled out because of surgical and prognostic implications. Positron emission tomography (PET)-CT has been shown to be more accurate than CT in the evaluation of high-grade salivary cancers. The diagnostic accuracy of predicting the pathological tumor extent is significantly higher for PET-CT (approximately 90%) than for CT alone (70%).

- Pleomorphic adenomas are thought to arise from the intercalated duct and have epithelial and myoepithelial components. More than half of the pleomorphic adenomas (51%) are classified as myxoid type, and of these, 71% often have a distinct focal absence of encapsulation in that tumors often merge into normal parotid gland tissue. The risk of malignant degeneration increases over time when observed. Surgical extirpation is recommended for all pleomorphic adenomas. The capsule can easily be disrupted when tumors are dissected from the facial nerve, which accounts for some of the potential for recurrence of these tumors. Capsular dissection and tumor spillage is associated with increased recurrence, and extracapsular dissection, at a minimum, is required. The surgical objective of a superficial parotidectomy is complete removal of the lesion, as well as identification and preservation of the facial nerve and its branches. A 38-year Ovid Medline search (1970-2008) recently reported tumor recurrence in 36 (3.0%) of 1183 extracapsular dissection (ECD) cases and in 1 (0.3%) of 340 partial superficial parotidectomy (PSP) cases. Permanent facial nerve dysfunction occurred in 22 (1.8%) of 1202 ECD cases and in 2 (0.2%) of 924 PSP cases.

- In patients with recurrent pleomorphic adenomas, greater surgical intervention is required and with that comes higher rates of facial nerve trauma and higher recurrence rates, despite aggressive surgical clearance.

- The majority of tumors of the deep lobe are benign. A pleomorphic adenoma within the deep lobe of the parotid (i.e., deep to the facial nerve) requires the lateral parenchyma of the parotid to be dissected from the nerve to facilitate mobilization of the nerve and excision of the tumor. Upon removal of the mass, the lateral lobe of the parotid gland, if not completely detached, may be returned to its anatomical position. This will reduce the soft tissue deficit deformity of total parotidectomy.

- In the malignant setting, the traditional teaching is that tumor grade rather than clinical stage is prognostically more significant. Lymph nodes at risk of primary malignant parotid tumors are located at the tail of the parotid, along the external jugular vein, and in the postauricular, jugulodigastric, upper posterocervical, and midjugular areas. If the malignant tumor is more anteriorly located, then nodes along the facial artery and submandibular triangle are also at risk.

- Patients with advanced T stages, high-grade tumors, positive surgical margins, perineural invasion, and lymph node metastasis usually receive postoperative radiation therapy. Adjuvant radiation therapy to the primary site maximizes the potential for locoregional control and adds a considerable survival advantage in high-stage cancers. In a 1990 study by Armstrong et al, a 5-year survival rate of 19% was reported at Memorial Sloan Kettering Cancer Center, which was increased to 49% with surgery and adjuvant radiation therapy. Furthermore, local control improved from 40% to 69% over a 5-year period.

- One of the largest radiation oncology studies in the literature by Terhaard et al (2005) examined 538 patients with salivary gland cancer. Postoperative radiation therapy improved 10-year local control rates significantly compared with surgery alone in patients with T3 to 4 tumors (84% versus 18%), close resection margins (95% versus 55%), incomplete resection (82% versus 44%), bone invasion (86% versus 54%), and perineural invasion (88% versus 60%). The authors also concluded that the decision to treat neck nodes electively should be based on both the T stage and the histological type of the tumor. A dose of at least 46 Gy at levels I through III was recommended.

- Elective dissection of the neck should eradicate micrometastatic occult disease and may possibly allow the patient to avoid radiation therapy. The strongest predictors of occult disease are histological type, pathological grade, T stage, and the size of the primary lesion. Because risk factors associated with the primary tumor indicate a strong possibility of occult disease, it is recommended that definitive management of the neck include dissection of levels I, II, and III. Therefore, in cases of high-grade tumors, even if the tumor is small and confined to the superficial lobe, elective neck dissection of an N0 neck should be considered.

- Malignant tumor extirpation may require removing part or all of the facial nerve. A functionally intact nerve should be preserved in meticulous fashion as long as all gross tumor is removed in a monobloc fashion. Microscopic positive margins in this setting will require postoperative radiation therapy. Gross intraoperative facial nerve involvement requires nerve sacrifice. This should be anticipated and always discussed with patients before surgery for malignant tumors so that all facial nerve reconstruction rehabilitation possibilities are available, given the excessive morbidity associated with functional loss.

- Most studies of minor salivary gland cancers have reported use of multimodality therapy with initial surgery and adjuvant radiation therapy. Nodal status is a major determinant of survival. Nodal metastases from mucoepidermoid carcinoma are more common than metastases from adenoid cystic carcinoma. Classic features of adenoid cystic carcinoma include extensive local infiltration and perineural invasion. The tumor grade is an adverse prognostic factor. Decreases in survival rates of 50% are seen with high-grade pathological features. Patients with advanced T stage, high-grade tumors, positive surgical margins, perineural invasion, and lymph node metastasis should receive postoperative radiation therapy. Many studies report better overall survival rates compared with disease-free survival rates, which demonstrates the indolent nature of these tumors. It also suggests that local recurrences do not necessarily portend decreased survival rates. Thus aggressive surgical intervention is warranted even if clear microscopic margins are not considered feasible. Overall, patients with minor salivary gland carcinoma have good survival statistics, and this should be kept in mind while choosing primary treatment and salvage options.

- The goals of reconstruction in facial paralysis include the following: facial symmetry at rest, a symmetrical smile, voluntary coordinated spontaneous facial movements, oral competence, eyelid closure with corneal protection, and an absence or limitation of synkinesis and mass movement. Facial nerve rehabilitation may be classified as either static or dynamic.

- Chemotherapy is reserved for palliative treatment of metastatic disease, but results are currently disappointing. At present, available drugs yield poor results, whether as single agents or in combination. Thus the role of systemic chemotherapy in salivary cancers remains investigational. Advanced salivary gland tumors continue to be a difficult problem in oncology and palliation, mainly because of their low chemosensitivity and protracted disease course.

## SUGGESTED READING

Armstrong JG, Harrison LB, Spiro RH, Fass DE, Strong EW, Fuks ZY. Malignant tumors of major salivary gland origin. A matched pair analysis of the role of combined surgery and postoperative radiotherapy. Arch Otolaryngol 1990;116:290–3.

Iseli T, Harris G, Dean N, Iseli CE, Rosenthal EL. Outcomes of static and dynamic facial nerve repair in head and neck cancer. Laryngoscope 2010;120:478–83.

Kelley DJ, Spiro RH. Management of the neck in parotid carcinoma. Am J Surg 1996;172:695–7.

Liu JC, Shah JP. Surgical technique refinements in head and neck oncologic surgery. J Surg Oncol 2010;101(8):661–8.

Loh KS, Barker M, Bruch G, O'Sullivan B, Brown D, Goldstein DP, et al. Prognostic factors of malignancy of the minor salivary glands. Head Neck 2009;31:58–63.

Pederson AW, Haraf DJ, Blair EA, Stenson KM, Witt ME, Vokes EE, et al. Chemoreirradiation for recurrent salivary gland malignancies. Radiother Oncol 2010;95(3):308–11.

Postema RJ, van Velthuysen ML, van den Brekel MW, Balm AJ, Peterse JL. Accuracy of fine-needle aspiration cytology of salivary gland lesions in the Netherlands cancer institute. Head Neck 2004;26(5):418–24.

Spiro RH. Salivary neoplasms: overview of a 35-year experience with 2,807 patients. Head Neck Surg 1986;8(3):177–84.

Terhaard CH, Lubsen H, Van der Tweel I, Hilgers FJ, Eijkenboom WM, Marres HA, et al. Salivary gland carcinoma: independent prognostic factors for locoregional control, distant metastases, and overall survival: results of the Dutch Head And Neck Oncology Cooperative Group. Head Neck 2004;8:681–92.

Terhaard CH, Lubsen H, Rasch CR, Levendag PC, Kaanders HH, Tjho-Heslinga RE, et al. The role of radiotherapy in the treatment of malignant salivary gland tumors. Int J Radiat Oncol Biol Phys 2005;61(1):103–11.

# 11 Neurogenic Tumors and Paragangliomas

## Questions

### TRUE/FALSE

1. The head and neck region is the most common location for benign peripheral nerve sheath tumors. (T/F)

2. Paraganglia are derived from embryonic neural crest and are found in vascular adventitia throughout the body. (T/F)

3. Schwannomas originate from microglial cells. (T/F)

4. Head and neck paragangliomas typically secrete catecholamines. (T/F)

5. Carotid body tumors are the most common paragangliomas in the head and neck. (T/F)

6. Carotid body tumors arise from the chemoreceptor cells located at the carotid bifurcation. (T/F)

7. Paragangliomas and schwannomas typically present as pulsatile neck masses. (T/F)

8. Schwannomas and neurofibromas are usually mobile along the long axis of the nerve involved and are immobile in the axis perpendicular to the long axis of the nerve. (T/F)

9. Paragangliomas are usually benign and grow slowly. (T/F)

10. Paragangliomas usually cause symptoms by invading surrounding structures. (T/F)

11. Approximately 40% of paragangliomas are reported to be malignant. (T/F)

12. Approximately 30% of paragangliomas are reported to be bilateral or multiple. (T/F)

13. Approximately 10% of paragangliomas are reported to be familial. (T/F)

14. The paraganglioma syndromes are associated with mutations in the *SDH* gene. (T/F)

15. *SDHB* and *SDHC* mutations are transmitted in an autosomal recessive manner, whereas an *SDHD* mutation is transmitted exclusively by the father. (T/F)

16. Paragangliomas/pheochromocytomas in patients with *SDHB* mutations tend to behave in a malignant fashion with a high rate of metastasis and therefore serve as a marker of malignant disease. (T/F)

17. Tissue diagnosis of paraganglioma is an essential part of the workup and should always be established. (T/F)

18. Paragangliomas frequently arise in the masticator space (Figure 11-1). (T/F)

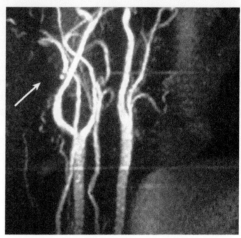

**Figure 11-1** (From Shah JP, Patel SG, Singh B. Jatin Shah's head and neck surgery and oncology. 4th ed. Philadelphia: Mosby; 2012 [Figure 14-28].)

19. Neurogenic tumors frequently arise in the masticator space. (T/F)

20. Plexiform neurofibromas are typically associated with familial neurofibromatosis type 1 (NF1). (T/F)

21. Multifocal presentation of schwannomas raises the suspicion for neurofibromatosis type 1 (NF1). (T/F)

22. Carotid body tumors originate within the carotid bifurcation and tend to splay the internal and the external carotid arteries, a finding described as a lyre sign. (T/F)

23. Glomus vagale tumors tend to displace the carotid artery posteriorly. (T/F)

24. Multiple low-signal flow voids on T1-weighted magnetic resonance imaging (MRI) are typically characteristic of paragangliomas. (T/F)

25. For observation of paragangliomas and schwannomas, MRI scanning only needs to be performed twice; once the tumor growth rate has been established, it can be relied on. (T/F)

26. Direct angiography is the only confirmatory radiographic test for a carotid body tumor.  (T/F)

27. Paragangliomas express somatostatin receptor.  (T/F)

28. An octreotide scan can be used to detect additional paragangliomas and to screen patients thought to be at risk of SDH mutations.  (T/F)

29. The management of neurogenic and neurovascular tumors in the head and neck has evolved significantly during the last decade because of a better understanding of the natural course of the tumors.  (T/F)

30. Surgery for carotid body tumors generally results in cranial nerve injury and deficit.  (T/F)

31. Surgery for paragangliomas and schwannomas arising from the cranial nerves inflicts considerable morbidity.  (T/F)

32. Longitudinal population-based studies have shown that the average rate of growth of paragangliomas is 1 mm/year.  (T/F)

33. Treatment selection of paragangliomas is based on balancing the risk of cranial nerve deficits resulting from surgery versus the potential benefit of nonsurgical treatment approaches.  (T/F)

34. Once the diagnosis is established, close observation of paragangliomas and schwannomas with serial radiographic imaging should only be considered in a carefully selected group of patients.  (T/F)

35. While under observation, a patient who develops symptoms or shows rapid tumor progression on clinical examination and/or imaging warrants consideration of intervention.  (T/F)

36. The appropriate measure of efficacy of radiation therapy in the management of a paraganglioma is tumor regression.  (T/F)

37. Radiation therapy is an effective modality in the management of paragangliomas and schwannomas and has 10-year local progression-free rates ranging from 92% to 100%.  (T/F)

38. The appropriate dose of radiation required in the management of paragangliomas is 60 to 70 Gy.  (T/F)

39. Radiation therapy in young patients with paragangliomas and schwannomas poses the risk of radiation-induced tumors at a later age; therefore alternative treatment approaches should be considered.  (T/F)

40. The diagnosis of malignant paraganglioma can be established with a histological examination.  (T/F)

41. Rapid growth, cervical lymph node metastasis, or radiographic features of local invasion of paragangliomas should raise the suspicion of malignancy.  (T/F)

42. If a schwannoma is enucleated with preservation of the surrounding fibers of the nerve, the involved nerve will generally retain function.  (T/F)

43. Schwannomas and neurofibromas of the lateral compartment of the neck can be treated with early surgical intervention because the resultant deficit is usually not significant.  (T/F)

44. Schwannomas and neurofibromas of the medial compartment of the neck can be treated with early surgical intervention because the resultant deficit is usually not significant.  (T/F)

45. Carotid body tumors are best treated by early surgical intervention if the patient is a safe surgical candidate.  (T/F)

46. If a paraganglioma is large and highly vascular, preoperative angiographic studies should be performed to demonstrate feeding vessels.  (T/F)

47. If preoperative embolization is considered, it should be performed within 72 hours of the planned surgical procedure.  (T/F)

48. Patients with functioning paragangliomas require preoperative management of hypertension with alpha blockade.  (T/F)

49. Balloon occlusion studies should be performed preoperatively in every patient undergoing surgical resection of carotid body tumor.  (T/F)

50. Dissection of carotid body tumors should be performed in a subadventitial plane.  (T/F)

## MULTIPLE CHOICE

51. Review the computed tomographic (CT) scan and MRI of a parapharyngeal space tumor shown in Figure 11-2. What features presented here allow one to make the correct diagnosis?
    i. Flow voids
    ii. Lyre sign
    iii. Cystic changes within the tumor
    iv. Anterior displacement of the carotid arteries
    v. Postgadolinium enhancement on T2 MRI
    vi. Intense enhancement on CT with contrast
    A. i, ii
    B. iii, iv
    C. i, ii, vi
    D. iv, v
    E. iii, vi

52. From the options shown below, choose the single most likely diagnosis for each of the scenarios below. Each option may be used once, more than once, or not at all.
    i. Carotid body tumor
    ii. Vagal paraganglioma
    iii. Schwannoma
    iv. Neurofibroma
    v. Malignant peripheral nerve sheath tumor
    vi. Malignant carotid body tumor
    vii. Neurofibromatosis type 1
    viii. Familial paraganglioma
    (a) A 50-year-old man presents with the complaint of a slowly growing pulsatile mass in the upper part of the neck on the right

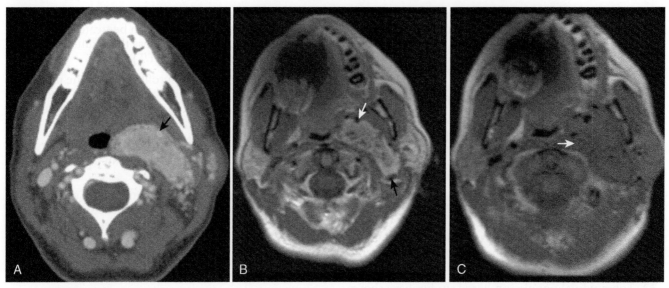

**Figure 11-2** (From Stambuk HE, Patel SG. Imaging of the parapharyngeal space. Otolaryngol Clin North Am 2008;41(1):77–101.)

side. MRI reveals a 5-cm mass at the carotid bifurcation splaying the internal and external carotid arteries.

(b) A 45-year-old man presents with the complaint of a slowly growing pulsatile neck mass in the upper part of the neck on the right side. A contrast-enhanced CT scan of the neck reveals splaying of the external and internal carotid arteries and a metastatic lymph node lateral to the submandibular gland.

(c) A 47-year-old man presents with the complaint of a slowly growing mass in the upper part of the neck on the right side. MRI reveals a 5-cm mass in the parapharyngeal space displacing the carotid artery anteriorly.

(d) A 45-year-old man presents with the complaint of a mass in the upper part of the left side of the neck. T2 MRI reveals a heterogeneous high-signal mass in the left carotid space without flow voids but with postcontrast enhancement.

(e) A 30-year-old woman with a family history of paraganglioma presents with the complaint of a pulsatile mass on the right side of the neck. MRI reveals a 3-cm mass at the carotid bifurcation splaying the internal and external carotid arteries; in addition, a 2-cm mass on the left side of the neck is displacing the carotid artery anteriorly.

53. Observation of paragangliomas and neurogenic tumors may be appropriate in any of the following circumstances:
    i. Newly diagnosed asymptomatic schwannoma.
    ii. Vagal paraganglioma with radiological features of local invasion.
    iii. A 3-cm carotid body tumor in a healthy 45-year-old man.
    iv. A 5-cm vagal paraganglioma that has grown 2 cm since a previous MRI 6 months ago.

v. A newly diagnosed 5-cm carotid body tumor with evidence of cervical lymph node metastasis on MRI.
vi. Newly diagnosed vagal paraganglioma.
A. i, ii, iii, vi
B. i, iii, v, vi
C. i, vi
D. ii, iv, v
E. ii, iii, iv

54. Which of the following are true regarding the role of radiation therapy in the management of paragangliomas and neurogenic tumors?
    i. The goal of radiation therapy is to arrest the growth of the tumor.
    ii. The recommended radiation dose is 45 to 54 Gy.
    iii. The 10-year local progression-free rate is 50%.
    iv. There is no risk of radiation-induced tumors after radiation therapy of paragangliomas and neurogenic tumors in younger patients.
    v. Radiation therapy is a treatment of choice in older patients who have larger tumors and a high risk of multiple cranial neuropathies with a surgical approach.
    vi. The goal of radiation therapy is to shrink the tumor.
A. ii, iii
B. iii, iv, vi
C. i, ii, v
D. iii, iv
E. i, ii, iv, vi

55. Which of the following are true regarding surgical management of paragangliomas and neurogenic tumors?
    i. Surgical resection is a treatment of choice in solitary carotid body tumors.
    ii. Surgical resection is a treatment of choice in asymptomatic vagal paraganglioma.
    iii. Consideration of surgical resection is warranted if malignancy is suspected.

iv. Preoperative embolization is required in all cases of paragangliomas and neurogenic tumors.

v. Infiltration of 1% lidocaine in the sub-adventitial plane of the carotid bulb will reverse the bradycardia and hypotension that frequently results from stimulation of the baroreceptors at the carotid bifurcation.

A. i, iii, v
B. i, ii, v
C. iii, iv, v
D. ii, iii, iv
E. i, iv, v

56. Which of the following are required in the diagnostic workup of paragangliomas?

i. History and physical examination
ii. CT with contrast
iii. MRI
iv. Octreotide scan
v. Genetic testing
vi. Angiography

A. i, iii, iv
B. i, ii, iii
C. i, ii, vi
D. i, ii, v, vi
E. i, iii, vi

57. What are the contents of the carotid space?

i. Carotid artery
ii. Fat
iii. Cranial nerves IX, XI, and XII and the sympathetic chain
iv. Deep lobe of the parotid gland
v. Lymph nodes
vi. Internal jugular vein

A. i, ii, iii, vi
B. i, iii, vi
C. i, iii, v, vi
D. i, iv
E. i, vi

58. Which statements are true regarding histological findings in paragangliomas (Figure 11-3)?

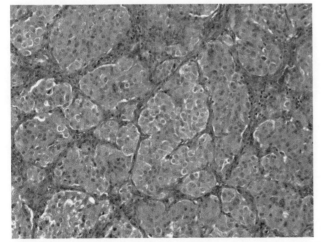

**Figure 11-3** (From Shah JP, Patel SG, Singh B. Jatin Shah's head and neck surgery and oncology. 4th ed. Philadelphia: Mosby; 2012 [Figure 14-10].)

i. A nested (Zellballen) pattern is present.
ii. The hematoxylin and eosin (H&E) section shown in Figure 3-11 is pathognomonic of paragangliomas.
iii. S-100 staining is positive.
iv. Chromogranin staining for the cytoplasm of chief cells reveals neurosecretory granules.
v. Pseudorosettes are present.
vi. Verocay bodies are present.
vii. Palisading nuclei are present.
viii. Antoni A areas are present.
ix. Malignant paragangliomas can be easily differentiated on H&E staining on the basis of aggressive nuclear features.

A. i, ii, iii, iv
B. i, iii, vi, viii
C. i, iii, v
D. i, ii, vii
E. i, ii, iii, iv, ix

59. What are the expected sequelae of surgical resection of the tumor presented in the MRI shown in Figure 11-4?

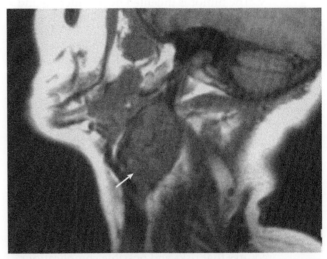

**Figure 11-4** (From Shah JP, Patel SG, Singh B. Jatin Shah's head and neck surgery and oncology. 4th ed. Philadelphia: Mosby; 2012 [Figure 14-46].)

i. Paralysis of the vagus nerve
ii. Hoarseness
iii. Aspiration
iv. Paralysis of the spinal accessory nerve
v. Paralysis of the hypoglossal nerve
vi. Paralysis of the glossopharyngeal nerve
vii. Sacrifice of the internal jugular vein
viii. Sacrifice of the external carotid artery

A. i, ii, iv
B. i, ii, v
C. i, ii, iii
D. vi, vii, viii
E. None of the above

60. The following is true regarding the paraganglioma seen in an axial view of the MRI scan shown in Figure 11-5.

i. This is a Shamblin type I tumor.
ii. This is a Shamblin type II tumor.

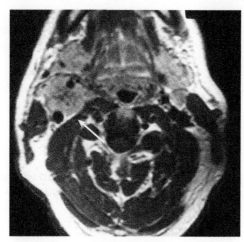

**Figure 11-5** (From Shah JP, Patel SG, Singh B. Jatin Shah's head and neck surgery and oncology, 4th ed. Philadelphia: Mosby; 2012 [Figure 14-27].)

  iii. This is a Shamblin type III tumor.
  iv. Arteries are simply displayed by the tumor and lie on its surface.
   v. The tumor is indented by the internal and external carotid arteries, making a deep groove within the tumor.
  vi. The arteries are encased by the tumor.
  A. i, v
  B. ii, v
  C. iii, vi
  D. i, iv
  E. ii, iv

61. Which of the following is true about observation of a glomus vagale tumor?
  A. It plays no role in the management of glomus vagale.
  B. MRI only needs to be performed twice to get a reliable assessment of the rate of growth of the tumor.
  C. Observation, like surgery or radiation therapy, requires that risks and possible complications be discussed with the patient.
  D. It may be used in older patients with symptomatic glomus vagale tumors.

62. A 25-year-old father of two is given a diagnosis of bilateral small carotid body tumors on MRI. Further evaluation and treatment includes
  A. Immediate bilateral surgical removal of the patient's tumors.
  B. Genetic counseling.
  C. Tissue diagnosis.
  D. Radiation therapy to arrest tumor growth.

63. A 55-year-old man presents with an asymptomatic 3-cm neck mass. This mass enhances intensely on CT and MRI and has flow voids on MRI. In addition, this mass displaces the internal carotid artery anteromedially. The most appropriate next step is
  A. A follow-up MRI in 6 months to establish the rate of tumor growth.
  B. Immediate surgical removal of the patient's tumor.
  C. Radiation therapy to arrest tumor growth.

  D. Genetic testing.
  E. Tissue diagnosis.

64. Paragangliomas often have demonstrable feeder vessels that most commonly arise from the
  A. External carotid artery.
  B. Internal carotid artery.
  C. Ascending pharyngeal artery.
  D. Lingual artery.
  E. Superior thyroid artery.

65. Which of the following statements is true about paraganglioma tumor growth?
  A. Paragangliomas often invade surrounding structures.
  B. Paragangliomas generally grow slowly at the rate of 1 to 2 mm per year.
  C. Nerve palsy is usually caused by tumor invasion.
  D. Paragangliomas frequently erode the skull base.
  E. All of the above are true.

66. Which of the following statements is true regarding the typical presentation of a carotid body tumor?
  A. A carotid body tumor usually presents as a pulsatile neck mass.
  B. A carotid body tumor usually is accompanied by cranial nerve palsies at the time of presentation.
  C. Bilateral tumors are usually sporadic.
  D. Benign and malignant carotid body tumors have a different histological picture.

67. Neurogenic tumors and paragangliomas are most frequently located in this space.
  A. Masticator space
  B. Carotid space
  C. Prevertebral space
  D. Retropharyngeal space

68. The parapharyngeal space is bounded by the following structures, except the
  A. Base of the skull.
  B. Lateral pharyngeal wall.
  C. Masseter muscle.
  D. Pterygoid muscles.
  E. Prevertebral muscles.

69. A 35-year-old man presents with a 6-year history of a slowly enlarging mass in the upper part of the neck. A contrast-enhanced CT scan reveals a tumor splaying the internal and external carotid arteries. In addition, a metastatic lymph node is noted just lateral to the submandibular salivary gland. What is the best next step?
  A. Tissue diagnosis to rule out malignancy
  B. Observation
  C. Radiation therapy
  D. Chemotherapy
  E. Excision of the carotid body tumor
  F. Excision of the carotid body tumor and modified radical neck dissection

70. Which of the following statements about malignant paragangliomas is NOT true?
  A. Malignant paragangliomas exhibit local invasion with development of cranial nerve palsies.
  B. Malignant paragangliomas exhibit invasion of the carotid artery.

C. Malignant paragangliomas have a distinct histological appearance when compared with benign paragangliomas.

D. Malignant paragangliomas exhibit destruction of the skull base and infiltration of soft tissues.

E. Malignant paragangliomas are seen with regional nodal metastasis.

F. Malignant paragangliomas are seen with distant metastasis.

71. The indications for surgical intervention for paragangliomas depend on the following, except the
   A. Symptomatic burden.
   B. Size and location of the lesion.
   C. Rate of tumor growth.
   D. Availability of intensity-modulated radiation therapy (IMRT).
   E. Multiplicity of lesions.
   F. Risk of surgical intervention.

72. A 35-year-old man presents with a 3-cm schwannoma of the cervical plexus. The best next step is
   A. Observation with repeated imaging in 6 months.
   B. Radiation therapy.
   C. Chemotherapy.
   D. Early surgical intervention.

73. If the nerve affected by a schwannoma is functioning preoperatively, which of the following is true about its postoperative function?
   A. Function can be retained if the tumor is carefully enucleated and the surrounding fibers of the nerve are preserved.
   B. Function cannot be retained even if the nerve is carefully enucleated and the surrounding fibers of the nerve are preserved.
   C. The nerve does not retain its function because it needs to be resected so that recurrence is prevented.
   D. The nerve does not retain its function because enucleation with preservation of the surrounding fibers of the nerve is not feasible.

74. Which of the following is NOT an important preoperative consideration in paraganglioma surgery?
   A. Although blood transfusions are seldom required, blood should be available in the event of unexpected hemorrhaging.
   B. For larger lesions in which integrity of the internal carotid artery is at risk, appropriate occlusion studies should be performed to demonstrate satisfactory intracranial crossover circulation.
   C. A vascular surgeon should be available in the event of the need for resection of a segment of internal carotid artery and its reconstruction.
   D. Preoperative angiographic studies demonstrating feeding vessels and preoperative embolization are necessary in all cases.

75. Functional loss due to the excision of a hypoglossal nerve schwannoma results in
   A. Paralysis of the ipsilateral half of the tongue.
   B. Paralysis of the contralateral half of the tongue.
   C. No paralysis.
   D. Paralysis of the ipsilateral half of the tongue, dysphagia, and hoarseness of the voice.

76. Functional loss due to the excision of a sympathetic chain schwannoma results in
   A. No sequelae.
   B. Horner syndrome.
   C. Dysphagia.
   D. Hoarseness of the voice.
   E. B, C, and D.

77. The diagnosis of paraganglioma is generally established by
   A. Fine-needle aspiration.
   B. A combination of CT and MRI.
   C. Angiography.
   D. Histological examination of the surgical specimen.

78. A 65-year-old man with a past medical history significant for atrial fibrillation, currently taking anticoagulants, is seen for a 6-month follow-up of his 5-cm glomus vagale tumor. Since his previous visit, he developed hoarseness in his voice, and a fiberoptic examination confirmed ipsilateral true vocal cord paralysis. The tumor had grown 0.5 cm since the previous examination. The most reasonable next step is
   A. Surgical resection, despite the patient being a high-risk surgical candidate.
   B. Radiation therapy to achieve tumor regression.
   C. Radiation therapy to arrest tumor growth.
   D. Chemotherapy.
   E. Continued observation.

79. A 65-year-old man with a past medical history significant for atrial fibrillation, currently taking anticoagulants, is seen for a 6-month follow-up of his 5-cm glomus vagale tumor. Since his previous visit, he remains asymptomatic, and the tumor had grown 0.2 cm since the previous examination. The most reasonable next step is
   A. Surgical resection, despite the patient being a high-risk surgical candidate.
   B. Radiation therapy to achieve tumor regression.
   C. Radiation therapy to arrest tumor growth.
   D. Chemotherapy.
   E. Continued observation.

80. Radiation therapy for paragangliomas is not recommended in younger patients
   A. Because paragangliomas are generally small and easily resectable in this patient population.
   B. Because recent studies have demonstrated an absence of response of paragangliomas to radiation therapy in this patient population as compared with older patients.
   C. Because of the risk of a radiation-induced second malignancy.
   D. Because paragangliomas generally respond to somatostatin analogue inhibitors in this patient population.

81. The contents of the carotid sheath include all of the following, except the
   A. Carotid artery.
   B. Vagus nerve.
   C. Internal jugular vein.
   D. Sympathetic chain.

82. Important considerations in preoperative preparation of the patient with a malignant carotid body tumor include all of the following, except
    A. Angiography with carotid artery occlusion.
    B. Informing the patient of the potential risks of cerebrovascular injury, stroke, and death.
    C. Requesting vascular surgery assistance.
    D. Appropriately designing the surgical incision to achieve the best cosmetic outcome.

83. Which of the following is NOT true regarding facial nerve schwannomas?
    A. Facial nerve schwannomas are rare.
    B. The surgical approach to a facial nerve schwannoma is achieved via a modified Blair incision.
    C. Facial nerve function can be preserved if the tumor is carefully enucleated and the surrounding fibers of the nerve are preserved.
    D. Extension of the tumor through the stylomastoid foramen may require a mastoidectomy to accomplish removal of the tumor.

84. Functional loss due to the excision of a glomus vagale tumor results in
    A. No sequelae.
    B. Hoarseness of voice due to true vocal cord paralysis.
    C. Aspiration due to loss of sensation in the supraglottic larynx.
    D. B and C.

85. Functional loss due to excision of a carotid body tumor results in
    A. No sequelae.
    B. Hoarseness of voice due to true vocal cord paralysis.
    C. Aspiration due to loss of sensation in the supraglottic larynx.
    D. B and C.
    E. Ipsilateral deviation of the tongue.
    F. Horner syndrome.

86. The surgical approach to schwannomas of the trigeminal nerve without intracranial extension requires
    A. A maxillary swing approach.
    B. A mandibulotomy approach.
    C. A craniotomy.
    D. A and C.
    E. B and C.

87. The surgical approach to schwannomas of the trigeminal nerve with extension through the foramen ovale in the floor of the middle cranial fossa requires
    A. A maxillary swing approach.
    B. A mandibulotomy approach.
    C. A craniotomy.
    D. A and C.
    E. B and C.

88. The prestyloid and poststyloid (carotid) compartments are divided by the
    A. Fascia between the styloid process and the tensor veli palatini.
    B. Lateral pterygoid.
    C. Medial pterygoid.
    D. Retromandibular vein.

89. The prestyloid compartment includes all of the following, except
    A. The maxillary artery.
    B. The inferior alveolar nerve.
    C. The lingual nerve.
    D. The deep lobe of the parotid.
    E. The vagus nerve.
    F. Fat.

90. A 45-year old man presents with a 4-cm upper neck mass consistent with schwannoma of the hypoglossal nerve. During the course of a 6-month initial observation period, the tumor grew in size by 2 cm. In addition, fasciculations of the ipsilateral tongue could be noted on the physical examination. The most appropriate next step is
    A. Surgical resection.
    B. Radiation therapy.
    C. Continued observation.
    D. Chemotherapy.

91. Which of the following statements regarding radiation therapy is NOT true?
    A. Removal of neurogenic tumors and paragangliomas after radiation therapy may be more difficult.
    B. Transient cranial nerve palsies after radiation therapy have been reported.
    C. The risk of permanent neuropathy after radiation therapy is high.
    D. The typical radiation dose is 45 to 54 Gy.

92. Head and neck paragangliomas are more prevalent among carriers of which of the following mutations?
    A. *SDHD*
    B. *SDHB*
    C. *SDHC*
    D. *SDHA*
    E. A and B

93. Intraabdominal and extraadrenal tumors are more frequent among the carriers of which of the following mutations?
    A. *SDHD*
    B. *SDHB*
    C. *SDHC*
    D. *SDHA*
    E. A and B

94. Which of the following is true regarding *SDHD* and *SDHB* mutation carriers?
    A. *SDHB* mutation carriers generally develop tumors at a relatively young age, whereas *SDHD* mutation carriers generally develop tumors at a relatively older age.
    B. *SDHB* mutation carriers generally are seen with multiple tumors, whereas malignant tumors are more prevalent in *SDHD* mutation carriers.

C. *SDHD* mutation carriers generally are seen with multiple tumors, whereas malignant tumors are more prevalent in *SDHB* mutation carriers.

D. Patients with head and neck paragangliomas should be targeted for *SDHB* mutation testing, whereas the patients with extraadrenal abdominal presentations should be targeted for *SDHD* mutation testing.

95. The differential diagnosis of a 3-cm mass on the right side of the neck located in the carotid space should include all of the following, except a
    A. Glomus vagale tumor.
    B. Carotid body tumor.
    C. Schwannoma of the vagus nerve.
    D. Pleomorphic adenoma of the deep lobe of the parotid gland.

96. Which of the following is NOT true regarding the first bite syndrome?
    A. First bite syndrome is a painful complication of upper neck surgery.
    B. First bite syndrome develops because of sympathetic denervation with parasympathetic hyperactivity.
    C. This unusual pain syndrome should be recognized promptly by the head and neck surgeon because it may have a significant impact on the patient's quality of life.
    D. Botulinum toxin injection into the parotid gland is a standard of care for the management of the first bite syndrome.

97. First bite syndrome is
    A. Excruciating pain triggered at the beginning of a meal by chewing or swallowing, waning on subsequent bites and recurring with identical features after pausing for several minutes or at the next meal.
    B. Dull pain persisting throughout meal intake.
    C. Excruciating pain associated with meal intake.
    D. Dull pain triggered at the beginning of a meal by chewing or swallowing, waning on subsequent bites and recurring with identical features after pausing for several minutes or at the next meal.

98. A 55-year-old man presents with an 8-cm neck mass. This mass enhances intensely on CT and MRI and has flow voids on MRI. CT imaging demonstrates significant skull base involvement. In addition, this mass displaces the internal carotid artery anteromedially. The most likely diagnosis is a
    A. Schwannoma of the sympathetic trunk.
    B. Glomus vagale tumor.
    C. Glomus tympanicum.
    D. Carotid body tumor.
    E. Schwannoma of the vagus nerve.

99. In the previous case scenario, the most appropriate next step is
    A. Follow-up MRI in 6 months to establish the rate of tumor growth.

B. Immediate surgical removal of the patent's tumor.
C. Radiation therapy to arrest tumor growth.
D. Radiation therapy to achieve complete tumor regression.
E. Genetic testing.
F. Tissue diagnosis.

100. Which of the following is NOT true regarding the surgical technique of carotid body tumor resection?
    A. The operative procedure can be performed under local anesthesia.
    B. Tumor dissection should be performed in the subadventitial plane.
    C. Level II lymph nodes should be excised to provide adequate exposure.
    D. Vagus and hypoglossal nerves need to be carefully identified.

## Answers

| | | |
|---|---|---|
| 1. T | 28. T | 54. C |
| 2. T | 29. T | 55. A |
| 3. F | 30. F | 56. B |
| 4. F | 31. T | 57. B |
| 5. T | 32. T | 58. A |
| 6. T | 33. T | 59. C |
| 7. F | 34. F | 60. B |
| 8. F | 35. T | 61. C |
| 9. T | 36. F | 62. B |
| 10. F | 37. T | 63. A |
| 11. F | 38. F | 64. C |
| 12. F | 39. T | 65. B |
| 13. T | 40. F | 66. A |
| 14. T | 41. T | 67. B |
| 15. F | 42. F | 68. C |
| 16. T | 43. T | 69. F |
| 17. F | 44. F | 70. C |
| 18. F | 45. T | 71. D |
| 19. F | 46. T | 72. D |
| 20. T | 47. F | 73. B |
| 21. F | 48. T | 74. D |
| 22. T | 49. F | 75. A |
| 23. F | 50. T | 76. B |
| 24. T | 51. C | 77. B |
| 25. F | 52. (a) i (b) vi (c) ii (d) iii (e) viii | 78. C |
| 26. F | | 79. E |
| 27. T | 53. C | 80. C |

| | | |
|---|---|---|
| 81. D | 88. A | 95. D |
| 82. D | 89. E | 96. D |
| 83. C | 90. A | 97. A |
| 84. D | 91. C | 98. B |
| 85. A | 92. A | 99. C |
| 86. A | 93. B | 100. A |
| 87. D | 94. C | |

## Core Knowledge

- Neurogenic tumors and paragangliomas form a very small percentage of neoplastic lesions of the head and neck region.

- These tumors are located in the parapharyngeal space (PPS), which is a potential space in the shape of an inverted cone whose base is at the base of skull and whose apex is at the level of the tip of the hyoid bone. The lateral pharyngeal wall and tonsillar fossa form its medial wall, and the pterygoid muscles, parotid muscles, parotid gland, and prevertebral muscles form its lateral boundary.

- The PPS is divided into two components separated by the styloid process and its attached muscles. The space anterior to the styloid process is called the *true PPS*. The parapharyngeal region posteromedial to the styloid process is called the *carotid space*. The most common neoplasms in this space are paragangliomas and neurogenic tumors arising from the lower cranial nerves.

### NEUROGENIC TUMORS

- The head and neck region is the most common location for benign peripheral nerve tumors. Neurogenic tumors of the medial compartment arise from the lower cranial nerves or the sympathetic chain, and lateral compartment tumors arise from the cutaneous or muscular branches of the cervical or the brachial plexus.

- Schwannomas originate from the neuroectodermal sheath surrounding peripheral nerves. Schwannomas are usually solitary neoplasms. Multifocal presentation should raise the suspicion for neurofibromatosis type 2 (resulting from mutations in the *NF2* suppressor gene) or nonfamilial schwannomas (resulting from somatic alteration of the *NF2* gene).

- Schwannomas are slowly growing tumors that can lead to a variety of symptoms and signs, depending on their nerve of origin and location.

- Neurofibromas are benign, unencapsulated tumors that may be localized, diffuse, or plexiform. They may be familial or sporadic.

- Plexiform neurofibromas are pathognomonic of familial neurofibromatosis (NF1).

- Malignant peripheral nerve sheath tumors (MPNST) originate from Schwann or perineurial cells and arise either de novo or from preexisting neurofibromas. The local recurrence rate is high. Distant metastases occur to the lung, bone, and liver.

- Schwannomas and neurofibromas are usually mobile in the axis perpendicular to the long axis of the nerve involved and do not involve the mobility along the long axis.

- On imaging, schwannomas are seen as well-encapsulated tumors with or without cystic degeneration and/or hemorrhage. Schwannomas are isointense on T1 magnetic resonance imaging (MRI), hyperintense on T2 MRI, and enhance with contrast.

### PARAGANGLIOMAS

- Paragangliomas arise from extraadrenal paraganglionic cells derived from the neural crest.

- Paragangliomas of the head and neck can arise in the jugulotympanic region, vagal body, carotid body, superior and inferior laryngeal paraganglionic tissue, nasal cavity, or the orbit.

- Paragangliomas are usually benign and grow slowly, causing symptoms by compressing adjacent structures.

- The rule of 10 is as follows: 10% of paragangliomas are multiple or bilateral, 10% are malignant, and 10% are familial.

- Carotid body tumors are the most common paragangliomas of the head and neck. Carotid body tumors arise from the chemoreceptors in the carotid sheath, located at the bifurcation of the carotid artery.

- Shamblin classified carotid body tumors into three categories based on the difficulty of resection. In type I tumors, the arteries are displaced by the tumor and lie on its surface. In type II, the tumor is indented by the internal and external carotid arteries, making a deep groove within the tumor; the hypoglossal and superior laryngeal nerves are on the tumor's surface. In type III, the arteries and the nerves are encased by the tumor (Figure 11-6).

- On histological examination, paragangliomas have a characteristic nested (Zellballen) pattern surrounded by spindled sustentacular cells (see Figure 11-3). Immunohistochemical analysis usually shows positivity for S-100 and chromogranin.

- Benign and malignant paragangliomas have a similar histological appearance. The diagnosis of a malignant paraganglioma is made on the basis of one of the following features: local invasion with development of cranial nerve paralysis, invasion of the carotid artery, destruction of the skull base or infiltration of the soft tissues, the presence of regional node metastasis, or distant metastasis.

- Three known genes associated with paragangliomas are succinate dehydrogenase (SDH) subunit D (*SDHD*), subunit B (*SDHB*), and subunit C (*SDHC*).

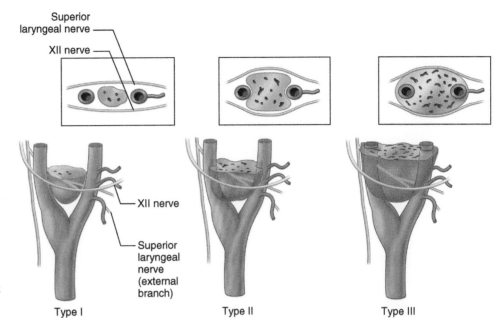

Superior
laryngeal nerve

XII nerve

XII nerve

Superior
laryngeal
nerve
(external
branch)

Type I          Type II          Type III

**Figure 11-6** (From Shah JP, Patel SG, Singh B. Jatin Shah's head and neck surgery and oncology. 4th ed. Philadelphia: Mosby; 2012 [Figure 14-9].)

*SDHB* and *SDHC* are inherited as autosomal dominant traits. *SDHD* is inherited as an autosomal dominant trait with maternal imprinting. Genetic testing is recommended for patients seen with multiple paragangliomas and a suggestive family history.

- Paragangliomas usually are seen with pulsatile neck masses.

- A computed tomographic (CT) scan with contrast provides an accurate diagnosis of paraganglioma by revealing hypervascular masses with avid contrast enhancement and splaying internal and external carotid arteries at the bifurcation.

- T2-weighted MRI of a paraganglioma typically demonstrates internal flow voids.

- An MRI angiogram is a noninvasive test that demonstrates both the characteristic lyre sign of carotid body tumors that appear to bow and displacement of the internal and external carotid arteries.

- The high density of somatostatin receptor provides the basis for octreotide scanning, recommended as a possible screening test for familial paragangliomas for patients at risk and for the purpose of detection of additional tumors when malignant paraganglioma is suspected.

## TREATMENT

- The indications for surgical intervention depend on the symptomatic burden, size and location of the lesion, and multiplicity of the lesions, weighted against the risk of surgical intervention.

- Close observation with serial imaging is recommended as an initial management strategy for paragangliomas and schwannomas.

- Surgery of carotid body tumors generally does not cause cranial nerve injury; therefore most patients with tumors as large as 6 to 7 cm without extension to the skull base should be treated surgically.

- Surgery for paragangliomas arising from the cranial nerves inflicts considerable morbidity. Given that paragangliomas grow very slowly (approximately 1 mm per year), the surgical intervention may be associated with more significant functional deficits than would be encountered with natural progression of the disease. Indications for surgery include malignancy, rapid tumor growth, local pressure effects, and the severity of symptoms.

- Radiation therapy has recently emerged as an effective treatment modality for controlling tumor growth. The short-term and late morbidity after moderate-dose intensity-modulated radiation therapy or stereotactic radiation therapy is low. As reported by Stambuk and Patel (2008), less than 10% of benign paragangliomas progress locally after radiation therapy.

## SUGGESTED READING

Everson LJ, Mendenhall WM, Parsons JT, Cassisi NJ. Radiotherapy in the management of chemodectomas of the carotid body and glomus vagale. Head Neck 1998;20:609–13.

Jansen JC, van den Berg R, Kuiper A, van der Mey AG, Zwinderman AH, Cornelisse CJ. Estimation of growth rate in patients with head and neck paraganglioma influences the treatment proposal. Cancer 2000;88:2811–6.

Krych AJ, Foote RL, Brown PD, Garces YI, Link MJ. Long-term results of irradiation for paraganglioma. Int J Radiat Oncol Biol Phys 2006;65:1063–6.

Mendenhall WM, Amdur RJ, Vaysberg M, Mendenhall CM, Werning JW. Head and neck paragangliomas. Head Neck 2011;33(10):1530–4.

Moukarbel RV, Sabri AN. Current management of head and neck schwannomas. Curr Opin Otolaryngol Head Neck Surg 2005;13(2):117–22.

Newmann HP, Erlic Z, Boedeker CC, Rybicki LA, Robledo M, et al. Clinical predictors for germline mutations in head and neck paraganglioma patients: cost reduction strategy in genetic diagnosis fall-out. Cancer Res 2009;69:3650–6.

Newmann HP, Pawlu C, Pecskowska M, Bausch B, McWhinney SR, et al. Distinct clinical features of paraganglioma syndromes associated with SDHB and SDHD gene mutations. JAMA 2004;292:943–51.

Shamblin WR, ReMine WH, Sheps SG, Harrison Jr EG. Carotid body tumor (chemodectoma). Clinicopathologic analysis of ninety cases. Am J Surg 1971;122:732–9.

Stambuk HE, Patel SG. Imaging of parapharyngeal space. Otolaryngol Clin North Am 2008;41:77–101.

van der Mey AG, Frijns JH, Cornelisse CJ, Brons EN, van Dulken H, Terpstra HL, et al. Does intervention improve the natural course of glomus tumors? A series of 108 patients seen in 32 year period. Ann Otol Rhinol Laryngol 1992;101:635–42.

# 12 Soft Tissue Tumors

## Questions

**TRUE/FALSE**

1. The *PAX3/FOXO1* fusion gene of chromosomes 2 and 13 is only seen in alveolar rhabdomyosarcomas (RMSs). (T/F)

2. Alveolar RMSs are more commonly seen in 3- to 10-year-old patients. (T/F)

3. The Intergroup Rhabdomyosarcoma Study-IV (IRS-IV) staging system is based on tumor size, invasiveness, nodal status, and the site of the primary tumor. (T/F)

4. RMSs are the most common soft tissue sarcoma in pediatric patients. (T/F)

5. Infants' and adolescents' poor outcomes are related to the higher frequency of undifferentiated or alveolar histiotypes of RMS. (T/F)

6. Schwannomas are hypointense on T1-weighted images and isointense on T2-weighted images (Figure 12-1). (T/F)

7. Schwannomas are hyperintense on T2-weighted images and have marked enhancement of the cystic component of the tumor after gadolinium administration. (T/F)

8. Malignant transformation of schwannomas is a controversial issue and is seldom thought to occur, if at all. (T/F)

9. Surgical excision is the treatment of choice for schwannomas; however, the recurrence rate is 15%. (T/F)

10. Approximately 25% to 45% of all extracranial schwannomas occur in the head and neck (Figure 12-2). (T/F)

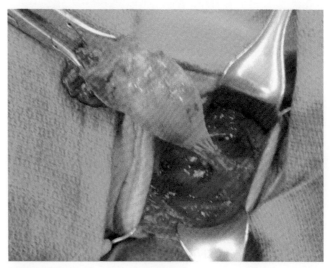

**Figure 12-2** (Courtesy of Memorial Sloan Kettering Cancer Center, New York.)

11. Malignant peripheral nerve sheath tumors are low to intermediate grade. (T/F)

12. The name *malignant peripheral nerve sheath tumor* was adopted by the World Health Organization (WHO) to unify the previously designated entities of malignant schwannoma, neurogenic sarcoma, and neurogenic fibrosarcoma. (T/F)

13. Malignant peripheral nerve sheath tumors have an increased incidence in neurofibromatosis type 1 (NF1). (T/F)

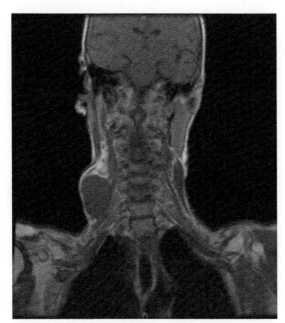

**Figure 12-1** (Courtesy of Memorial Sloan Kettering Cancer Center, New York.)

14. A malignant peripheral nerve sheath tumor is a large, fusiform, irregular, invasive tumor with areas of necrosis and hemorrhaging. (T/F)

15. Malignant peripheral nerve sheath tumors constitute 5% to 10% of all soft tissue sarcomas. (T/F)

16. The noncontrast computed tomographic (CT) scan in Figure 12-3 shows the classic "sunburst" appearance of malignant osteoid formation. (T/F)

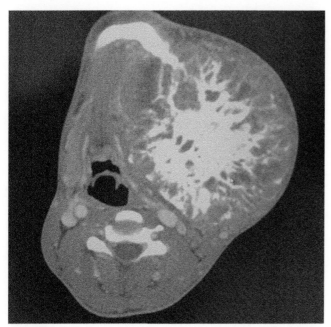

**Figure 12-3** (Courtesy of Memorial Sloan Kettering Cancer Center, New York.)

17. Silent pulmonary micrometastases are present in at least 80% of patients with extremity osteosarcomas at the time of diagnosis. (T/F)

18. Predisposition to osteosarcoma is related to overexpression of chromosomal region 13q14. (T/F)

19. With osteosarcoma, a positive margin carries with it a significant decrease in the survival rate from 75% to 35%. (T/F)

20. Osteosarcomas do not metastasize to the cervical lymph nodes. (T/F)

21. No treatment consensus exists for angiosarcoma; only scattered phase II and no phase III trials are reported in the literature. (T/F)

22. Approximately 10% of patients with angiosarcomas have distant metastases on presentation. (T/F)

23. With angiosarcomas, negative margins correlate with an improved survival rate. (T/F)

24. Angiosarcomas are insensitive to radiation therapy. (T/F)

25. Angiosarcomas respond to taxane chemotherapy. (T/F)

26. IRS-IV emphasized that therapy for children with RMS should be risk directed and based primarily on tumor site, histological type, and extent of the disease. (T/F)

27. Patients younger than 10 years with metastatic embryonal RMS are included within the intermediate-risk category. (T/F)

28. Outcomes in adults with RMS have improved; the 5-year survival rate is approximately 60%. (T/F)

29. Embryonal cell RMSs are low grade. (T/F)

30. Positivity of the *PAX3/FOXO1* fusion gene has a negative impact on failure-free survival rates. (T/F)

31. Chondrosarcomas are predominantly low-grade sarcomas. (T/F)

32. Immunohistochemical and cytogenetic studies have identified similarities in Ewing sarcoma. (T/F)

33. Chondrosarcomas are insensitive to radiation therapy. (T/F)

34. A number of chondrosarcoma subtypes exist, including mesenchymal, myxoid, small cell, and clear cell. (T/F)

35. Myxoid and small cell chondrosarcoma subtypes constitute a substantial portion of head and neck cases. (T/F)

36. Liposarcomas metastasize to cervical lymph nodes. (T/F)

37. A number of liposarcoma subtypes exist and include well-differentiated, round cell, myxoid, and pleomorphic tumors. (T/F)

38. Pleomorphic and round cell liposarcomas are high-grade tumors. (T/F)

39. Liposarcoma round cell tumors have the worst survival outcome. (T/F)

40. Adjuvant radiation therapy is only used for liposarcomas that are large or that have a high grade or positive margins. (T/F)

41. Malignant fibrous histiocytomas (MFHs) constitute as many as 40% of all head and neck sarcomas. (T/F)

42. MFHs are all high-grade tumors. (T/F)

43. MFHs have a strong association with NF2. (T/F)

44. Radiation-induced MFHs account for almost 50% of radiation-associated soft tissue sarcomas. (T/F)

45. The classic behavior of MFH is to recur in distant sites. (T/F)

46. Madelung disease is a benign collection of lipomas. (T/F)

47. In Madelung disease, fatty collections are enclosed within a membranous capsule. (T/F)

48. In Madelung disease, fatty collections are highly vascular. (T/F)

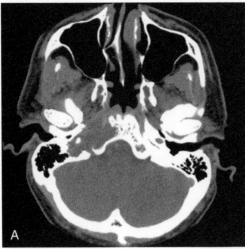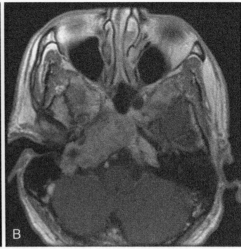

**Figure 12-4** (Courtesy of Memorial Sloan Kettering Cancer Center, New York.)

49. Madelung disease is radiosensitive. (T/F)

50. Type 2 Madelung disease is associated with fat deposition within the head and neck. (T/F)

## MULTIPLE CHOICE

51. Which of the following pathological types are included within the differential for the CT and T1 postcontrast magnetic resonance imaging (MRI) scans in Figure 12-4?
    i. Chondrosarcoma
    ii. Schwannoma
    iii. Lipoma
    iv. Cholesteatoma
    v. Branchial cleft cyst
    vi. Chordoma
    A. ii, iii, vi
    B. i, iv, vi
    C. i, iv
    D. iv, vi
    E. i, vi
    F. ii, iii, v

52. Which of the following pathological types commonly metastasize to cervical lymph nodes?
    i. Liposarcoma
    ii. Synovial sarcoma
    iii. Clear cell sarcomas
    iv. Osteosarcomas
    v. Angiosarcomas
    vi. RMSs
    vii. Epithelioid sarcomas
    viii. Fibrosarcomas
    A. ii, iii, v, vi
    B. ii, iii, v, vi, vii
    C. i, iii, v, vi, vii
    D. i, iv, v, vi, viii
    E. ii, iv, v, vi

53. What are the most common five sarcomas in the adult head and neck?
    i. Liposarcoma
    ii. Osteosarcoma

iii. Epithelioid
iv. Chondrosarcoma
v. Angiosarcoma
vi. Clear cell
vii. Synovial
viii. MFH
ix. Fibrosarcoma
A. ii, v, vi, viii, ix
B. i, ii, iv, viii, ix
C. ii, iii, iv, viii, ix
D. i, ii, v, vii, viii
E. i, ii, v, viii, ix

54. What are the key sarcoma prognostic indicators?
    i. Neoadjuvant chemotherapy
    ii. Size greater than 5 cm
    iii. Age older than 45 years
    iv. Positive margins
    v. Lymph node metastases
    vi. Female sex
    vii. Anatomical location
    viii. High grade
    ix. Hyperfractionated adjuvant radiation therapy
    A. iii, iv, v
    B. ii, iv, vii
    C. ii, iv, viii
    D. iii, iv, vi
    E. i, ii, v, ix

55. Which of the following are common sites of sarcoma metastases?
    i. Spleen
    ii. Lungs
    iii. Peritoneum
    iv. Thyroid
    v. Bone
    vi. Central nervous system
    vii. Maxilla
    viii. Liver
    ix. Bladder
    A. ii, v, vi, viii
    B. ii, iii, v, vi
    C. v, vi, vii, ix

D. i, ii, v, viii
E. ii, iii, iv, viii

56. From the following options, choose the single most likely diagnosis for each of the scenarios given. Each option may be used once, more than once, or not at all.
    i. Chondrosarcoma
    ii. Esthesioneuroblastoma
    iii. Osteosarcoma
    iv. RMS
    v. Nephroblastoma
    vi. Teratoma
    vii. Schwannoma
    viii. Lipoma
 (a). A 19-year-old pregnant woman reaches 38 weeks' gestation and is due to deliver. Ultrasonography of the baby shows a large complex mass of the neck with secondary tracheal compression.
 (b). A 56-year-old woman has a T1-weighted MRI. The report states that a homogenously enhancing tumor with intermediate signal intensity was identified. Angiography identified "tumor blush."
 (c). A 44-year-old woman presents with a tumor histologically similar to adrenal, sympathetic ganglionic neuroblastomas and retinoblastomas.
 (d). A 65-year-old man with a lateral neck mass had a T2-weighted MR image demonstrating a mildly heterogeneous lesion with a signal intensity greater than that of fat.
 (e). On immunohistochemical evaluation, positive staining of neoplastic cells with antibodies against desmin was noted.

57. Which of the following statements regarding RMS are correct?
    i. According to the Surveillance, Epidemiology, and End Results program, between 1973 and 2007 the incidence of RMS of the head and neck has increased significantly with an annual percentage change of 5.16%.
    ii. Survival rates for RMS in the pediatric age group have dramatically improved from 25% in the early 1970s to 71% by 2001.
    iii. The two main entities, embryonal and alveolar, are pathologically distinct.
    iv. Success in pediatric management has been largely credited to intensity-modulated radiation therapy (IMRT).
    v. The many drugs that have been used include vincristine, dactinomycin, doxorubicin, cisplatin, ifosfamide, and 5-fluorouracil.
 A. i, iii
 B. i, ii
 C. iii, iv
 D. iii, v
 E. ii, iii

58. Which of the following statements regarding lymphatic malformations are correct?

i. They occur in 1 in 10,000 live births.
ii. The operative approach must include all of the lymphatic malformation in a monobloc fashion.
iii. OK-432 (Picibanil) is Group A *Staphylococcus pyogenes*.
iv. OK-432 (Picibanil) is Group A *Streptococcus pyogenes*.
v. Approximately 75% of all lymphatic malformations occur in the head and neck region.
 A. i, iv
 B. ii, iii
 C. iv, v
 D. ii, iv
 E. i, iii

59. From the following options, choose the single most likely diagnosis for each of the scenarios given. Each option may be used once, more than once, or not at all.
    i. Stage I
    ii. Stage II
    iii. Stage III
    iv. Stage IV
    v. Stage V
 (a) Bilateral infrahyoid lymphatic malformation
 (b) Unilateral suprahyoid
 (c) Bilateral infrahyoid and suprahyoid
 (d) Unilateral infrahyoid
 (e) Unilateral infrahyoid and suprahyoid

60. Which of the following statements regarding osteosarcoma are true?
    i. Conventional osteosarcoma can be categorized into osteoblastic, chondroblastic, and fibroblastic subtypes.
    ii. Li-Fraumeni syndrome due to germline *TP53* mutations predisposes to osteosarcoma as does Rothmund-Thomson syndrome.
    iii. Head and neck osteosarcoma has a reduced likelihood of distant metastases compared with extremity osteosarcoma.
    iv. The most common sites of metastases are the brain and the lungs.
    v. A threefold improvement in the disease-free survival rate was realized in the 1980s with the introduction of neoadjuvant chemotherapy in the treatment of extremity osteosarcoma in the pediatric population.
 A. i, ii, iii
 B. i, iii, iv, v
 C. i, iii, iv
 D. i, ii, iii, iv, v
 E. ii, iii, iv, v

61. Lipoblastomas are best described as
 A. Rare malignant tumors of brown fat.
 B. Rare benign tumors of embryonic brown fat.
 C. Rare benign tumors of embryonic white fat.
 D. Rare malignant tumors of embryonic brown fat.

62. Lipoblastomas are best treated with
    A. IMRT alone.
    B. Complete surgical excision alone.
    C. Induction chemotherapy followed by complete surgical excision.
    D. Complete surgical excision and adjuvant radiation therapy.

63. Lipoblastomas commonly present in which age group category?
    A. 0 to 20 years
    B. 21 to 40 years
    C. 41 to 60 years
    D. 61 to 80 years

64. Which of the following statements about lipomas of the neck is correct?
    A. Lipomas of the neck usually present in the posterior triangle.
    B. The anatomical presentation of lipomas of the neck is between the superficial and middle layers of the deep cervical fascia.
    C. Lipomas of the neck can arise in any part of the head and neck region.
    D. The anatomical presentation of lipomas of the neck is between the middle and deep layers of the deep cervical fascia.

65. Which statement about surgical excision of lipomas is correct?
    A. Surgery should be performed in a compartmental piecemeal approach.
    B. Surgery should be performed in a meticulous monobloc fashion.
    C. Lipomas have low recurrence rates regardless of the surgical strategy.
    D. Lipomas rarely have vascular feeding vessels.

66. Low-grade liposarcomas
    A. Often require only surgical excision.
    B. Always require surgical excision and adjuvant radiation therapy.
    C. Can be treated with radiation therapy alone.
    D. Can be treated with concurrent chemoradiation therapy.

67. Which statement about high-grade sarcomas is most accurate?
    A. In general, high-grade sarcomas and other sarcomas exceeding 4 to 5 cm require adjunctive postoperative radiation therapy.
    B. All high-grade sarcomas require adjunctive concurrent chemoradiation therapy.
    C. All high-grade sarcomas require postoperative radiation therapy to improve the overall survival rate.
    D. All high-grade sarcomas require postoperative radiation therapy to reduce distant metastases.

68. Dermatofibrosarcoma protuberans
    A. Is a tumor of the thyroid cartilage.
    B. Is a tumor of the larynx.
    C. Is a tumor of the salivary glands.
    D. Is a tumor of the skin.

69. Dermatofibrosarcoma protuberans
    A. Is predominantly a high-grade sarcoma.
    B. Is predominantly an intermediate-grade sarcoma.
    C. Is predominantly a low-grade sarcoma.
    D. Is predominantly a mixed-grade sarcoma.

70. Risk factors for dermatofibrosarcoma protuberans include
    A. Heredity.
    B. A scar that develops after a burn or surgery.
    C. Smoking.
    D. Chronic sialadenitis.

71. A ranula is a
    A. Lipoma.
    B. Mucocele.
    C. Granuloma.
    D. Minor salivary gland.

72. Ranula formation is thought to be due to a blockage in the
    A. Submaxillary gland.
    B. Minor salivary gland of the floor of the mouth.
    C. Sublingual gland.
    D. Floor of the mouth lymphatics.

73. A plunging ranula
    A. Involves the oral cavity and oropharynx.
    B. Involves the oral cavity and buccal space.
    C. Involves the oral cavity and the neck.
    D. Involves the oral cavity and the masticator space.

74. Which surgical strategy for a plunging ranula is associated with the lowest recurrence rates?
    A. Marsupialization with placement of a silk suture
    B. Excision of the ranula and ipsilateral sublingual gland
    C. Marsupialization with a $CO_2$ laser
    D. Excision of the ranula and ipsilateral submandibular gland

75. In lymphatic malformations, the sclerosing agent OK-432 is a
    A. Lyophilized incubation mixture of group A *Streptococcus pyogenes* of human origin.
    B. Lyophilized incubation mixture of group B *Streptococcus pyogenes* of human origin.
    C. Lyophilized incubation mixture of group C *Streptococcus pyogenes* of human origin.
    D. Lyophilized incubation mixture of group D *Streptococcus pyogenes* of human origin.

76. In lymphatic malformations, the sclerosing agent OK-432 is effective for
    A. Microcystic lymphatic malformations.
    B. Mixed lymphatic malformations.
    C. Lymphatic malformations outside of the head and neck.
    D. Macrocystic lymphatic malformations.

77. Liposarcoma
    A. Is the most common of the soft tissue sarcomas.
    B. Is the rarest of the soft tissue sarcomas.

C. Most commonly presents within the head and
   neck region.
D. More commonly presents in female patients.

78. The WHO describes what three forms of
    liposarcoma?
    A. Atypical lipomatous/well-differentiated
       myxoid/round cell and pleomorphic
    B. Well-differentiated/medullary/anaplastic
    C. Atypical lipomatous tumor/well-differentiated
       myxoid/round cell and anaplastic
    D. Well-differentiated/round cell/adenoid

79. The most common subtype of liposarcoma is
    A. Anaplastic.
    B. Myxoid/round cell.
    C. Atypical lipomatous/well-differentiated.
    D. Medullary.

80. Metastases are most commonly seen in which
    subtypes?
    A. Atypical lipomatous/well-differentiated
    B. Myxoid and pleomorphic
    C. Medullary
    D. Adenoid

81. What organ is the most common site of metastases
    in liposarcoma?
    A. Bone
    B. Liver
    C. Brain
    D. Lung

82. MFHs
    A. Are undifferentiated high-grade pleomorphic
       sarcomas.
    B. Are predominantly low-grade sarcomas of the
       extremities.
    C. Are predominantly pediatric high-grade sarcomas.
    D. Rarely metastasize.

83. Immunohistochemical analysis identifies
    A. Vimentin-positive cells.
    B. S-100 negative cells.
    C. Ki-67 positive cells.
    D. All of the above.

84. Risk factors for MFHs include
    A. Smoking.
    B. Female sex.
    C. Ionizing radiation.
    D. Graves' disease.

85. Dendritic cell sarcoma
    A. Is a high-grade sarcoma of the parotid.
    B. Has similarities in presentation and
       immunohistochemical markers to lymphoma.
    C. Rarely metastasizes.
    D. Is associated with human papillomavirus
       (HPV) type 16 oropharyngeal infection.

86. A cavernous hemangioma
    A. Is also known as a strawberry nevus and
       regresses with time.
    B. Fails to regress with time.
    C. May be treated with OK-432.
    D. May dedifferentiate to hemangiopericytoma.

87. A capillary hemangioma
    A. Is also known as a strawberry nevus and
       regresses with time.
    B. Predominantly occurs in the extremities.
    C. More commonly presents in male patients.
    D. Fails to regress with time.

88. Hemangiopericytomas
    A. Arise from Zimmermann pericytes.
    B. Are commonly seen in the head and neck.
    C. Are predominantly pediatric tumors.
    D. May be treated with cetuximab (Erbitux)
       alone.

89. The IRS-IV staging system is based on several
    factors including
    A. Tumor histological type.
    B. Site.
    C. Age.
    D. All of the above.

90. Alveolar RMS
    A. Is pathologically and clinically distinct from
       embryonal RMS.
    B. Has similar histopathological characteristics to
       embryonal RMS.
    C. Presents in the 0 to 10-year-old age group.
    D. Has an improved prognosis compared with
       embryonal RMS.

91. Success in treatment of RMS is largely attributed to
    A. The introduction of multiagent chemotherapeutic
       regimens.
    B. IMRT.
    C. Transnasal endoscopic skull base surgery.
    D. Positron emission tomography (PET)-CT.

92. The *PAX3/FOXO1* fusion gene in RMS
    A. Is identified only in embryonal RMS.
    B. Is identified only in alveolar RMS.
    C. Is identified in both alveolar and embryonal RMS.
    D. Is identified in extremity osteosarcomas.

93. The *PAX3/FOXO1* fusion gene in RMS
    A. Is a negative prognostic indicator.
    B. Is a positive prognostic indicator.
    C. Has no bearing on outcome.
    D. Is identified in extremity osteosarcomas.

94. The most common site of presentation of
    osteosarcomas of the head and neck is the
    A. Vertebral column.
    B. Zygoma.
    C. Maxilla.
    D. Mandible.

95. Neoadjuvant chemotherapy in head and neck
    osteosarcomas
    A. Reduces the size of the tumor before surgery.
    B. Treats silent pulmonary micrometastases.
    C. Has no role in osteosarcoma management.
    D. Is administered before radiation therapy to
       radiosensitize the tumor.

96. The "best" management for adult head and neck
    osteosarcomas is
    A. Surgery/chemotherapy.

B. Chemotherapy/surgery/chemotherapy.
C. Chemotherapy/surgery/chemoradiation therapy.
D. Still to be decided; no formal consensus exists on what constitutes "best" treatment for adult osteosarcoma.

97. Angiosarcomas are malignant
A. Vascular tumors.
B. Endothelial tumors of the vascular system.
C. Endothelial tumors of lymphatic or vascular origin.
D. Epithelial tumors of lymphatic or vascular origin.

98. Angiosarcomas mainly present in what age category?
A. Patients older than 10 years
B. Patients older than 20 years
C. Patients older than 40 years
D. Patients older than 60 years

99. Which of the following statements about angiosarcomas of the head and neck is correct?
A. A negative margin correlates with an improved chance of survival.
B. Irradiation improves local recurrence but not overall survival rates.
C. Approximately 20% to 45% of patients present with distant metastases.
D. High-dose methotrexate with leucovorin is the chemotherapy drug of choice.

100. What is the 10-year survival rate for angiosarcomas of the head and neck?
A. 60% to 80%
B. 40% to 60%
C. 20% to 40%
D. 10% to 20%

## Answers

| | | |
|---|---|---|
| 1. T | 19. T | 37. T |
| 2. F | 20. T | 38. T |
| 3. T | 21. T | 39. T |
| 4. T | 22. F | 40. T |
| 5. T | 23. F | 41. T |
| 6. F | 24. F | 42. T |
| 7. F | 25. T | 43. F |
| 8. F | 26. T | 44. T |
| 9. F | 27. T | 45. F |
| 10. T | 28. F | 46. T |
| 11. F | 29. F | 47. F |
| 12. T | 30. T | 48. T |
| 13. T | 31. T | 49. F |
| 14. T | 32. T | 50. F |
| 15. T | 33. F | 51. E |
| 16. F | 34. T | 52. B |
| 17. T | 35. F | 53. E |
| 18. F | 36. F | 54. C |

| | | |
|---|---|---|
| 55. A | 69. C | 85. B |
| 56. (a) vi (b) ii (c) ii (d) vii (e) iv | 70. B | 86. B |
| | 71. B | 87. A |
| 57. E | 72. C | 88. A |
| 58. C | 73. C | 89. A |
| 59. (a) iv (b) ii (c) v (d) i (e) iii | 74. B | 90. A |
| | 75. A | 91. A |
| | 76. D | 92. B |
| 60. D | 77. A | 93. A |
| 61. C | 78. A | 94. D |
| 62. B | 79. C | 95. B |
| 63. A | 80. B | 96. D |
| 64. C | 81. D | 97. C |
| 65. B | 82. A | 98. D |
| 66. A | 83. D | 99. C |
| 67. A | 84. C | 100. D |
| 68. D | | |

## Core Knowledge

- Sarcomas are classified according to their tissue of origin, which can be bone or soft tissue, whether the tumor is high-grade or low-grade, and the anatomical subsites of presentation within the head and neck.

- Head and neck sarcomas account for approximately 2% to 15% of all sarcomas, which represents approximately 1% of head and neck malignancies. In the United States, more than 10,000 new cases are now reported yearly, and the mortality rate yearly includes 4000 patients.

- Malignant fibrous histiocytoma (MFH), osteosarcoma, fibrosarcoma, angiosarcoma, rhabdomyosarcoma (RMS), and liposarcoma are the most frequently reported sarcoma pathological types in the head and neck.

- Sarcoma surgery demands extirpation of the tumor, including pseudocapsule margins, in an effort to succeed in gross disease removal with free microscopic margins. This can be challenging in an anatomically confined region such as the head and neck.

- Sarcoma types that metastasize to lymph nodes are clear cell, RMS, epithelioid, angiosarcoma, and synovial. When these pathological types are identified, this information must be considered within the operative strategy or adjunctive radiation fields.

- Distant metastases occur in approximately 25% to 30% at diagnosis or during follow-up. The common sites of metastases are lung, bone, central nervous system, and liver.

- MFHs, osteosarcomas, RMSs, angiosarcomas, synovial sarcomas, and Ewing sarcomas are all considered to be high-grade tumors.

- Dermatofibrosarcoma protuberans, atypical lipomatous tumors, and desmoid tumors are predominately low-grade. Chondrosarcomas, fibrosarcomas, liposarcomas, leiomyosarcomas, neurogenic sarcomas, and hemangiopericytomas require individualized grade characterization.

- Adjuvant radiation therapy should be considered for patients with locally recurrent lesions or intermediate- to high-grade tumors and for those with close or positive margins.

- Neoadjuvant chemotherapy and radiation therapy may be considered on an individual histopathological and staging basis.

## MALIGNANT FIBROUS HISTIOCYTOMA

- This tumor largely presents in the fifth and sixth decades, and as many as 40% of all sarcomas in the head and neck are of this type. Surgery is the main treatment modality for MFH, and chemotherapy and radiation therapy are used in the adjuvant setting. The main negative prognostic variables for MFH include positive margins, tumors found in the head and neck anatomical region, tumor size greater than 5 cm, and high stage.

## OSTEOSARCOMA

- This tumor represents approximately 1% of head and neck cancers and less than 10% of all osteosarcomas. Subtypes include osteoblastic, chondroblastic and fibroblastic, multifocal, telangiectatic, small cell, intraosseous well-differentiated, intracortical, periosteal, parosteal, high-grade surface, and extraosseous. Predisposition to this tumor is related not only to deletion of chromosomal region 13q14, which inactivates the retinoblastoma gene, but also to Paget disease, fibrous dysplasia, enchondromatosis, Li-Fraumeni syndrome, and Rothmund-Thomson syndrome. The Codman triangle and a sunburst appearance are the classic radiological features. The posterior body of the ramus is the classic mandibular location. The alveolar ridge, sinus floor, and palate are classic maxillary tumor locations. Extremity osteosarcomas metastasize early, and there is good evidence that neoadjuvant chemotherapy, surgery, and adjuvant chemotherapy improves disease-free survival and overall survival rates. Neoadjuvant chemotherapy in the pediatric population has resulted in a threefold improved survival rate. No formal consensus exists on the treatment of adult osteosarcoma. Complete surgical excision to achieve negative surgical margins is the main goal of therapy. A positive margin carries with it a significant decrease in survival rate from 75% to 35%. Memorial Sloan Kettering Cancer Center reports 3-year overall, disease-specific, and recurrence-free survival rates of approximately 81%, 81%, and 73%, respectively.

## RHABDOMYOSARCOMA

- This tumor type is the most common soft tissue sarcoma in children. The Intergroup Rhabdomyosarcoma Study-IV (IRS-IV) emphasized that therapy for children with RMSs should be risk directed and based primarily on tumor site, histological type, and extent of the disease. The course of RMS in pediatric age groups has changed with a dramatic improvement in survival rates from 25% in the early 1970s to 71% by 2001. The two distinct pathological entities are alveolar and embryonal. IRS-V used the concept of risk stratification to conduct studies based on clinical and biological prognostic factors. The clinical group is based on the extent of residual tumor after surgery with consideration of regional lymph node status. The IRS staging system is based on tumor size, invasiveness, nodal status, and site of the primary tumor. In adolescents and adults, there is a greater predilection for alveolar and pleomorphic histopathological subtypes and anatomical presentation within truncal or extremity sites. The PAX3/FOXO1 fusion gene was discovered in 1993. The presence of PAX3/7-FOXO1 translocation in adult patients is significantly associated with a higher frequency of metastatic disease. As such, outcomes in adult patients with RMSs are poor, with a 5-year survival rate of approximately 30%.

## ANGIOSARCOMA

- These are malignant endothelial cell tumors of lymphatic or vascular origin that are found primarily in elderly patients. Men are affected twice as frequently as women. No treatment consensus exists. Known risk factors include radiation exposure; chronic lymphedema; Milroy disease; exogenous toxins including vinyl chloride, arsenic, and anabolic steroids; and familial syndromes including the BRCA1 and BRCA2 genes, NF1 gene, Maffucci syndrome, and Klippel-Trénaunay syndrome. Diffuse tumor margins often inhibit satisfactory oncological excision. Combined modality therapies are applied, including surgical extirpation with a wide 2-cm margin and adjunctive radiation therapy of 60 to 66 Gy to wide treatment fields. Neoadjuvant or adjuvant taxane chemotherapy can also be considered in select cases.

## LIPOSARCOMA

- Approximately 2% of liposarcomas present within the head and neck region. Etiological factors include the NF1 gene, trauma, and irradiation. Well-differentiated and myxoid types are considered low-grade, whereas pleomorphic and round cell types are high-grade tumors. Survival probability is determined by the subtype of tumor, grade, size, and anatomical site of presentation. Radiation therapy has been shown to improve local recurrence rates; however, it may not affect overall survival rates.

# FIBROSARCOMA

- Fibrosarcomas appear in the fourth and fifth decades, and most commonly present as a painless mass. Patients with low-grade lesions and adequate surgical margins receive surgery alone. Patients with high-grade lesions or positive surgical margins should receive adjuvant radiation therapy.

# CHONDROSARCOMAS

- Myxoid and mesenchymal chondrosarcoma subtypes constitute the majority of head and neck cases. The majority of chondrosarcomas are low-grade tumors. High-grade tumors may also have histopathological similarities to tumors such as chondroblastic osteosarcoma, fibrosarcoma, or MFH. Contrary to earlier beliefs, these tumors are radiosensitive. Intensity-modulated radiation therapy allows for the delivery of high-dose conformal photons with the use of either standard fractionation, as with protons, or hypofractionated regimens. Chemotherapy has no current role in the management of these tumors.

## SUGGESTED READING

Brockstein B. Management of sarcomas of the head and neck. Curr Oncol Rep 2004;6(4):321–7.

Crist WM, Anderson JR, Meza JL, Fryer C, Raney RB, Ruymann FB, et al. Intergroup rhabdomyosarcoma study-IV: results for patients with nonmetastatic disease. J Clin Oncol 2001;19(12):3091–102.

Guadagnolo BA, Zagars GK, Araujo D, Ravi V, Shellenberger TD, Sturgis EM. Outcomes after definitive treatment for cutaneous angiosarcoma of the face and scalp. Head Neck 2011;33(5):661–7.

Jaffe N. Osteosarcoma: review of the past, impact on the future. The American experience. Cancer Treat Res 2009;152:239–62.

Koch BB, Karnell LH, Hoffman HT, Apostolakis LW, Robinson RA, Zhen W, et al. National cancer database report on chondrosarcoma of the head and neck. Head Neck 2000;22(4):408–25.

O'Neill JP, Bilsky M, Shah JP, Kraus D. Head and neck sarcomas. epidemiology, pathology, and management. Neurosurg Clin N Am 2013;24(1):67–78.

Patel SG, Meyers P, Huvos AG, Wolden S, Singh B, Shaha AR, et al. Improved outcomes in patients with osteogenic sarcoma of the head and neck. Cancer 2002;95(7):1495–503.

Perkins J, Manning SC, Tempero R, Cunningham MJ, Edmonds Jr JL, Hoffer FA, et al. Lymphatic malformations: current cellular and clinical investigations. Otolaryngol Head Neck Surg 2010;142:789–94.

Sturgis EM, Potter BO. Sarcomas of the head and neck region. Curr Opin Oncol 2003;15(3):239–52.

Turner JH, Richmon JD. Head and neck rhabdomyosarcoma: a critical analysis of population-based incidence and survival data. Otolaryngol Head Neck Surg 2011;145(6):967–73.

Zagars GK, Ballo MT, Pisters PW, Pollock RE, Patel SR, Benjamin RS, et al. Prognostic factors for patients with localized soft-tissue sarcoma treated with conservation surgery and radiation therapy: an analysis of 1225 patients. Cancer 2003;97(10):2530–43.

# 13 Bone Tumors and Odontogenic Tumors

## Questions

### TRUE/FALSE

1. Dentigerous cysts occur around impacted teeth. (T/F)

2. Dentigerous cysts occur at the apical region of the tooth. (T/F)

3. Dentigerous cysts frequently involve the maxillary canine and mandibular third molar. (T/F)

4. Dentigerous cysts develop when fluid accumulates between the reduced enamel epithelium and tooth crown. (T/F)

5. Dentigerous cysts have the ability to transform into malignant neoplasms. (T/F)

6. Odontogenic keratocysts are multiloculated and radiolucent lesions. (T/F)

7. Odontogenic keratocysts occur only in the setting of basal cell nevus syndrome. (T/F)

8. Odontogenic keratocysts are the same as keratinizing odontogenic cysts. (T/F)

9. Odontogenic keratocysts have parakeratin in their cystic spaces. (T/F)

10. Odontogenic keratocysts have a low recurrence rate after enucleation. (T/F)

11. Odontogenic keratocysts may recur many years after initial treatment. (T/F)

12. Odontogenic keratocysts have been renamed *keratocystic odontogenic tumors.* (T/F)

13. Basal cell nevus syndrome is associated with keratinizing odontogenic cysts. (T/F)

14. Basal cell nevus syndrome is associated with odontogenic keratocysts. (T/F)

15. Basal cell nevus syndrome is an autosomal dominant disease. (T/F)

16. Basal cell nevus syndrome often presents with odontogenic keratocysts as the initial presenting component of the syndrome. (T/F)

17. Basal cell nevus syndrome is associated with multiple basal cell carcinomas, odontogenic keratocysts, and skeletal abnormalities. (T/F)

18. Radicular cysts are associated with the crown of the tooth. (T/F)

19. The rests of Malassez are a common source for odontogenic neoplasms. (T/F)

20. The rests of Serres are a common source for odontogenic neoplasms. (T/F)

21. Most odontogenic cysts are surfaced by keratinized epithelium. (T/F)

22. Ghost cells are pathognomonic of calcifying odontogenic cysts. (T/F)

23. Ameloblastoma is an uncommon benign, locally aggressive odontogenic neoplasm. (T/F)

24. Ameloblastomas occur in men and women with equal frequency. (T/F)

25. Ameloblastomas occur more frequently in the mandible. (T/F)

26. Ameloblastomas are usually multilocular. (T/F)

27. Ameloblastomas generally infiltrate cortical bone. (T/F)

28. Ameloblastomas do not have malignant potential. (T/F)

29. Multicystic ameloblastomas are best treated with enucleation and curettage. (T/F)

30. Malignant ameloblastomas are defined by metastatic spreading to lymph nodes, distant sites, or both. (T/F)

31. Malignant ameloblastomas most commonly metastasize to the lungs. (T/F)

32. Ameloblastic carcinomas have cytopathological features similar to those of benign ameloblastomas. (T/F)

33. Malignant transformation of odontogenic cysts is a rare occurrence. (T/F)

34. Peripheral ameloblastomas do not infiltrate the underlying bone. (T/F)

35. Ameloblastic fibromas are associated with developing teeth. (T/F)

36. Ameloblastic fibromas can produce enamel, dentin, and cementum. (T/F)

37. Calcifying epithelial odontogenic tumors (Pindborg tumors) contains foci of amyloid material that may become calcified. (T/F)

38. Pindborg tumors can have a mixed radiolucent and radiopaque radiographic appearance. (T/F)

39. Odontomas are the most common odontogenic tumors. (T/F)

40. Odontomas have a high recurrence rate. (T/F)

41. Osteosarcomas of the head and neck account for less than 10% of all osteosarcomas. (T/F)

42. Osteosarcomas of the head and neck have a high propensity for distant metastasis. (T/F)

43. Osteosarcomas of the head and neck are usually low grade. (T/F)

44. Osteosarcomas of the head and neck have a genetic association with retinoblastoma at chromosomal region 13q14. (T/F)

45. Osteosarcomas of the head and neck require radiation therapy after resection to achieve better local control than surgery alone. (T/F)

46. A majority of chondrosarcomas of the craniofacial skeleton involve the jaws. (T/F)

47. Primary intraosseous squamous cell carcinoma develops from the usual carcinogenic factors associated with mucosal squamous cell carcinoma. (T/F)

48. Primary intraosseous squamous cell carcinoma develops from odontogenic epithelial remnants. (T/F)

49. Fibrous dysplasia may involve single or multiple bones. (T/F)

50. Fibrous dysplasia may be part of the McCune-Albright syndrome. (T/F)

51. Fibrous dysplasia involves the mandible more commonly than the maxilla. (T/F)

52. Fibrous dysplasia has three radiographic patterns: cystic, sclerotic, and mixed radiolucent and radiopaque. (T/F)

53. Fibrous dysplasia may develop into osteosarcoma. (T/F)

54. Ossifying fibromas mainly occur in the posterior mandible. (T/F)

55. Ossifying fibromas are well demarcated and/or encapsulated compared with fibrous dysplasia. (T/F)

56. Ossifying fibromas are best managed with observation. (T/F)

57. Aneurysmal bone cysts commonly occur in the jaws. (T/F)

58. Aneurysmal bone cysts are expansile, osteolytic, multiloculated, blood-filled spaces with fibrous septa. (T/F)

59. Aneurysmal bone cysts have a radiographic "soap bubble" appearance. (T/F)

60. Aneurysmal bone cysts may be treated with curettage. (T/F)

61. Aneurysmal bone cysts may be treated primarily with radiation therapy. (T/F)

## MULTIPLE CHOICE

62. What are the Vickers and Gorlin criteria that describe ameloblastomas?
    i. Columnar basilar cells
    ii. Palisading of basilar cells
    iii. Polarization of basilar layer nuclei away from the basement membrane
    iv. Hyperchromatism of basal cell nuclei in the epithelial lining
    v. Subnuclear vacuolization of the cytoplasm of the basal cells
    A. i, ii
    B. i, ii, iii
    C. ii, iii, iv
    D. i, ii, iv, v
    E. All of the above

63. Which of the following odontogenic tumors are uniloculated?
    i. Ameloblastoma
    ii. Calcifying epithelial odontogenic tumor
    iii. Keratocystic odontogenic tumor
    iv. Adenomatoid odontogenic tumor
    v. Odontogenic ghost cell tumor
    vi. Calcifying cystic odontogenic tumor
    vii. Odontogenic fibroma
    A. i, ii, iii
    B. i, iii
    C. i, ii, iii, iv
    D. i, iii, iv, v, vi
    E. All of the above

64. Which of the following odontogenic tumors are multiloculated?
    i. Ameloblastoma
    ii. Calcifying epithelial odontogenic tumor
    iii. Keratocystic odontogenic tumor
    iv. Adenomatoid odontogenic tumor
    v. Odontogenic ghost cell tumor
    vi. Calcifying cystic odontogenic tumor
    vii. Odontogenic fibroma
    A. i
    B. i, ii
    C. i, iii
    D. i, ii, iii
    E. All of the above

65. Which of the following tumors appear as radiolucent lesions on a computed tomographic (CT) scan?
    i. Ameloblastoma
    ii. Calcifying epithelial odontogenic tumor
    iii. Keratocystic odontogenic tumor
    iv. Adenomatoid odontogenic tumor

v. Odontogenic ghost cell tumor
vi. Calcifying cystic odontogenic tumor
vii. Odontogenic fibroma
A. i, iii, iv, vii
B. i, iii, iv, v
C. i, iii, iv, v, vii
D. ii, vi
E. All of the above

66. Which of the following tumors appear as radiopaque lesions on a CT scan?
    i. Ameloblastoma
    ii. Calcifying epithelial odontogenic tumor
    iii. Keratocystic odontogenic tumor
    iv. Adenomatoid odontogenic tumor
    v. Odontogenic ghost cell tumor
    vi. Calcifying cystic odontogenic tumor
    vii. Odontogenic fibroma
    A. ii
    B. i, ii, vi
    C. ii, v, vi
    D. ii, iii, iv, v, vi
    E. ii, iv, v, vi, vii

67. Which of the following lesions can be treated with enucleation?
    i. Ameloblastoma
    ii. Calcifying epithelial odontogenic tumor
    iii. Keratocystic odontogenic tumor
    iv. Adenomatoid odontogenic tumor
    v. Odontogenic ghost cell tumor
    vi. Calcifying cystic odontogenic tumor
    vii. Odontogenic fibroma
    A. i, ii, iii, iv
    B. ii, iii, iv, v
    C. v, vi, vii
    D. vi, vii
    E. iii, vi, vii

68. Which of the following odontogenic lesions have a "soap bubble" appearance on a CT scan?
    i. Odontogenic keratocyst
    ii. Ameloblastoma
    iii. Odontogenic myxoma
    iv. Calcifying epithelial odontogenic tumor
    v. Aneurysmal bone cyst
    A. ii
    B. ii, iii
    C. ii, iii, iv
    D. ii, iii, iv, v
    E. ii, iii, v

69. Which odontogenic tumors are of mesenchymal origin?
    i. Odontogenic fibroma
    ii. Odontogenic myxoma
    iii. Cementoblastoma
    iv. Odontoma
    v. Calcifying cystic odontogenic tumor
    A. i, ii
    B. i, ii, iii
    C. i, ii, iii, iv
    D. iii, iv
    E. All of the above

70. Which of the following are considered fibro-osseous lesions?
    i. Ossifying fibroma
    ii. Fibrous dysplasia
    iii. Osseous dysplasia
    iv. Central giant cell lesion
    v. Cherubism
    vi. Aneurysmal bone cyst
    vii. Simple bone cyst
    A. i, ii
    B. i, ii, iii
    C. i, ii, iii, iv
    D. i, ii, iii, iv, v
    E. All of the above

71. Odontogenic tumors and cysts are best identified based on the
    A. Patient's age.
    B. Histological components.
    C. Location and imaging.
    D. History, histological components, and location.

72. Which of the following is a possible source of inflammatory odontogenic cysts?
    A. Rests of Serres
    B. Rests of Malassez
    C. Enamel organ
    D. Rests of Serres and rests of Malassez

73. Which of the following is a possible source of odontogenic tumors?
    A. Rests of Serres
    B. Rests of Malassez
    C. Rests of Serres and the enamel organ
    D. Rests of Serres and rests of Malassez

74. Which are the most common odontogenic cysts?
    A. Dentigerous cyst, radicular cyst, residual cyst
    B. Dentigerous cyst, radicular cyst, eruption cyst
    C. Dentigerous cyst, radicular cyst, Gorlin cyst
    D. Dentigerous cyst, radicular cyst, nasopalatine cyst

75. What is the most common odontogenic tumor?
    A. Ameloblastoma
    B. Calcifying epithelial odontogenic tumor
    C. Odontoma
    D. Adenomatoid odontogenic tumor

76. A radicular cyst is best described as a
    A. Unilocular radiolucency at the apical portion of a nonvital tooth.
    B. Unilocular radiolucency at the crown portion of a nonvital tooth.
    C. Multilocular radiolucency at the apical portion of a vital tooth.
    D. Multilocular radiolucency at the crown portion of a vital tooth.

77. Radicular cysts are treated with
    A. Tooth extraction.
    B. Enucleation.
    C. Tooth extraction and enucleation.
    D. Tooth extraction and curettage.

78. Which of the following are inflammatory cysts?
    A. Radicular cyst, lateral radicular cyst, eruption cyst
    B. Radicular cyst, lateral radicular cyst, residual cyst
    C. Radicular cyst, residual cyst, dentigerous cyst
    D. Radicular cyst, dentigerous cyst, Gorlin cyst

79. A dentigerous cyst is best described as a
    A. Unilocular radiolucency associated with the apical portion of an unerupted tooth.
    B. Unilocular radiolucency associated with the crown portion of an unerupted tooth.
    C. Unilocular radiolucency associated with the apical portion of an erupted tooth.
    D. Unilocular radiolucency associated with the crown portion of an erupted tooth.

80. Dentigerous cysts are treated by
    A. Tooth extraction.
    B. Enucleation.
    C. Tooth extraction and enucleation.
    D. Tooth extraction, enucleation, and curettage.

81. Keratinizing odontogenic cysts are associated with
    A. Orthokeratin.
    B. Parakeratin.
    C. Basal cell nevus syndrome.
    D. Multilocular radiolucency.

82. Odontogenic keratocysts
    A. Behave like cysts rather than neoplasms.
    B. Mostly involve the mandible.
    C. Are generally asymptomatic.
    D. Have a low recurrence rate.

83. Which of the following is true about odontogenic keratocysts?
    A. They may develop in all areas of odontogenesis.
    B. They are radiolucent lesions.
    C. They are associated with basal cell nevus syndrome.
    D. All of the above are true.

84. Basal cell nevus syndrome
    A. Is an autosomal dominant disease with multiple odontogenic keratocysts.
    B. Is an autosomal dominant disease with multiple odontogenic keratocysts and skeletal abnormalities.
    C. Has no genetic linkage but has multiple odontogenic keratocysts.
    D. Has no genetic linkage but has multiple odontogenic keratocysts and skeletal abnormalities.

85. Odontogenic keratocysts are best treated with
    A. Simple enucleation.
    B. Enucleation and curettage.
    C. Enucleation, curettage, and cryosurgery.
    D. Wide local resection.

86. Calcifying odontogenic cysts (Gorlin cysts) typically
    A. Contain ghost cells, occur in the anterior jaw, and are radiolucent.
    B. Contain ghost cells, occur in the anterior jaw, and are mixed radiolucent and radiopaque.

C. Contain ghost cells, occur in the posterior jaw, and are radiolucent.
D. Contain ghost cells, occur in the posterior jaw, and are mixed radiolucent and radiopaque.

87. Malignant transformation can occur in which of the following odontogenic cysts?
    A. Odontogenic keratocysts
    B. Dentigerous cysts
    C. Odontogenic keratocysts and dentigerous cysts
    D. Odontogenic keratocysts, dentigerous cysts, and Gorlin cysts

88. Most ameloblastomas occur in the
    A. Maxilla.
    B. Mandible.
    C. Sinonasal cavity.
    D. Gingiva.

89. Radiographically, ameloblastomas have a
    A. Salt and pepper appearance.
    B. Ground-glass appearance.
    C. Moth-eaten appearance.
    D. Soap bubble or honeycomb appearance.

90. The local spreading of ameloblastoma of the mandible is limited by
    A. Medullary bone
    B. Cortical bone
    C. Periosteum
    D. Cortical bone and periosteum

91. Mandibular ameloblastomas are managed with
    A. Enucleation.
    B. Enucleation and curettage.
    C. Resection with 1-cm bone margins.
    D. Resection with 1-cm bone and soft tissue margins.

92. Peripheral ameloblastomas are managed with
    A. Enucleation and curettage.
    B. Resection with 1-cm soft tissue margins.
    C. Resection with 1-cm soft tissue margins and neck dissection margins.
    D. Resection with 1-cm soft tissue margins and resection of adjacent bone.

93. Malignant ameloblastomas
    A. Have pathological features of benign ameloblastomas.
    B. Have pathological features of sarcoma.
    C. Demonstrate local invasion.
    D. Metastasize mainly to regional lymph nodes.

94. Malignant ameloblastomas most commonly metastasize to the
    A. Regional lymph nodes.
    B. Bones.
    C. Brain.
    D. Lungs.

95. Ameloblastic carcinomas
    A. Have pathological features of benign ameloblastomas.
    B. Have pathological features of malignancy.
    C. Occur more commonly than malignant ameloblastoma.
    D. Do not metastasize distantly.

96. Ameloblastic fibromas
    A. Can form enamel, dentin, or cementum.
    B. Contain mesenchymal and ameloblastic cells.
    C. Are radiopaque.
    D. Are associated with the apical portion of an unerupted tooth.

97. Calcifying epithelial odontogenic tumors (Pindborg tumors) are
    A. Characterized by foci of amyloid and mineralization.
    B. Occur mainly in the maxilla.
    C. Associated with erupted tooth roots.
    D. Radiopaque.

98. Odontomas
    A. Are rare odontogenic tumors.
    B. Contain toothlike elements.
    C. Have no impact on surrounding dentition.
    D. Have the radiographic appearance of an unerupted tooth.

99. Ossifying fibromas typically have the following characteristics:
    A. Benign, epithelial origin, radiolucent appearance.
    B. Benign, epithelial origin, radiopaque appearance.
    C. Benign, mesenchymal origin, radiolucent appearance.
    D. Benign, mesenchymal origin, radiopaque appearance.

100. Fibrous dysplasia
    A. Is a rapidly growing lesion.
    B. Has a ground-glass appearance on a CT scan.
    C. Has well-defined borders.
    D. Is best treated surgically.

## Answers

| | | | |
|---|---|---|---|
| 1. T | 18. F | 35. T | |
| 2. F | 19. F | 36. F | |
| 3. T | 20. T | 37. T | |
| 4. T | 21. F | 38. T | |
| 5. T | 22. F | 39. T | |
| 6. T | 23. T | 40. F | |
| 7. F | 24. T | 41. T | |
| 8. F | 25. T | 42. F | |
| 9. T | 26. T | 43. F | |
| 10. F | 27. F | 44. T | |
| 11. T | 28. F | 45. T | |
| 12. T | 29. F | 46. F | |
| 13. F | 30. T | 47. F | |
| 14. T | 31. T | 48. T | |
| 15. T | 32. F | 49. T | |
| 16. T | 33. T | 50. T | |
| 17. T | 34. T | 51. F | |

| | | |
|---|---|---|
| 52. T | 69. B | 86. B |
| 53. T | 70. E | 87. C |
| 54. T | 71. D | 88. B |
| 55. T | 72. B | 89. D |
| 56. F | 73. C | 90. D |
| 57. F | 74. A | 91. C |
| 58. T | 75. C | 92. B |
| 59. T | 76. A | 93. A |
| 60. T | 77. C | 94. D |
| 61. T | 78. B | 95. B |
| 62. E | 79. B | 96. B |
| 63. E | 80. C | 97. A |
| 64. D | 81. A | 98. B |
| 65. A | 82. B | 99. D |
| 66. C | 83. D | 100. B |
| 67. D | 84. B | |
| 68. E | 85. B | |

## Core Knowledge

- Odontogenic cysts are cysts derived from odontogenic epithelium and may be classified as either inflammatory or developmental.

- Odontogenic tumors may be derived from odontogenic epithelium, ectomesenchyme, or mesenchymal tissue.

- Radicular cysts are the most common odontogenic cysts and develop at the apex of an erupted tooth. Radiographically, the cysts are round and involve the apex of the tooth. Treatment involves extraction of the affected tooth and enucleation of the cyst.

- Dentigerous cysts develop around the crown of an unerupted tooth, usually the third maxillary molars or maxillary canines. Radiographically, they appear as unilocular radiolucencies surrounding the crown of an unerupted tooth. Treatment involves extraction of the affected tooth and enucleation of the cyst.

- Odontogenic keratocysts (keratocystic odontogenic tumors) contain parakeratinizing epithelium. They may be single or multiple and generally involve the angle of the mandible. Multiple lesions are seen in the setting of basal cell nevus syndrome. They may appear as unilocular or multilocular radiolucencies. Treatment generally entails enucleation and curettage with regular long-term follow-up because these tumors are associated with a reasonable risk of recurrence or secondary tumors in the setting of basal cell nevus syndrome.

- Ameloblastoma is an uncommon benign, locally aggressive odontogenic neoplasm that generally develops in the mandible in the region of the molars and ramus.

Central ameloblastomas occur within the jawbone, whereas peripheral lesions involve the adjacent gingiva but not the bone. Most ameloblastomas are multicystic and have a greater tendency for recurrence compared with unicystic lesions. Rarely, ameloblastomas have malignant potential and are classified as malignant ameloblastoma or ameloblastic carcinoma. Unicystic ameloblastomas may be treated conservatively with enucleation and curettage, but multicystic ameloblastomas are best managed with wide surgical resection and at least 1-cm bone margins.

- Calcifying epithelial odontogenic tumors (Pindborg tumors) are locally invasive epithelial tumors containing amyloid material and calcifications. They are unilocular or multilocular and, in general, have a mixed radiolucent and radiopaque appearance. Treatment entails local resection, although enucleation may be adequate for smaller tumors.

- Adenomatoid odontogenic tumors are called *two-third tumors* and are seen in female patients and teenagers and in the setting of impacted teeth or in the maxilla. They appear as unilocular radiolucencies involving the crown and root of an unerupted tooth. Treatment involves local excision.

- Odontomas (complex and compound types) are the most common odontogenic neoplasms and contain enamel, dentin, cementum, and other tooth elements. They appear as a central radiopacity with a thin radiolucent zone. Treatment involves simple enucleation. Recurrence has never been reported.

- Calcifying cystic odontogenic tumors (Gorlin cyst) contain ameloblastoma-like epithelium, ghost cells, and calcifications. In general, they appear as unilocular radiolucencies, and half contain some amount of radiopaque material. Treatment involves simple enucleation.

- Odontogenic ghost cell tumors contain ameloblastoma-like epithelium, ghost cells, and dysplastic dentin. Most lesions are unilocular and have a mixed radiolucent and radiopaque appearance. Treatment generally involves wide resection.

- Ossifying fibromas are well-demarcated, encapsulated fibro-osseous lesions mainly involving the posterior mandible. Lesions have a mixed radiopaque and radiolucent appearance. Treatment involves local excision.

- Fibrous dysplasia causes replacement of medullary bone with fibrous tissue mixed with irregular trabecular bone. It can occur in a single bone (monostotic) or in multiple locations (polyostotic). Polyostotic lesions occur in McCune-Albright syndrome. Lesions have a ground-glass appearance on computed tomography (CT). Surgery is generally reserved for correcting cosmetic deformities or functional deficits.

- Aneurysmal bone cysts (ABCs) are expansile osteolytic lesions with blood-filled spaces separated with fibrous septa. They are generally unilocular or multilocular radiolucencies in the posterior region of the mandible. ABCs can be treated with curettage.

## SUGGESTED READING

Barnes L, Eveson JW, Reichart P, Sidransky D. World Health Organization classification of tumors. Pathology and genetics. Head and neck tumours. Lyon, France: International Agency for Research on Cancer Press; 2005. p. 283–328.

Flint PW, Haughey BH, Lund VJ, Niparko JK, Richardson MA, Robbins KT, et al. Cummings otolaryngology–head and neck surgery. 5th ed. Philadelphia: Mosby; 2010. p. 1259–78.

Reichart PA, Philipsen HP, Sonner S. Ameloblastoma: biological profile of 3677 cases. Eur J Cancer B Oral Oncol 1995;31B:86–99.

Som PM, Curtin HD. Head and neck imaging. Philadelphia: Mosby; 2003. p. 930–94.

# 14 Reconstructive Surgery

## Questions

### TRUE/FALSE

1. In advancement flaps, the ratio of flap to defect should be approximately 4:1.  (T/F)

2. Bilobed flaps are a good option when the surrounding skin is not mobile enough to achieve primary closure of a surgical defect.  (T/F)

3. Rotation flaps are best suited for triangular defects.  (T/F)

4. Transposition flap design enables the surgeon to bring tissue from some distance away from the defect.  (T/F)

5. Rhomboid flaps are a good option for reconstructing cheek and temple defects.  (T/F)

6. The main blood supply to the pectoralis major is located medial to the tendon of pectoralis minor.  (T/F)

7. A proximal (cephalad) skin island flap will permit a greater arc of rotation of the pectoralis major myocutaneous flap.  (T/F)

8. When the pectoralis major flap is harvested, the nerves to the muscle should be identified and divided.  (T/F)

9. The pectoralis major muscle flap shares a common blood supply with the deltopectoral flap.  (T/F)

10. The superior trapezius flap and the lower trapezius island flap have the same blood supply.  (T/F)

11. Radical neck dissection is a contraindication to use of the superior trapezius flap.  (T/F)

12. In oral cavity tumors, the need for a thorough level I dissection might preclude the use of a submental island flap based on the ipsilateral side.  (T/F)

13. The palatal island flap is a good choice in cases of salvage of the oropharynx.  (T/F)

14. The primary blood supply to the temporalis muscle is from the superficial temporal artery.  (T/F)

15. In facial reanimation, it is important to divide the nerve to the temporalis muscle.  (T/F)

16. The deltopectoral flap receives its blood supply from the internal mammary artery.  (T/F)

17. The paramedian forehead flap is based on the supraorbital artery.  (T/F)

18. Paramedian forehead flap reconstruction is usually done in one step.  (T/F)

19. The anterior limit of dissection of the temporoparietal fascia is marked by the course of the frontal branch of the facial nerve (approximately 1.5 cm lateral to the orbital rim).  (T/F)

20. The temporoparietal fascia flap and the temporalis flap share the same blood supply.  (T/F)

21. The temporoparietal fascia flap is not a good choice for use in contaminated fields because it is very thin and not resistant to infection.  (T/F)

22. The Allen test is not a reliable test in determining adequate blood supply to the hand after harvest of a radial forearm free flap.  (T/F)

23. Up to 60% of the radius diameter can be harvested in an osteocutaneous radial forearm free flap.  (T/F)

24. The cephalic vein can be used as venous drainage of the radial forearm free flap.  (T/F)

25. Both the palmaris longus tendon and the lateral antecubital sensory nerve can be harvested with a radial forearm free flap.  (T/F)

26. Hypoesthesia/anesthesia of the anatomical snuffbox is an unavoidable sequela of harvesting a radial forearm free flap because of sacrifice of the sensory branches of the radial nerve.  (T/F)

27. Occlusion of the superficial femoral artery is a contraindication to harvesting of the anterolateral thigh flap.  (T/F)

28. The most common cutaneous perforators for the anterolateral thigh flap are within 3 cm of the midpoint between the anterosuperior iliac spine and the superolateral corner of the patella.  (T/F)

29. Donor site defects as wide as 8.5 cm can be closed primarily after harvesting of the anterolateral thigh flap.  (T/F)

30. A cuff of the rectus femoris can be raised with the anterolateral thigh flap.  (T/F)

31. The anterolateral thigh flap cannot be raised as a sensate flap.  (T/F)

32. The rectus abdominis muscle flap is based on the deep superior epigastric artery.  (T/F)

33. The abdominal skin around the umbilicus has the most reliable blood supply for the musculocutaneous rectus abdominis flap. (T/F)

34. The deep superior epigastric artery is larger than the deep inferior epigastric artery. (T/F)

35. The most consistent cutaneous perforators are located at the junction of the proximal third and mid third of the skin on the lateral side of the calf. (T/F)

36. Cutaneous perforators travel through posterior intermuscular septa or through the soleus muscle. (T/F)

37. During insetting, the peroneal artery should be placed on the lingual surface of the neomandible. (T/F)

38. Leaving 6 to 7 cm of fibula proximally reduces the risk of injury to the posterior tibial artery. (T/F)

39. The fibula is preferred for reconstruction of an anterior mandible defect. (T/F)

40. The scapular tip free flap is based on the angular branch of the thoracodorsal artery. (T/F)

41. Regardless of the extent of the flap, the parascapular flap base should be centered over the triangular space (between the teres major, minor, and long head of the triceps). (T/F)

42. Up to 10 cm of lateral scapular border can be harvested based on the angular branch. (T/F)

43. Latissimus dorsi, scapular tip, and serratus flaps cannot be raised based on one pedicle. (T/F)

44. The parascapular flap can be raised as a fasciocutaneous flap without disrupting any of the shoulder musculature. (T/F)

45. Donor site defects as wide as 7 cm can be closed primarily after harvesting of a musculocutaneous latissimus dorsi flap. (T/F)

46. The ascending branch of the deep circumflex iliac artery supplies the internal oblique muscle. (T/F)

47. When an iliac crest flap is harvested, the external oblique muscle is harvested with the bone. (T/F)

48. The skin paddle for the iliac crest can be extended from the anterosuperior iliac spine to approximately 9 cm posteriorly. (T/F)

49. The main blood supply to the gracilis is from the adductor artery, a branch of the profunda femoris. (T/F)

50. The nerve supply to the gracilis is from the anterior branch of the obturator nerve, which enters the muscle distal to the entry point of the vascular pedicle. (T/F)

## MULTIPLE CHOICE

51. The lesions in Figures 14-1 and 14-2 are diagnosed as squamous cell carcinoma (SCC) on biopsy.

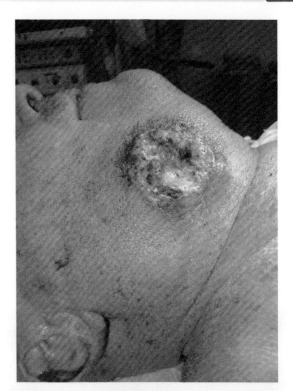

**Figure 14-1**

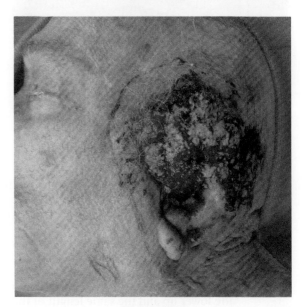

**Figure 14-2**

Patient 1 is undergoing wide local excision and comprehensive neck dissection (modified radical neck dissection, Type II). Patient 2 is undergoing temporal bone resection, parotidectomy, and comprehensive neck dissection. Which of the following are true regarding reconstruction options?
    i. Anterior neck skin defects can be reconstructed with pectoralis major musculocutaneous pedicle flaps.
    ii. Both of these defects can be reconstructed with parascapular fasciocutaneous free flaps.
    iii. Deltopectoral flaps are the best option.

iv. Split-thickness skin grafts are an option for the anterior neck skin defects.

v. Good options for these defects are lower trapezius musculocutaneous island flaps.

vi. Anterolateral thigh flaps will give the best color match

vii. Anterolateral thigh flaps are a good option for filling lateral temporal bone defects because they have adequate bulk and are associated with low donor site morbidity.

A. i, iii, vii
B. iii, v, vi
C. iv, v, vi
D. i, ii, vii
E. ii, iv, v

52. Figure 14-3 shows SCC of the lower lip. Which of the following statements are true?

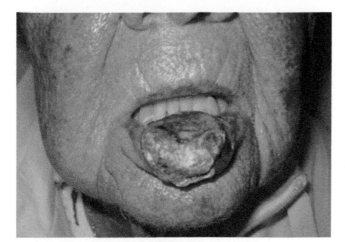

**Figure 14-3**

i. Lower lip defects up to half the length of the lip can be repaired with primary closure.

ii. The Karapandzic flap is a good option for this defect.

iii. The Abbe flap is ideal for central defects of the lip.

iv. The size of the Abbe flap should be designed as half the width of the defect for the lower lip and the same length of the defect for the upper lip reconstruction.

v. The Estlander flap reconstruction is performed in one stage.

vi. The Gillis fan flap will result in superior functional results compared with the Karapandzic flap.

A. i, ii
B. iii, v
C. ii, iv
D. i, iii
E. v, vi

53. In reconstruction of oral cavity and oropharynx defects,
i. Very large defects of buccal mucosa are better left to granulate to avoid trismus.

ii. Muscle-only flaps are better options for tongue reconstruction.

iii. Providing adequate bulk and providing epithelial coverage are equally important goals in reconstruction of the tongue.

iv. The pectoralis major flap is a good choice for oral cavity reconstruction.

v. The radial forearm free flap is the preferred free flap for oral tongue reconstruction in most situations.

vi. Defects larger than half of the soft palate are better served by secondary intention healing than reconstruction.

vii. Most oropharyngeal defects after transoral resection of the tonsil and tumors of the base of the tongue can be left to granulate without the need for reconstruction.

A. i, ii, iv
B. iii, v, vii
C. ii, iii, iv
D. v, vi, vii
E. i, ii, vi

54. The patient shown in Figure 14-4 with SCC of the lower alveolus will require segmental mandibulectomy to remove the entire tumor. Which of the following statements are true?

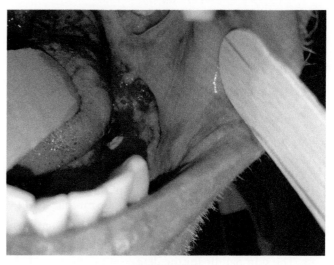

**Figure 14-4**

i. The resultant defect can be reconstructed with primary closure with equally good functional results.

ii. This defect cannot be repaired with a scapular free flap.

iii. The radial forearm osteocutaneous free flap is the best option for bony reconstruction.

iv. For left-sided defects, the left fibula is the better option in terms of the position of the skin paddle and the pedicle.

v. Iliac crest bone is amenable to an osteotomy to form the bone to the defect.

vi. A fibula osteocutaneous free flap and an iliac crest free flap will give the best chance for placement of dental implants and dental rehabilitation.

A. i, ii
B. iii, iv
C. v, vi
D. iv, v
E. i, vi

55. A sagittal view of a patient diagnosed with hypopharyngeal SCC (Figure 14-5) shows complete obstruction. The patient is undergoing a laryngopharyngectomy. The extent of pharyngectomy is not possible to determine before the operation because an endoscope could not be passed through the lesion into the distal esophagus. Which of the following statements are true?

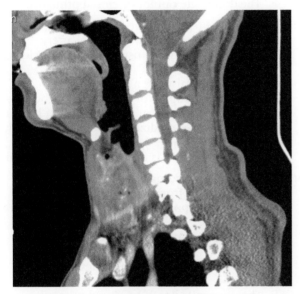

**Figure 14-5**

i. Gastric pull-up is the only option for circumferential defects of the pharynx.
ii. A jejunal free flap will be the best option for voice rehabilitation via tracheoesophageal puncture.
iii. One-stage reconstruction (without controlled pharyngostomy) is not possible in circumferential defects.
iv. The pectoralis major flap is not an option in repair of pharyngeal defects.
v. The anterolateral thigh flap can be used in circumferential defects.
vi. The radial forearm free flap can be used as a patch for repair of large pharyngeal defects.

A. i, ii
B. iii, iv
C. v, vi
D. iv, v
E. i, iii

56. In facial reanimation,
i. Eye rehabilitation is best done with a gold weight.

ii. The gracilis flap can provide dynamic rehabilitation to the orbicularis oris.
iii. It is best to do nerve grafting from the stump of the facial nerve to all the branches.
iv. The nerve to masseter cannot be used as a donor to the gracilis free flap.
v. Delayed nerve grafting is better than immediate nerve grafting.
vi. Nerve XII to nerve VII jump grafting is not an option in midface rehabilitation.

A. i, ii
B. iii, iv
C. v, vi
D. iv, v
E. i, iii

57. In maxillary reconstruction,
i. A deep circumflex iliac crest bone free flap cannot be used to restore the alveolus because the bone is too thick.
ii. If more than one wall of the orbit is missing, reconstruction is required to preserve good function in the eye.
iii. The orbital rim can be restored with a scapular free flap.
iv. Soft tissue–only free flaps such as the rectus flap are not an option in maxillary reconstruction.
v. Hard palate defects should be reconstructed with bony free flaps.
vi. The oral surface of maxillary defects should be restored with cutaneous flaps.

A. i, ii
B. iii, iv
C. v, vi
D. ii, iii
E. i, iv
F. iii, v

58. Which of the following statements are true about reconstructive choices for the surgical defect in the nasal dorsum after removal of SCC (Figure 14-6)?
i. Nasal tip defects are best reconstructed with a transposition flap.
ii. The V-Y advancement flap is a good option for cephalad nasal dorsum defects larger than 2 cm.
iii. The bilobed flap is a good option for the repair of this defect.
iv. The dorsal nasal flap is a good option for younger patients with tighter skin.
v. Large defects of the nasal tip are best reconstructed with a paramedian forehead flap.
vi. A melolabial interpolated flap is a good option for repair of alar defects.

A. i, ii, iii
B. ii, iv, vi
C. i, iii, v
D. iii, v, vi
E. i, ii, iv

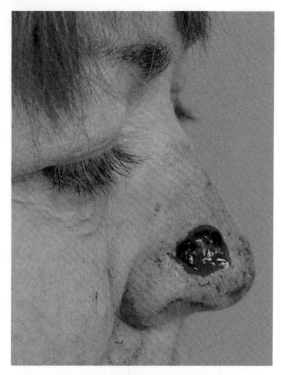

**Figure 14-6**

59. Which vein is not a reliable recipient for venous drainage of a free flap?
    A. External jugular vein
    B. Internal jugular vein
    C. Facial vein
    D. Anterior jugular vein
    E. Middle thyroid vein

60. Which nerve is used in the sensate anterolateral thigh flap?
    A. The medial cutaneous nerve of the thigh is used.
    B. The lateral cutaneous nerve of the thigh is used.
    C. The anterior cutaneous nerve of the thigh is used.
    D. The anterolateral thigh flap cannot be raised as a sensate flap.
    E. Sensory branches of the obturator nerve are used.

61. Which nerve is used in the sensate radial forearm free flap?
    A. The lateral antecubital cutaneous nerve is used.
    B. The sensory branch of the radial nerve is used.
    C. The radial forearm flap cannot be raised as a sensate flap.
    D. The medial antecubital cutaneous nerve is used.
    E. The posterior cutaneous nerve of the forearm is used.

62. Which is true regarding the deltopectoral flap?
    A. The donor site can be closed primarily.
    B. It is the preferred choice for pharyngeal reconstruction.
    C. The blood supply is from the axillary artery.
    D. It should be raised as a musculocutaneous flap to preserve the blood supply.
    E. The distal end of the flap has the most tenuous blood supply.

63. The blood supply to the iliac crest osteocutaneous flap
    A. Is from the external iliac artery.
    B. Travels between the external oblique and internal oblique muscles.
    C. Runs deep to the transversus abdominis muscle.
    D. Travels in a posterior to anterior direction.
    E. Is located on the external surface of the iliac bone.

64. Which is true regarding the lower trapezius island musculocutaneous flap?
    A. It has the same blood supply as the superior trapezius flap.
    B. The blood supply is from the transverse cervical and dorsal scapular arteries.
    C. The blood supply is deep to the scapula.
    D. It has a very short arc of rotation.
    E. The donor site cannot be closed primarily.

65. Which is true regarding the lateral arm flap?
    A. It is based on the recurrent radial artery.
    B. The donor site defect usually cannot be closed primarily.
    C. It cannot be raised as a sensate flap.
    D. The vascular supply of the arm has to be tested before raising the flap to ascertain that harvesting will not jeopardize the blood supply to the arm.
    E. The blood supply is from the profunda brachii.

66. Which is true regarding the palatal island flap?
    A. The pedicle is from the facial artery.
    B. The blood supply from both sides must be preserved.
    C. The blood supply is from the greater palatine artery.
    D. The blood supply is from the lesser palatine artery.
    E. The donor site has to be closed primarily.

67. The blood supply to the skin paddle of the fibula osteocutaneous flap
    A. Is highly unreliable.
    B. Is always anterior to the fibula.
    C. Is always in the posterior intermuscular septum.
    D. Is usually located in the proximal one third of the bone.
    E. Can be better protected with harvesting of a cuff of soleus or flexor hallucis longus muscle.

68. Which is true regarding the parascapular flap?
    A. It is based on the circumflex scapular artery.
    B. It is a musculocutaneous flap.
    C. The blood supply is from the thoracodorsal artery.
    D. It can be raised as a sensate flap.
    E. The donor site is associated with significant morbidity.

69. Which statement is correct in palatal reconstruction?
    A. Larger palatal defects are better fit for a palatal obturator than are smaller defects.

B. Canine teeth are the preferred anchors for obturators.

C. Bony flaps are required for palate reconstruction.

D. The radial forearm free flap is not a good option for reconstruction of the hard palate.

E. Palate reconstruction requires epithelial coverage by the flap.

70. Which is true regarding the fibula free flap?
    A. The blood supply is from the peroneal artery.
    B. The blood supply is from the posterior tibial artery.
    C. The blood supply is from the anterior tibial artery.
    D. Imaging studies to determine the arterial anatomy of the extremity are not necessary before harvesting.
    E. The peroneal artery runs anterior to the interosseous membrane.

71. Which statement is correct in lip reconstruction?
    A. Using local tissue is discouraged because of the increased risk of microstomia.
    B. In V wedge resection, an angle wider than 45 degrees will give better aesthetic results.
    C. Limiting the wedge resection to the limits of lip tissue will achieve better aesthetic results.
    D. The advancement flaps in the Karapandzic flap are designed to be full-thickness.
    E. The Estlander flap will change the position of the oral commissure.

72. Which statement is correct?
    A. The latissimus dorsi flap cannot be raised as a pedicled flap for head and neck reconstruction because the pedicle will not reach to most sites.
    B. The serratus anterior muscle flap is based on the circumflex scapular artery.
    C. Both latissimus dorsi and serratus anterior muscle flaps can be raised based on the thoracodorsal artery.
    D. The distal portion of the latissimus dorsi muscle has the best blood supply for designing the skin paddle.
    E. To reduce shoulder morbidity, the surgeon should preserve the lower portion of the serratus anterior muscle when harvesting the serratus flap.

73. Which is true regarding the rotation flap?
    A. It is not a good options in reconstructing scalp defects.
    B. Chin defects are not good candidates for this flap.
    C. It is better to design a superiorly based flap for face reconstruction.
    D. The length of a rotation flap should be approximately four times the width of the defect in face reconstruction.
    E. It cannot be used in nasal reconstruction.

74. The blood supply to the temporoparietal fascial flap comes from the
    A. Internal maxillary artery.
    B. Deep temporal artery.
    C. Supraorbital artery.
    D. Superficial temporal artery.
    E. Posterior auricular artery.

75. Which is true regarding the submental island flap?
    A. It is preferred for skin grafting the donor site defect.
    B. The blood supply is from the lingual artery.
    C. The blood supply is from the facial artery.
    D. The vascular pedicle is deep to the anterior belly of the digastric.
    E. Bilateral blood supply to the flap should be preserved.

76. Which is true regarding the gracilis flap?
    A. The loss of function of the muscle will cause a noticeable functional deficit in adduction of the thigh.
    B. The nerve supply is from the posterior branch of the obturator nerve.
    C. Peripheral vascular disease in the superficial femoral artery is a contraindication to use of this flap.
    D. The blood supply to the gracilis enters the muscle at the junction of the upper two thirds and lower one third.
    E. The nerve supply is from the anterior branch of the obturator nerve.

77. Advancement flaps
    A. Work better in areas of skin with less elasticity.
    B. Have the greatest tension perpendicular to the proximal border of the flap (the base).
    C. Are not good options for reconstructing cheek defects.
    D. Work well in dorsal nasal defects.
    E. Are good options for repair of forehead defects.

78. Which is true regarding the pectoralis major muscle?
    A. The blood supply is from the pectoral branch of the thoracoacromial artery.
    B. The nerve supply is from the long thoracic nerve.
    C. The main blood supply to the muscle is from the internal mammary artery.
    D. The lateral thoracic artery should be preserved.
    E. The nerve supply is from the axillary nerve.

79. Regarding the osteocutaneous radial forearm flap,
    A. Prophylactic plating is usually not necessary.
    B. Up to 50% of the radial bone can be harvested safely.
    C. The risk of a pathological fracture can be significantly reduced with prophylactic plating.
    D. The harvested bone is usually thick enough to accept dental implants in oromandibular reconstruction.
    E. Not more than 6 cm of bone length can be safely harvested.

80. The blood supply to the superior trapezius flap
    A. Is from the transverse cervical artery.
    B. Is from the dorsal scapular artery.
    C. Is from the paraspinal perforators.
    D. Is from the occipital artery.
    E. Is random.

81. The blood supply to the parascapular flap
    A. Is from the dorsal scapular artery.
    B. Is shared between the parascapular flap and latissimus dorsi flap.
    C. Is not distinct from the serratus anterior flap.
    D. Runs between the teres major and minor muscles.
    E. Is from the angular branch of the thoracodorsal artery.

82. Which one of these defects requires bony reconstruction?
    A. An inferior orbital wall defect after maxillectomy with orbital exenteration
    B. The defect after maxillectomy with orbital preservation without an inferior orbital wall defect
    C. The defect after maxillectomy with orbital preservation and loss of the inferior orbital wall
    D. A purely hard palate defect
    E. A posterior upper alveolar defect

83. In facial reanimation,
    A. Synkinesis can happen if all the branches of the facial nerve are reanastomosed to the main trunk.
    B. Nerve grafting works better in the older patient population.
    C. If a zonal approach to facial reconstruction is used, the upper branch is rehabilitated with nerve grafts.
    D. The midface cannot be dynamically rehabilitated.
    E. The lower face can only be rehabilitated with dynamic reanimation.

84. Which one is not a transposition flap?
    A. Rhombic flap
    B. Bilobed flap
    C. Note flap
    D. Dorsal nasal flap
    E. Z-plasty

85. Which is true regarding the rectus abdominis flap?
    A. The skin island can only be designed vertically.
    B. The skin island can only be designed transversely.
    C. This flap is not a good option for large skull base defects.
    D. The flap can be used in a contaminated field.
    E. This flap is not a good option for total glossectomy defect reconstruction.

86. Which is true regarding repair of laryngectomy defects?
    A. The myocutaneous pectoralis muscle flap is not as good of an option as a patch.
    B. In salvage laryngectomy after definitive chemoradiation therapy failure, primary closure is the most successful method in limiting occurrence of fistulas.
    C. The anterolateral thigh flap is not a viable option for circumferential pharyngeal defects.
    D. If the skin of the neck has to be excised with the tumor, the pectoralis major myocutaneous flap with split-thickness skin grafts is a viable option.
    E. In salvage laryngectomy after chemoradiation therapy failure, free flaps or pectoralis major flaps are only recommended if there is not enough tissue for primary closure.

87. Which one is not a pivotal flap?
    A. Bilobed flap
    B. Rhombic flap
    C. V-Y flap
    D. Z-plasty
    E. Paramedian forehead flap

88. Which is true regarding interpolated flaps?
    A. They cannot have a random blood supply.
    B. The pedicle can pass over but not under the intervening tissues.
    C. Reconstruction using these flaps cannot be performed in one stage.
    D. They can be harvested in regions of redundant tissue.
    E. The base is contiguous with the defect.

89. In reconstruction of oropharynx defects,
    A. Most defects after transoral resection of the base of the tongue or tonsil will require reconstruction with a flap.
    B. A palatal island flap can be used to reconstruct the soft palate in salvage situations.
    C. The radial forearm free flap is not a good option in reconstructing soft palate defects larger than 50%.
    D. Tonsil and lateral pharyngeal wall defects in salvage situations are better repaired with free tissue transfer.
    E. An obturator is a good option for large soft palate defects.

90. Which one of these defects is better reconstructed with a free flap?
    A. A glossectomy defect less than 30%
    B. A lateral marginal mandibulectomy defect in a nonirradiated patient with more than 1 cm of thickness of remaining mandible
    C. A mucosal defect of the floor of the mouth
    D. A mucoperiosteal defect of the hard palate
    E. A hemiglossectomy defect

91. In scalp defect repair,
    A. Advancement flaps are good options.
    B. A split-thickness skin graft can be safely applied to the skull without periosteal coverage.
    C. A split-thickness skin graft will achieve the best aesthetic results.
    D. Rotation flaps are a good option.
    E. Primary closure can be achieved in defects as large as 6 cm.

92. Melolabial flaps
    A. Are a very good option for repair of alar defects.
    B. Can only be superiorly based.
    C. Can only be inferiorly based.
    D. Have the best match for skin on the dorsum of the nose.
    E. Cannot be used as advancement flaps.

93. Which is true regarding repair of buccal mucosal defects?
    A. Secondary intention healing is the best option for defects as large as 5 cm.

B. Full-thickness large defects of the mucosa and buccinator muscle are better treated with acellular collagen matrix (AlloDerm) or split-thickness skin grafts.
C. Buccal mucosa defects should always be reconstructed with distant tissues to avoid trismus.
D. The parotid gland duct (Stensen duct) should be found and marsupialized if the parotid gland is preserved.
E. The parotid gland duct can be safely ligated.

94. Which vessel is not a first choice option in microvascular anastomosis in the neck?
A. Superior thyroid artery
B. Facial artery
C. Lingual artery
D. Transverse cervical artery
E. Occipital artery

95. Which flap is the better option in reconstruction of large full-thickness (>10 cm) scalp defects?
A. An anterolateral thigh flap
B. A latissimus dorsi flap and a split-thickness skin graft
C. A lower trapezius island flap
D. A vertical rectus abdominis musculocutaneous flap
E. A parascapular flap

96. Which is true regarding the jejunal free flap?
A. It can only be used as a tubed graft.
B. The vascular pedicle can be severed after the graft has established blood supply from surrounding neck tissue.
C. Any portion of the jejunum from the ligament of Treitz to the ileum can be used.
D. The orientation of the segment of the intestine is not an important factor.
E. The plicae circularis of the jejunum will disappear after some time.

97. Which is true regarding the supraclavicular island flap?
A. It is based on the supraclavicular artery, which is a branch of the thoracoacromial artery.
B. Radical neck dissection is not a contraindication to use of this flap.
C. The donor site cannot be closed primarily in most cases.
D. It is not an option for pharyngeal reconstruction.
E. It is based on a branch of the transverse cervical artery.

98. Which is true regarding cheek reconstruction?
A. The flap incisions should be designed perpendicular to the relaxed skin tension lines.
B. If more than 50% of an aesthetic unit is lost, the other half should be used to reconstruct the defect.
C. For lesions with a high risk of recurrence, it is better to use skin grafting or primary closure.
D. A cervicofacial rotation advancement flap is not a good option for zygomatic cheek defects.
E. Small- to medium-sized medial cheek defects are not good candidates for primary closure.

99. Which statement is true regarding the use of skin grafts in head and neck reconstruction?
A. Split-thickness skin grafts should always be meshed to improve graft uptake.
B. Full-thickness skin grafts cannot be harvested from the neck.
C. If no periosteum is left on the skull, the outer table can be drilled to expose cancellous bone to improve the take of split-thickness skin grafts.
D. Acellular matrix grafts such as Alloderm (Lifecell, Bridgewater, NJ) achieve better results than skin grafts in the resurfacing of oral cavity defects.
E. Use of a wound V.A.C. system is not safe on skin grafts on the skull.

100. Which statement is correct?
A. Split-thickness skin grafts are more resistant to contraction than full-thickness skin grafts.
B. Skin grafts are more appropriate for reconstruction of areas of the face with thicker skin.
C. Full-thickness skin grafts are less likely to fail in a poorly vascularized recipient bed.
D. Full-thickness skin grafts provide better color match than split-thickness skin grafts.
E. Full-thickness skin grafts are not appropriate for reconstruction of concave surfaces/defects.

## Answers

| | | |
|---|---|---|
| 1. F | 23. F | 45. T |
| 2. T | 24. T | 46. T |
| 3. T | 25. T | 47. F |
| 4. T | 26. F | 48. T |
| 5. T | 27. F | 49. T |
| 6. T | 28. T | 50. F |
| 7. F | 29. T | 51. D |
| 8. T | 30. F | 52. C |
| 9. F | 31. F | 53. B |
| 10. F | 32. F | 54. C |
| 11. F | 33. T | 55. C |
| 12. T | 34. F | 56. A |
| 13. F | 35. F | 57. D |
| 14. F | 36. T | 58. D |
| 15. F | 37. T | 59. D |
| 16. T | 38. F | 60. B |
| 17. F | 39. T | 61. A |
| 18. F | 40. T | 62. E |
| 19. T | 41. T | 63. C |
| 20. F | 42. T | 64. B |
| 21. F | 43. F | 65. E |
| 22. F | 44. T | 66. C |

| | | |
|---|---|---|
| 67. E | 79. C | 91. D |
| 68. A | 80. C | 92. A |
| 69. B | 81. D | 93. D |
| 70. A | 82. C | 94. E |
| 71. C | 83. A | 95. B |
| 72. C | 84. D | 96. C |
| 73. C | 85. D | 97. E |
| 74. D | 86. D | 98. C |
| 75. E | 87. C | 99. C |
| 76. E | 88. D | 100. D |
| 77. E | 89. D | |
| 78. A | 90. E | |

# Core Knowledge

## LOCAL FLAPS

- Advancement flaps have a linear configuration. They work by sliding adjacent tissues toward the defect. The greatest tension is perpendicular to the distal border of the flap. This flap works best in areas of skin with greater elasticity. Advancement flaps can be unipedicled, bipedicled, V-Y, Y-V, or island. Unipedicled flaps work well for the forehead, helical rim, upper and lower eyelids, and medial cheek. Mucosal advancement flaps work well for vermilion reconstruction. The flap-to-defect ratio is usually around 3:1 for unipedicled flaps.

- Rotation flaps are pivotal flaps with a curvilinear configuration. They are best suited for the repair of a triangular defect. When a rotation flap is designed for the face, the length of incision should be four times the width of the defect. Rotation flaps are good options for small- to medium-sized scalp defects, large cheek defects, and dorsal nasal defects.

- Transposition flaps are pivotal flaps that have a linear configuration. They can be designed with the borders of the flap away from the defect (in contrast to rotation flaps). Transposition flaps are some of the most common flaps used in the reconstruction of head and neck skin defects. Bilobed, rhombic, Z-plasty, and note flaps are all different types of transposition flaps.

- A bilobed flap is a double transposition flap that shares a single base. Bilobed flaps are good options for lateral nasal reconstruction and can also be used in cheek defects.

- A rhombic flap is an advancement and pivotal transposition flap. A rhombus is a square tilted to one side. Hiding the scars of the flap is not always easy. Rhombic flaps are most commonly used in cheek and temple defects.

- Melolabial flaps are flaps harvested from the skin of the cheek (nasolabial fold) lateral to the melolabial crease. Because of rich vascularity, they can be superiorly or inferiorly based. Because of excellent color and texture match, they are ideal for repair of the lips, lateral region of the nose, and alar defects. The skin of the flap can be too thick for superior dorsal nasal defects and is not the best option. They can be used as advancement flaps, pivotal flaps (rotational or transposition), or interpolated flaps.

- The paramedian forehead flap is one of the most widely used flaps in nasal reconstruction. This flap is based on the surpratrochlear artery and is usually used as an axial, interpolated flap for reconstruction of the nasal tip. The pedicle can be divided safely after 2 to 3 weeks. The disadvantages of this flap are the need for a two-stage operation and the donor site scar.

- The cervicofacial flap (Mustardé) is an advancement, pivotal flap that is usually used in the repair of large facial defects. The flap is designed with an incision in the preauricular region toward the posterior part of the neck to utilize the skin of the neck. This flap is always inferiorly based so that the use of neck skin is maximized and lymphatic drainage is facilitated.

## REGIONAL FLAPS

- The pectoralis major flap is one of the most reliable and versatile flaps used in head and neck surgery. This flap is based on the pectoral branch of the thoracoacromial artery, which is a branch of the axillary artery. The pedicle is located medial to the tendon of the pectoralis minor muscle. This flap can be raised as a muscle only or as a musculocutaneous flap. When it is used as a musculocutaneous flap, a more distal (caudal) skin paddle will provide a larger arc of rotation. The pectoralis major flap is a very good option for reconstructing large skin defects of the neck and providing coverage to the major vessels after radical neck dissection or in postirradiated neck tissue because it is not part of the radiation field. The pectoralis major flap is commonly used for repair of pharyngeal defects after total laryngectomy, especially in the settings of salvage laryngectomy after definitive chemoradiation failure. This flap is not an ideal option for the reconstruction of oral cavity defects.

- The trapezius flap can be designed as two distinct musculocutaneous flaps. The superior trapezius flap is based on the paraspinal perforators. It is a highly reliable flap but has a short arc of rotation. The blood supply to this flap is not affected by prior neck dissection. This flap can be used in the repair of posterolateral defects of the neck that do not extend more medially than the midline. The lower musculocutaneous trapezius island flap is designed over the inferior aspect of the muscle between midline and the medial border of the scapula. The blood supply for the flap is from the transverse cervical artery and the dorsal scapular artery. This flap is thin and pliable and has a large arc of rotation. It can be used in reconstruction of lateral skull, midface, neck, and oral cavity defects. If a prior neck dissection is performed on the side of the flap, the surgeon must verify the patency of the transverse cervical and dorsal scapular arteries before harvesting. In most cases, radical neck dissection is a contraindication to the use of the lower trapezius island flap.

- The deltopectoral flap is a medially based fasciocutaneous flap. The blood supply to this flap comes from the parasternal perforators that branch off the internal mammary artery. The deltopectoral flap has been utilized in the reconstruction of pharyngeal, neck, cheek, and even oral cavity defects. The disadvantages of this flap include unreliable distal flap viability, a multistage procedure, and the need for skin grafting of the donor site. The availability of free flaps has significantly reduced the use of this flap.

- The submental island flap is a fasciocutaneous flap based on the submental artery and vein, branching off the facial artery and vein. This flap provides a good color and texture match for the repair of lower and midfacial skin defects. In addition, the donor site can be well camouflaged by primary closure. The submental island flap can also be used in the repair of oral cavity, oropharynx, and larynx mucosal defects. Because of the proximity of the vascular pedicle to level I lymph nodes, if these nodes have to be dissected for oncological reasons, the use of this flap is not recommended. During the harvest of the flap, it is important to avoid injury to the marginal mandibular branch of the facial nerve.

- The palatal island flap is mucoperiosteal flap based on the greater palatine artery, a branch of the internal maxillary artery. Almost the entire mucosa of the hard palate can be harvested with the use of only one arterial pedicle. The exposed bone of the donor site is left open to granulate by secondary intention. This flap has been used for the repair of retromolar trigone and tonsillar fossa defects. It is also a good option for soft palate repair after resection of minor salivary gland tumors. The use of this flap is not recommended in postirradiation and salvage situations because of the possibility of development of osteoradionecrosis of the exposed bone of the hard palate.

- The temporalis flap has a wide variety of uses in head and neck reconstruction. The temporalis flap is a pedicled flap that uses different parts of the temporalis muscle for different reconstructive purposes. The blood supply to the temporalis muscle is from the deep temporal artery, a branch of the internal maxillary artery. The nerve supply to the muscle is from V3. Temporalis muscle can be used as a turnover flap for reconstructing defects of the lateral skull base, orbit, and maxilla and for repair of oroantral fistulas. Because it readily accepts split-thickness skin grafts, it can also be used in reconstructing skin defects of the midface or full-thickness buccal mucosal defects. Temporalis muscle is also used in facial rehabilitation.

In this capacity, a portion of the muscle or its tendon is transferred and inserted into the nasolabial fold or orbicularis oris. For dynamic facial rehabilitation to be achieved, it is important to preserve the nerve supply to the muscle.

- The suprascapular island flap is a fasciocutaneous pedicled flap based on the supraclavicular branch of the transverse cervical artery. The flap can be raised as large as 15 × 7 cm, and the donor site can be primarily closed. This flap has been used in a variety of head and neck defects, such as pharyngeal, oral cavity, neck skin, and temporal bone defects. Prior neck dissection and radical neck dissection with injury to the transverse cervical arteries are contraindications to the use of this flap.

## FREE FLAPS

- The temporoparietal fascia flap is an ultrathin, pliable, highly vascular fascial flap based on the superficial temporal artery and vein. This flap is resistant to infection, which makes it a good choice for use in postirradiated and infected fields. During the harvest of the flap, the surgeon must avoid injuring the frontal branch of the facial nerve. Meticulous dissection and preservation of hair follicles will reduce the risk of temporal alopecia after harvesting. This flap has been used for a variety of defects as a pedicled or free flap. It can be used in auricular, orbital, and temporal bone reconstruction. It has also been used to drape over cartilage grafts in auricular and laryngeal reconstruction and to create a bed on which split-thickness skin grafts can be attached.

- The lateral arm flap is a fasciocutaneous flap based on the posterior radial collateral artery, which is one of the two terminal branches of the profunda brachii. This donor site has the advantages of being able to be closed primarily in most cases and avoidance of compromise to the perfusion of the upper extremity when the flap is harvested. The dissection can be more difficult than the radial forearm flap. This flap can be raised as a sensate flap if the posterior cutaneous nerve of the arm is used. This flap can be used in the repair of a variety of head and neck defects such as those in the oral cavity, midface, and neck. With the increased use of the anterolateral thigh flap, this donor site has been used less frequently.

- The radial forearm free flap is one of the most widely used free flaps in head and neck reconstruction. It can be raised as a fasciocutaneous or osteocutaneous flap. The palmaris longus tendon and lateral antecubital cutaneous nerve can also be harvested with the flap for use as a sensate flap. The flap is based on the radial artery and vena comitanes; however, the cephalic vein, if patent, can be used for venous drainage. Before the flap is harvested, an Allen test is mandatory to ascertain the adequacy of blood flow to the hand after disruption of the radial artery. As much as 40% of the radius can be harvested safely with the flap. Most surgeons recommend prophylactic plating after bone harvest so that pathological fractures do not occur. During harvesting, the sensory branches of the radial nerve should be identified and preserved to avoid numbness in the area of the anatomical snuffbox. The radial forearm flap is used in a variety of head and neck defects. It is the preferred choice for repair of glossectomy defects. Other oral cavity defects for which this flap can be used include large lip defects and those involving the gingiva, buccal mucosa, floor of the mouth, and hard and soft palates. Repair of defects of the pharynx and neck and face skin and orbital cavity resurfacing are other examples of the utility of the radial forearm flap. The osteocutaneous flap can be used in total nose reconstruction and mandibular and maxillary reconstruction. The bone is very thin, and it is unlikely to successfully accept dental implants, particularly in women.

- The anterolateral thigh flap is one of the most versatile free flaps in the armamentarium of head and neck reconstruction. The anterolateral thigh flap can be raised as a fasciocutaneous or musculofasciocutaneous flap. A cuff of the vastus lateralis muscle can be harvested with the flap when more volume is needed. This flap can also be raised as a sensate flap by harvesting the lateral femoral cutaneous nerve. The anterolateral thigh flap is based on the cutaneous perforators of the descending branch of the lateral circumflex femoral artery, which is a branch of the profunda femoris. The most common site for the cutaneous perforators is around 3 cm from the midpoint of the line between the anterosuperior iliac spine and the superolateral border of the patella. The profunda femoris system is preserved even in cases of severe superficial femoris artery (peripheral vascular) disease. This flap can be raised with a width of 8 to 9 cm for circumferential pharyngeal repair, and the donor site can still be primarily closed. The anterolateral thigh flap has been widely used in the repair of a variety of head and neck defects. Oral cavity defects, total glossectomy defects, large pharyngeal defects, and defects of the maxilla, temporal bone, and lateral skull base can all be repaired with the use of this flap. Donor site morbidity is extremely low; however, in some individuals as a result of body habitus, the flap might be thick. In addition, the color match between the thigh and head and neck and facial skin is inferior to other cutaneous flaps (e.g., the parascapular flap).

- The rectus abdominis free flap is a versatile flap for the reconstruction of a variety of head and neck defects. This flap can be harvested as a muscle only or as a musculocutaneous flap. The rectus muscle receives its blood supply from the superior and inferior deep epigastric vessels. The deep inferior epigastric vessels are larger and are the preferred pedicle for this flap. The skin around the umbilicus has the most robust blood supply and is usually used as the skin paddle in musculocutaneous flaps. The skin paddle can be oriented transversely (transverse rectus abdominis musculocutaneous [TRAM] flap) or vertically (vertical rectus abdominis musculocutaneous [VRAM] flap). The rectus abdominis can be used in a wide variety of situations. Most commonly it is used in repairing

defects of the skull base when a watertight cerebral spinal fluid (CSF) seal is needed and a large cavity is created after resection of the tumor. It can also be used in maxillary reconstruction, facial and neck skin reconstruction, and in defects resulting from a total glossectomy. This flap is very reliable and also can be used in infected, contaminated fields.

- The gracilis flap is primarily used for dynamic facial rehabilitation after facial paralysis. The gracilis muscle is a long, thin muscle that receives its blood supply from the adductor artery, a branch of the profunda femoris. The vascular pedicle enters the muscle at the junction of its upper third and lower two thirds (8 to 10 cm inferior to the pubic tubercle). The nerve supply is from the anterior branch of the obturator nerve, which enters the muscle 2 to 3 cm cephalad to the entry point of the vascular pedicle. The muscle is usually sutured between the temporalis fascia and the orbicularis oris at the corner of the mouth. The muscle is reinnervated with the use of a cross facial nerve graft from the contralateral side of the face or with the use of the nerve to the masseter.

- The jejunal free flap is based on the mesenteric branches of the superior mesenteric artery. Any portion of the jejunum can be harvested from the ligament of Treitz to the ileum. This flap can be used as a tube conduit for circumferential pharyngeal defects or as a patch if the antimesenteric side of the jejunum is opened. The jejunum is unique in that the viability of the flap will always remain dependent on the vascular pedicle. Therefore interruption of the pedicle at any time will result in flap necrosis. Unlike gastric rugae in gastric pull-up cases, the plicae circularis of the jejunum will never disappear and can cause food trapping and halitosis. The voice rehabilitation results of the jejunal free flap are conspicuously lower than other free flaps. Although this is a reliable flap, the use of the jejunal free flap has decreased with the advent of the tubed anterolateral thigh flap, which is associated with less morbidity.

- The fibula free flap is the most widely used bony flap for reconstruction of large mandibular defects. This flap can be raised as a bone only or as an osteocutaneous flap. Approximately 22 to 25 cm of bone can be harvested, which is adequate for the reconstruction of the entire mandible. This flap is based on the peroneal artery and vein. Because of the variation in anatomy and also because of the possibility of peripheral vascular disease, preoperative imaging such as angiography or magnetic resonance angiography is highly recommended. Leaving approximately 6 cm of bone proximally and distally will maintain the stability of the knee and ankle joint and also reduces the risk of injury to the common peroneal nerve. The most reliable cutaneous perforators to the skin of the calf are located around the junction of the middle and lower third of the fibula. The skin perforators can run through the posterior septum (septal) or soleus muscle (musculocutaneous). Harvesting a cuff of soleus and flexor hallucis longus will reduce the risk of injury to the cutaneous perforators. The main use of the fibula free flap in the head and neck is for mandibular reconstruction. Osteotomies can be safely performed in the fibula, and the bone has adequate height and bicortical strength to receive dental implants. The fibula is the preferred method for long segment and anterior mandibular defects. The fibula has also been used in maxillary gingival reconstruction.

- Scapular and subscapular system free flaps include a variety of muscular, musculocutaneous, and osteo-musculocutaneous flaps. All of these flaps are based on the scapular artery and vein; therefore more than one flap can be raised on one pedicle. Latissimus dorsi and serratus anterior flaps are based on the thoraco-dorsal artery and are usually raised as muscle-only flaps, but they can also be raised as musculocutaneous and osteomusculocutaneous flaps (a rib with the serratus flap and scapula with the latissimus flap). Because of the large size of the latissimus muscle, this flap is a good option for large scalp defects. Donor site defects as wide as 7 cm can be closed primarily, which is one of the advantages of this flap. The parascapular flap is based on the circumflex scapular artery. Regardless of the extent of the flap, it should always be centered over the infraspinatus fossa (the triangular space between the teres major, teres minor, and long head of the triceps). The parascapular flap is purely fasciocutaneous and does not cause any disruption of the shoulder muscles. In addition, the color match is better than with use of the anterolateral thigh flap. The scapular tip bony flap is based on the angular branch of the thoracodorsal artery. Up to 10 to 14 cm of bone can be harvested from the lateral border of the scapula. The scapular tip can also be harvested to repair total palatectomy defects. The scapula is not as thick as the fibula and is more suitable for the repair of lateral mandibular defects. Dental implants can usually be placed in the scapula. Because of the versatility of this system, scapula and parascapular system flaps have been used in most head and neck defects. The positioning of the patient during the operation can be a disadvantage as can be the fact that, in most cases, simultaneous harvesting of the flap cannot be performed.

- The iliac crest osteocutaneous and osteomusculocutaneous flaps are based on the deep circumflex iliac artery and vein, which are branches of the internal iliac artery and vein, respectively. The iliac crest provides the thickest stock of vascularized bone for oromandibular reconstruction. In addition to the bone, the internal oblique muscle and skin of the groin can be harvested based on the same pedicle. The extent of skin paddle can extend from the anterosuperior iliac spine to 9 cm posterior. The main use of the iliac crest flap is in mandibular and maxillary reconstruction. Because of the thickness of the bone, dental implants can be more effectively placed in this flap than in all other bony flaps. The major disadvantage of this flap lies in its donor site morbidity (e.g., abdominal wall hernias, donor site pain, and disability).

## RECONSTRUCTION TOPICS

- Facial nerve reanimation is one the challenging topics in head and neck reconstruction. The goal is to restore critical functions (e.g., eye closure and oral competence) and symmetry as much as possible. If simple, immediate interposition nerve grafting is not possible, a variety of reconstruction techniques are available. In general, immediate nerve reanastomosis or nerve interposition grafting (e.g., greater auricular or sural), especially in younger patients, will give the best results. If the proximal facial nerve is not available, a hypoglossal-to-facial-nerve graft is often used. A downside of anastomosing all branches of the facial nerve to the main trunk is the development of synkinesis. In the zonal approach to facial rehabilitation, the upper face is rehabilitated with a brow lift for the frontal branch and a gold weight or lateral tarsorrhaphy for the palpebral branch. The gold weight will give a very satisfactory result and better eyelid closure. For the midface, static slings, a temporalis tendon transfer, and a gracilis dynamic free flap can be used. For reinnervation of the gracilis flap, either a cross-facial nerve graft from the contralateral facial nerve or anastomosis to the nerve to the masseter can be used. For the lower face, chemodenervation of the contralateral side (e.g., with botox) can achieve symmetry. Digastric muscle transfer to strengthen the affected side has also been used.

- Nasal reconstruction has undergone significant recent evolution. The main principles are the use of color- and texture-matched skin, restoration of the contour of the nose with cartilage and bone grafts, and restoration of the inner lining with an epithelial surface. Attention to aesthetic units in the nose is very important. If most of the skin of one unit is missing, it is better to replace the entire unit. Incisions for local flaps are best placed in the borders of aesthetic units rather than in the middle of one. A variety of local and regional flaps can be used with a combination of cartilage grafts from auricular or septal cartilages. Alar defects are best restored with cartilage grafts or composite skin–cartilage grafts from the ear. Lateral defects can be repaired with bilobed flaps. Medial defects can be repaired with nasal advancement flaps. For bigger defects, the paramedian forehead flap is a good, time-tested option. For a total rhinectomy defect, an osteocutaneous free flap or sometimes a full prosthesis will achieve satisfactory results.

- Lip reconstruction is based on the preservation of oral competence, the avoidance of microstomia, and the preservation of aesthetics. Local tissues are strongly preferred because they provide a better color match, better function, and superior cosmetic results. For small superficial defects, primary closure or mucosal advancement flaps will suffice. Full-thickness defects, depending on the location and extent, can be repaired by a variety of techniques. Full-thickness defects up to one third of the lower lip can be reconstructed by wedge resection and primary closure. When the wedge is designed, the angle should not be wider than 30 degrees and the wedge should not extend beyond the lip tissue. For defects larger than one third, a variety of local flaps are used. For central defects, the Karapandzic flap is a popular choice. The advantage of this flap is that it preserves neurovascular bundles to the flap, thus achieving superior functional results. For lateral defects, the Abbe or Estlander flaps can be used. Abbe flap reconstruction is done in one stage, but Estlander flap reconstruction has to be performed in two stages because the pedicle must be preserved for 2 to 3 weeks. When the Abbe and Estlander flaps are designed, the size of the flap is measured as half of the defect for lower lip reconstruction and the same size as the defect for upper lip reconstruction. Very large, full-thickness lip defects might require free flap reconstruction (e.g., from the radial forearm).

- For cheek reconstruction, the cheek is divided into four separate aesthetic subunits: medial, lateral, zygomatic, and buccal. If more than 50% of a subunit is missing, it is usually better to reconstruct the entire unit. The incisions are best placed at the borders of each subunit or, if not possible, parallel to the relaxed tension skin lines. For small to midsize medial defects, primary closure can give very good aesthetic results. Rhombic flaps can be used for a variety of cheek defects. For larger zygomatic or lateral defects, the cervicofacial rotation flap is a good option.

- In oral cavity reconstruction, the main principle is to preserve the functions of swallowing and speech. In general, for large, deep defects, it is better to provide adequate epithelial coverage to prevent orocutaneous fistulas and also excessive scarring that can result in trismus and a tethered tongue. For oral tongue defects larger than 30%, most surgeons advocate the radial forearm free flap. It provides enough bulk and epithelial coverage and a very pliable skin paddle. For floor of the mouth, buccal mucosa, soft palate, and gingival defects without bony defects, the radial forearm is again a very good choice. In repair of the buccal mucosa, small defects in patients who have not received radiation therapy can be repaired primarily or with split-thickness skin grafts or acellular collagen matrix (AlloDerm). For larger defects, the radial forearm free flap is a good option. For through-and-through defects, rectus abdominis, pectoralis major, or other musculocutaneous or myogenous flaps can be used. Attention to the parotid gland duct is necessary. If the duct is in the field of resection, it should be found and reanastomosed to the mucosa (marsupialized), otherwise the risk of salivary complications (e.g., sialocele or sialadenitis) will be increased. For palatal defects, one can use soft tissue–only flaps to avoid oroantral fistulas; however, for total palatectomy defects, it might be necessary to perform bony reconstruction. Obturators can be used effectively in smaller defects, especially in dentate patients. The canine teeth are the most secure anchor for obturators. Mandibular reconstruction is best achieved with bony replacement. The best options are from the fibula and iliac crest, which provide the best bone stock for possible dental implant placement. For lateral defects, the scapula can also be used. The radial forearm

osteocutaneous flap has the thinnest bone and is better for older patients in whom dental rehabilitation is not a priority. Lack of bony reconstruction or delayed reconstruction will cause mandibular swing, malocclusion, and inferior functional results. Maxillary reconstruction is more complex, depending on the type and extent of the defect. If more than one wall of the orbit is missing, reconstruction is required. The orbital floor is best reconstructed with a bony reconstruction technique. The orbital rim can be reconstructed with a scapula, radial forearm osteocutaneous, or fibula flap. The maxillary alveolus can also be reconstructed with bone from the scapula, fibula, or iliac crest. Soft tissue–only repair is still used in large maxillary defects (e.g., with use of the rectus abdominis); however, the long-term results might not be as encouraging as with bony reconstruction.

- Pharyngeal reconstruction has become more common now that the incidence of salvage laryngectomy after chemoradiation therapy failure has increased. In salvage cases, most centers report superior results in terms of avoidance of pharyngocutaneous fistulas and the return of swallowing function with the use of free flaps or the pectoralis major flap. The radial forearm or anterolateral thigh are the preferred flaps for reconstruction of the neopharynx. For circumferential defects, jejunum, gastric pull-up, tubed anterolateral thigh, or tubed radial forearm can be used. If the level of the defect extends to the entire cervical esophagus or past the thoracic inlet, the gastric pull-up might be a better option. The use of jejunum or gastric conduit is associated with poorer quality voice rehabilitation after tracheoesophageal puncture. In contrast, most defects after transoral resection of oropharynx cancers or laryngeal cancers can be left open to granulate without the need for reconstruction.

## SUGGESTED READING

Baker SR. Local flaps in facial reconstruction. Philadelphia: Mosby; 2007.

Brown JS, Shaw RJ. Reconstruction of the maxilla and midface: introducing a new classification. Lancet Oncol 2010;11(10):1001–8.

Chiu ES, Liu PH, Friedlander PL. Supraclavicular artery island flap for head and neck oncologic reconstruction: indications, complications, and outcomes. Plast Reconstr Surg 2009;124(1):115–23.

Miles BA, Gilbert RW. Maxillary reconstruction with the scapular angle osteomyogenous free flap. Arch Otolaryngol Head Neck Surg 2011;137(11):1130–5.

Shah JP, Haribhakti V, Loree TR, Sutaria P. Complications of the pectoralis major myocutaneous flap in head and neck reconstruction. Am J Surg 1990;160(4):352–5.

Shah JP, Patel SG, Singh B. Jatin Shah's head and neck surgery and oncology. 4th ed. Philadelphia: Mosby; 2012.

Stern SJ, Goepfert H, Clayman G, Byers R, Wolf P. Orbital preservation in maxillectomy. Otolaryngol Head Neck Surg 1993;109(1):111–5.

Urken ML. Multidisciplinary head & neck reconstruction: a defect-oriented approach. Philadelphia: Wolters Kluwer Health/Lippincott Williams & Wilkins; 2010.

Urken ML. Atlas of regional and free flaps for head and neck reconstruction: flap harvest and insetting. Philadelphia: Wolters Kluwer Health/Lippincott Williams & Wilkins; 2012.

Yu P, Hanasono MM, Skoracki RJ, Baumann DP, Lewin JS, Weber RS, et al. Pharyngoesophageal reconstruction with the anterolateral thigh flap after total laryngopharyngectomy. Cancer 2010;116(7):1718–24.

# 15 Oncological Dentistry: Maxillofacial Prosthetics and Implants

## Questions

### TRUE/FALSE

1. The mucosal surfaces of the oral cavity are exposed to significant doses of radiation therapy during treatment of most tumors, except those of the larynx, hypopharynx, and thyroid. (T/F)

2. Major salivary glands are permanently altered at doses greater than 25 Gy. (T/F)

3. The risk of developing osteoradionecrosis of the jaw is greatly increased at doses greater than 55 Gy. (T/F)

4. Numerous metallic restorations in a patient's mouth can cause increased mucositis from scatter radiation. (T/F)

5. Ideally, dental extractions should occur at least 21 days before radiation therapy. (T/F)

6. After radiation therapy to any of the major salivary glands, patients should use a fluoride supplement for the rest of their lives. (T/F)

7. Dental implants in the radiation therapy treatment field must be removed before commencement of therapy. (T/F)

8. Dental implants are absolutely contraindicated after radiation therapy. (T/F)

9. After radiation therapy, hyperbaric oxygen must be used before extraction or placement of implants to eliminate the risk of osteoradionecrosis. (T/F)

10. The accepted hyperbaric oxygen therapy regimen after radiation therapy but before oral surgery consists of 20 "dives," the oral surgical procedure, then 10 dives. (T/F)

11. Osteoradionecrosis is more common in the mandibular arch than in the maxillary arch. (T/F)

12. Radiation therapy treatment fields including muscles of mastication can result in trismus. (T/F)

13. Osteoradionecrosis can occur spontaneously. (T/F)

14. The risk of osteoradionecrosis is lifelong. (T/F)

15. Advanced osteoradionecrosis that is unresponsive to curettage and antibiotics may require segmental resection and reconstruction. (T/F)

16. Patients should be instructed to see their dentist/hygienist more frequently than every 6 months after receiving radiation therapy. (T/F)

17. Osteoradionecrosis seen on radiographs can mimic persistent or recurrent disease. (T/F)

18. When prosthetic rehabilitation is chosen, maxillary defects are best rehabilitated in three phases: surgical, interim, and definitive obturator. (T/F)

19. The surgical obturator is intended to stabilize surgical packing, aid in wound isolation, and allow the patient to speak and swallow, usually without a nasogastric tube. (T/F)

20. Successful fabrication of a functional maxillary obturator is based on the principles of retention, stability, and support. (T/F)

21. Dental implants placed at the time of ablative surgery are preferable because 6 to 8 weeks of healing are necessary before the start of radiation therapy, if needed. (T/F)

22. Obturators are not designed to restore speech or swallowing or improve cosmetic appearance by providing lip and cheek support. (T/F)

23. Obturators cannot replace the orbital floor because the distance is too great, and the normal interincisal opening will not permit it. (T/F)

24. Despite the best possible fit, obturators will always have some leakage because they do not provide a hermetic seal. (T/F)

25. Flap reconstruction can make wearing a prosthesis impossible if there is too much bulk. (T/F)

26. Electing prosthetic rehabilitation over flap reconstruction allows for direct visual examination of the defect for recurrence. (T/F)

27. The palatopharyngeal sphincter is formed by the soft palate, lateral pharyngeal walls, and posterior pharyngeal wall. (T/F)

28. The inability of the palatopharyngeal sphincter to separate the nasopharynx from the oropharynx is known as velopharyngeal inadequacy. (T/F)

29. The inability of the soft palate to elevate superiorly to form the palatopharyngeal sphincter is known as velopharyngeal incompetency. (T/F)

30. When the soft palate is anatomically deficient and results in an incomplete velopharyngeal sphincter, it is known as velopharyngeal insufficiency. (T/F)

31. Patients with acquired defects of the soft palate can potentially be affected by velopharyngeal incompetency and velopharyngeal insufficiency. (T/F)

32. Bulky flaps will not impede access to the acquired soft palate defect, which makes prosthetic rehabilitation easier. (T/F)

33. Completely edentulous patients needing soft palate obturators fare much better than dentate/partially dentate patients. (T/F)

34. Implants can greatly increase stability, thereby increasing the efficacy of a soft palate obturator for partially dentate or completely edentulous patients. (T/F)

35. The Passavant ridge can be seen in Figure 15-1 protruding from the lateral pharyngeal walls. (T/F)

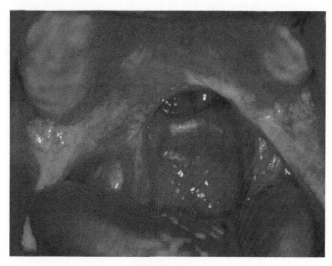

**Figure 15-1**

36. Initial acquired defects of the soft palate are rehabilitated with the same sequence as hard palate defects, that is, with surgical, interim, and definitive obturators. (T/F)

37. After a segmental resection without reconstruction, the remaining mandible deviates away from the resection. (T/F)

38. After a segmental resection without reconstruction, patients can sometimes train the mandible to seat in full occlusion with stretching and practice. (T/F)

39. Mandibular defects often result in obliteration of the buccal and lingual vestibules, thereby improving the fit and function of a prosthesis. (T/F)

40. Fibula free flaps are typically too small in width and height for the placement of dental implants and thus should be avoided. (T/F)

41. Hair can sometimes grow from the flap and must be removed as it is detrimental to the patient's health. (T/F)

42. The use of intraoperative wire fixation during a mandibulectomy and fibula free flap reconstruction can aid in maintaining the patient's existing occlusion. (T/F)

43. Facial prostheses can be retained with adhesives or mechanically via either the nature of the surgical defect or craniofacial implants. (T/F)

44. Facial prostheses are typically made of medical-grade silicone. (T/F)

45. Craniofacial implants provide superior retention when compared with conventional adhesives. (T/F)

46. Craniofacial implants prohibit the patient from undergoing postoperative magnetic resonance imaging. (T/F)

47. Facial prostheses using craniofacial implants will be attached via magnets or clips. (T/F)

48. Auricular prostheses have been shown to provide near preoperative levels of hearing for patients undergoing a total auriculectomy. (T/F)

49. Sun and chemical exposure will degrade the color and surface of a facial prosthesis. (T/F)

50. Skin grafts are recommended around craniofacial implants to reduce the amount of tissue movement and facilitate ease of cleaning. (T/F)

## MULTIPLE CHOICE

51. The *short-term* effects of radiation on the dentition, periodontium, and mucosal surfaces include the following:
    i. Mucositis.
    ii. Dysgeusia.
    iii. Dysphagia.
    iv. Loss of teeth.
    v. Ropy saliva.
    vi. Broken or chipped fillings or teeth
    A. ii, iii, vi
    B. i, ii, iii, v
    C. i, iii, iv, v
    D. iv, v, vi
    E. i, vi
    F. i, ii, iii, iv, v, vi

52. The *long-term* effects of radiation on the dentition, periodontium, and mucosal surfaces include the following:
    i. Osteoradionecrosis.
    ii. Xerostomia.
    iii. Caries.
    iv. Trismus.
    v. Mucositis.
    vi. Dysgeusia.

A. ii, iii, v, vi
B. ii, iii, iv, vi
C. i, ii, iii, iv
D. i, iv, v, vi
E. ii, iv, v, vi

53. Indications for dental extraction before radiation therapy include
    i. A history of poor dental compliance indicated by poor oral hygiene and multiple missing and decayed teeth.
    ii. Symptomatic impacted or incompletely erupted teeth not fully covered by alveolar bone.
    iii. Residual root tips incompletely covered by alveolar bone.
    iv. Dark stained teeth.
    v. Crooked teeth.
    vi. Advanced, symptomatic periodontal disease.
A. i, ii, iii
B. i, ii, iii, iv
C. ii, iii, iv, v, vi
D. i, ii, iii, vi
E. i, ii, iv, v

54. Common trismus prevention or treatment devices include the following:
    i. Commercial devices (e.g., TheraBite).
    ii. Tongue depressors.
    iii. Forceps.
    iv. Fingers.
    v. Acrylic resin "corkscrew."
A. i, ii, iii
B. i, ii, iii, iv
C. i, iii, iv, v
D. i, ii, iv, v
E. iii, iv, v

55. The following surgical issues are relevant to palatal resection so that the functional outcome of an obturator is maximized:
    i. Split-thickness skin grafting.
    ii. Keratinized mucosal coverage of the medial cut margin of the hard palate.
    iii. Enlargement of the defect to ease insertion of the obturator.
    iv. Removal of as many teeth as possible to facilitate insertion.
    v. Retention of as much premaxilla as possible.
    vi. Placement of bony resection lines through the socket of an extracted tooth.
A. i, ii, iii, iv
B. ii, iii, v, vi
C. i, ii, v, vi
D. ii, iii, iv, v
E. i, iii, iv

56. Depending on the dimensions and location of the defect of the palate and/or maxilla, the following may occur:
    i. Hypernasality and unintelligible speech.
    ii. Difficulty chewing.
    iii. Difficulty swallowing.
    iv. Nasal regurgitation.

    v. Facial asymmetry and disfigurement.
    vi. Desiccation of nasal mucous membranes.
    vii. Difficulty controlling nasal and/or sinus secretions.
A. i, ii, iii, iv, v, vi, vii
B. i, ii, iii, vi, vii
C. ii, iii, iv, v
D. ii, iv, v, vi
E. ii, iii, iv, v, vi, vii

57. The differential diagnosis for this lesion on the right lateral border of the tongue (Figure 15-2) includes

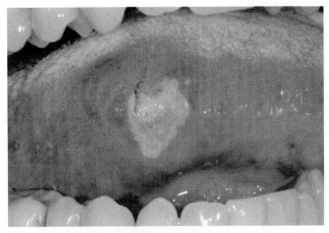

**Figure 15-2**

    i. Trauma from an occlusion.
    ii. An abrasion from toothbrushing.
    iii. Acute mucositis during radiation therapy.
    iv. Trauma from an ill-fitting prosthesis or rough restoration.
    v. Squamous cell carcinoma.
A. i, ii, iii
B. i, iii, iv, v
C. i, ii, iii, iv, v
D. ii, iii, iv
E. iii, iv, v

58. The differential diagnosis for this lesion of the right mandibular buccal vestibule (Figure 15-3) includes

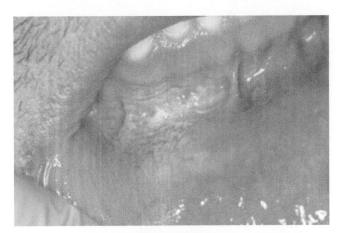

**Figure 15-3**

    i. Leukoplakia from smokeless tobacco use.
    ii. An abrasion from toothbrushing.
    iii. Chemical trauma (e.g., holding an aspirin tablet in the vestibule).
    iv. A herpetic outbreak.
A. i, iv
B. ii, iii
C. i, iii
D. ii, iv
E. i, ii, iii, iv

59. The differential diagnosis of this incidentally found asymptomatic lesion of the gum (Figure 15-4) includes

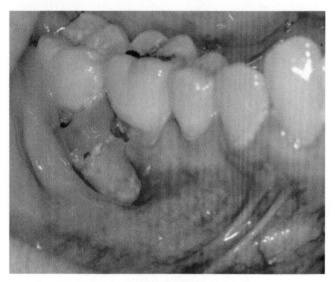

**Figure 15-4**

    i. Squamous cell carcinoma.
    ii. Osteoradionecrosis.
    iii. Bisphosphonate-induced osteonecrosis of jaw.
    iv. A herpetic outbreak.
    v. An aphthous ulcer.
A. i, ii
B. i, ii, iii
C. i, iv, v
D. ii, iii, iv
E. i, ii, iii, iv, v

60. A 35-year-old woman who recently had dental implants placed has lost one on the right side of the mandible. The area in question is otherwise asymptomatic, but she and her dentist are concerned. The differential diagnosis of this radiolucency (Figure 15-5) includes
    i. Squamous cell carcinoma.
    ii. Osteonecrosis.
    iii. Bisphosphonate-induced osteonecrosis of the jaw.
    iv. Osteomyelitis secondary to lack of integration of the implant.
    v. Severe periodontal disease.
A. i, ii, iii
B. i, ii, iii, iv

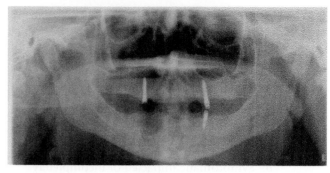

**Figure 15-5**

C. i, iii, iv
D. i, ii, iii, iv, v
E. ii, iii, iv, v

61. The palatopharyngeal sphincter is formed by the
A. Posterior and superior movement of the middle third of the soft palate, the anterior movement of the posterior pharyngeal wall, and the medial movement of the lateral pharyngeal walls.
B. Posterior and inferior movement of the middle third of the soft palate, the anterior movement of the posterior pharyngeal wall, and the medial movement of the lateral pharyngeal walls.
C. Posterior and superior movement of the middle third of the soft palate, the posterior movement of the posterior pharyngeal wall, and the medial movement of the lateral pharyngeal walls.
D. Posterior and superior movement of the middle third of the soft palate, the anterior movement of the posterior pharyngeal wall, and the inferior movement of the lateral pharyngeal walls.
E. Passavant ridge.

62. The muscles of the soft palate and fauces are the
A. Levator veli palatini, palatoglossus, palatopharyngeus, and uvula.
B. Tensor veli palatini, levator veli palatini, palatoglossus, palatopharyngeus, and uvula.
C. Tensor veli palatini, levator veli palatini, palatopharyngeus, and uvula.
D. Tensor veli palatini, levator veli palatini, and palatoglossus.

63. The components of speech are
A. Respiration, resonance, articulation, and neurological integration.
B. Respiration, phonation, resonance, and articulation.
C. Respiration, phonation, resonance, articulation, and neurological integration.
D. Respiration, phonation, articulation, and neurological integration.

64. The phases of swallowing are
A. Oral preparatory, salivatory, oral transit, and pharyngeal.
B. Oral preparatory, salivatory, oral transit, and esophageal.

C. Oral preparatory, salivatory, oral transit, pharyngeal, and esophageal.
D. Oral preparatory, oral transit, pharyngeal, and esophageal.

65. Maxillofacial prostheses are retained in place with any one or more of the following:
A. Adhesives, implants, the geometry of the defect, and physical straps/hooks.
B. Adhesives, implants, and the geometry of the defect.
C. Adhesives, implants, and physical straps.
D. Adhesives and implants.

66. The appropriate sequence from start to finish of prosthetic restoration of a maxillary defect would be
A. Definitive obturator, surgical obturator, and interim obturator.
B. Interim obturator, surgical obturator, and definitive obturator.
C. Surgical obturator, interim obturator, and definitive obturator.
D. Surgical obturator, definitive obturator, and interim obturator.

67. Obturator prostheses are retained in the oral cavity with
A. Adhesives, remaining teeth, and implants.
B. Adhesives, remaining teeth, the geometry of the defect, and implants.
C. Remaining teeth, the geometry of the defect, and implants.
D. Remaining teeth and implants.

68. The surgical obturator is intended to
A. Prevent infection, reduce physical postoperative discomfort, and allow for nutrition by mouth.
B. Prevent infection, allow for nutrition by mouth, and provide intelligible speech.
C. Allow for nutrition by mouth, provide intelligible speech, and stabilize surgical packing.
D. Prevent infection, provide intelligible speech, and stabilize surgical packing.

69. A nonreconstructed maxillectomy defect causes
A. Nasal regurgitation.
B. Nasal regurgitation and difficulty chewing.
C. Nasal regurgitation and hypernasal speech.
D. Nasal regurgitation, hypernasal speech, and difficulty chewing.

70. After radiation therapy, patients are advised to
A. Have frequent dental examinations/prophylactic treatment, use a fluoride supplement, and use water for relief of xerostomia.
B. Have frequent dental examinations/prophylactic treatment, decrease sucrose intake, and use water for relief of xerostomia.
C. Use a fluoride supplement, decrease sucrose intake, and use water for relief of xerostomia.
D. Have frequent dental examinations/prophylactic treatment, use a fluoride supplement, decrease sucrose intake, and use water for relief of xerostomia.

71. If hyperbaric oxygen is to be used to prevent osteoradionecrosis after a surgical procedure in the oral cavity of a patient who had previously received irradiation, the preferred protocol is for the patient to "take"
A. 20 dives, undergo the surgical procedure, and complete 10 additional dives.
B. 20 dives, undergo the surgical procedure, and complete 20 additional dives.
C. 30 dives, undergo the surgical procedure, and complete 10 additional dives.
D. 30 dives and undergo the surgical procedure.

72. A standard hyperbaric oxygen dive is usually
A. 80% oxygen at two to three times atmospheric pressure for 60 minutes.
B. 90% oxygen at two to three times atmospheric pressure for 30 minutes.
C. 100% oxygen at one to two times atmospheric pressure for 90 minutes.
D. 100% oxygen at two to three times atmospheric pressure for 90 minutes.

73. The initial treatment of osteoradionecrosis begins with
A. Curettage of the area, chlorhexidine gluconate rinses, 30 dives of hyperbaric oxygen, and systemic antibiotics.
B. Curettage of the area, 30 dives of hyperbaric oxygen, and systemic antibiotics.
C. Curettage of the area, chlorhexidine gluconate rinses, and systemic antibiotics.
D. Curettage of the area, chlorhexidine gluconate rinses, and 50 dives of hyperbaric oxygen.

74. After having a maxillectomy that created posterior hard and soft palate defects, a patient is rehabilitated with an obturator. If the patient complains of an earache and hearing disturbances, the following should be considered as causes for these symptoms:
A. Infection and edema of the maxillectomy defect.
B. Infection, edema, and prosthetic impingement of the torus tubarius.
C. Infection, edema, prosthetic impingement of the torus tubarius, and trismus.
D. Infection, prosthetic impingement of the torus tubarius, and trismus.

75. A patient presents with a 0.7-cm × 0.5-cm, firm, raised, pedunculated submucosal lesion on the right buccal mucosa adjacent to the occlusal plane. What is the most likely diagnosis?
A. Irritation fibroma
B. Lipoma
C. Mucocele
D. Parulis

76. If the radiology report of the panoramic x-ray film of a patient reads "cotton-wool appearance of the right mandible" the diagnosis should include
A. Cementoosseous dysplasia, Paget disease, and Gardner syndrome.

B. Cementoosseous dysplasia, Paget disease, and osteosarcoma.

C. Cementoosseous dysplasia, Gardner syndrome, and osteoradionecrosis.

D. Cementoosseous dysplasia, aneurysmal bone cyst, and ameloblastoma.

77. If the radiology report on the panoramic x-ray film of a patient reads "sunburst appearance of the anterior mandible," the diagnosis should include
A. Periodontitis, osteosarcoma, and intraosseous hemangioma.
B. Osteosarcoma, intraosseous hemangioma, and Paget disease.
C. Osteosarcoma and intraosseous hemangioma.
D. Fibrous dysplasia and Gardner syndrome.

78. A patient is referred by a local dentist who finds a lesion in the midline of the upper neck. The differential diagnosis should include
A. Thyroid tumor, thyroglossal duct cyst, and Kaposi sarcoma.
B. Thyroid tumor, thyroglossal duct cyst, and dermoid cyst.
C. Thyroid tumor, thyroglossal duct cyst, and pyogenic granuloma.
D. Thyroid tumor, thyroglossal duct cyst, and leukemic infiltrate.

79. A local dentist refers a patient with a fluctuant swelling of the anterior midline of the hard palate; the diagnosis is
A. Nasopalatine duct cyst.
B. Ranula/mucocele.
C. Irritation fibroma.
D. Congenital epulis.

80. A patient presents with a 6-mm lesion on the inner aspect of the lower lip, with intact overlying mucosa. It is pale blue in color and increases and decreases in size. The most likely diagnosis is
A. Mucocele.
B. Lipoma.
C. Irritation fibroma.
D. Kaposi sarcoma.
E. Epulis.

81. The following have been associated with an increased frequency of osteomyelitis of the jaws:
A. Tobacco use, alcohol abuse, diabetes mellitus, exanthematous fevers, and malaria.
B. Alcohol abuse, intravenous drug abuse, diabetes mellitus, exanthematous fevers, malaria, and acquired immunodeficiency syndrome (AIDS).
C. Intravenous drug abuse, diabetes mellitus, exanthematous fevers, malaria, and AIDS.
D. Tobacco use, alcohol abuse, intravenous drug abuse, diabetes mellitus, exanthematous fevers, malaria, and AIDS.

82. The treatment of acute osteomyelitis of the mandible comprises
A. Microbiological study of the infection and appropriate antibiotics.

B. Drainage, microbiological study of the infection, and appropriate antibiotics.
C. Drainage, microbiological study of the infection, appropriate antibiotics, and resection.
D. Drainage, microbiological study of the infection, appropriate antibiotics, resection, and immediate reconstruction.

83. Titanium implants placed before radiation therapy should be
A. Left alone because they pose no contraindication to radiation therapy.
B. Removed because they pose a threat to the surrounding bone.
C. Removed because they increase the risk of infection in the bone.
D. Removed because they are a source for osteoradionecrosis.

84. A patient presents emergently with difficulty breathing, a protruding tongue, and a swollen neck. The most likely diagnosis is
A. Cavernous sinus thrombosis.
B. Ludwig angina.
C. Leukemia.
D. Parulis.

85. Treatment of Ludwig angina consists of
A. Maintenance of the airway and antibiotic therapy.
B. Maintenance of the airway, incision and drainage, and antibiotic therapy.
C. Maintenance of the airway, incision and drainage, and elimination of focal infection.
D. Maintenance of the airway, incision and drainage, antibiotic therapy, and elimination of focal infection.

86. A patient presents to the emergency department with a 3-day history of pain in the left cheek, increased swelling, and periorbital edema with involvement of the eyelids and conjunctiva. Proptosis and fixation of the eyeball are evident. The most likely diagnosis is
A. Ludwig angina.
B. Lupus.
C. Psoriasis.
D. Cavernous sinus thrombosis.

87. A 33-year-old male patient is referred for a painless diffuse swelling at the angle of the mandible. A panoramic x-ray film of the mandible shows a multilocular, radiolucent lesion resembling a soap bubble and slight expansion of the buccal plate in the posterior mandible. The most likely diagnosis is
A. Cementoblastoma.
B. Odontogenic fibroma.
C. Ameloblastoma.
D. Complex odontoma.

88. A 40-year-old woman presents emergently with a history of loss of muscular control on the left side of the face on waking, asymmetry of the lips on smiling, and an inability to close the eye, wink, or raise the eyebrow. The most likely diagnosis is

A. Glossopharyngeal neuralgia.
B. Migrainous neuralgia.
C. Bell palsy.
D. Horner syndrome.

89. After a parotidectomy a year ago, a patient complains of flushing and sweating in the area of surgery when eating. The most likely diagnosis is
A. Frey syndrome.
B. Horner syndrome.
C. Behçet syndrome.
D. Bloom syndrome.

90. After a recent obturator adjustment after maxillectomy, a patient complains of constant clear drainage from the nostril on the side of the surgery. What is the next best step?
A. Recommend an antihistamine because it is caused by seasonal allergies.
B. Adjust the height of the obturator because the prosthesis is most likely irritating a turbinate.
C. Prescribe an antihistamine and antibiotic for a secondary infection.
D. Remove the obturator for 7 days, and prescribe an antihistamine and antibiotic.

91. The best option for rehabilitation of an infrastructure maxillectomy defect in an edentulous patient with complete atrophy of the alveolar process is
A. An obturator prosthesis alone.
B. An osteocutaneous fibula free flap.
C. A skin graft and obturator prosthesis.
D. A soft tissue and skin free flap.

92. Before radiation therapy of the oral cavity, patients should be educated about the following acute sequelae:
A. Mucositis, dysgeusia, dysphagia, and tooth abscess.
B. Mucositis, dysgeusia, ropy saliva, and tooth abscess.
C. Mucositis, dysgeusia, dysphagia, and ropy saliva.
D. Mucositis, dysgeusia, dysphagia, and tooth fracture.

93. Secondary to radiation therapy, the following long-term sequelae are expected in most patients:
A. Osteoradionecrosis, trismus, xerostomia, and an increased risk of caries.
B. Osteoradionecrosis, xerostomia, an increased risk of caries, and tooth abscess.
C. Xerostomia, trismus, an increased risk of caries, and tooth abscess.
D. Xerostomia and an increased risk of caries.

94. After surgery and/or radiation therapy that could potentiate trismus, the following prophylactic/therapeutic options could be considered:
A. Commercial devices, tongue depressors, fingers, and an acrylic "corkscrew."
B. Commercial devices, a physical therapist, and massage.
C. Commercial devices, botulinum toxin type A (Botox) injections, and "releasing" surgery.

D. Commercial devices, tongue depressors, fingers, an acrylic "corkscrew," and a physical therapist.

95. The following muscles elevate the mandible:
A. Temporalis, masseter, and medial pterygoid.
B. Temporalis, lateral pterygoid, medial pterygoid, and salpingopharyngeus.
C. Temporalis, lateral pterygoid, medial pterygoid, and superior constrictor.
D. Temporalis, masseter, medial pterygoid, and buccinators.

96. Symptomatic treatment of acute radiation/chemotherapy-induced mucositis may involve
A. Viscous lidocaine, ice, low-energy laser therapy, topical steroids, and sodium bicarbonate rinses.
B. Viscous lidocaine, ice, low-energy laser therapy, and topical steroids.
C. Viscous lidocaine, topical steroids, and sodium bicarbonate rinses.
D. Viscous lidocaine, ice, low-energy laser therapy, antibiotics, and narcotic analgesics.

97. Intraoral hair growth on a fibula free flap can be removed by the following:
A. A laser, scissors, and chemical depilatory creams.
B. A laser, scissors, and antibiotics.
C. A laser and scissors.
D. A laser.

98. What is the reason for removal of intraoral hair growth on a fibula free flap?
A. The hair retains food and is a source of infection to the patient.
B. The hair retains food and could result in loss of the flap.
C. The hair retains food and causes chronic halitosis.
D. It is not necessary to remove the hair if there is good hygiene, unless the patient requests it.

99. On removing surgical packing after a maxillectomy, you encounter significant bleeding. What is the cause and what is the best course of action?
A. The bleeding is from the internal maxillary artery; use high-volume suction and replace the packing or use cauterization.
B. The bleeding is from the lesser palatine artery; it will clot on its own, and no treatment is necessary.
C. The bleeding is from the internal maxillary artery; use high-volume suction and apply pressure. It will clot on its own, and no further treatment is necessary.
D. The bleeding is from the lesser palatine artery; use high-volume suction and cauterization.

100. When considering a segmental mandibulectomy, what should be the treatment of choice for the best prosthetic and functional outcome?
A. Intermaxillary wire fixation without reconstruction because the patient still has a residual mandible
B. Reconstruction with a titanium plate

C. Delayed reconstruction with a titanium plate
D. Immediate bony and soft tissue free flap reconstruction and grafting

## Answers

| | | |
|---|---|---|
| 1. T | 35. F | 69. D |
| 2. T | 36. T | 70. D |
| 3. T | 37. F | 71. A |
| 4. T | 38. T | 72. D |
| 5. T | 39. F | 73. A |
| 6. T | 40. F | 74. B |
| 7. F | 41. F | 75. A |
| 8. F | 42. T | 76. A |
| 9. F | 43. T | 77. C |
| 10. T | 44. T | 78. B |
| 11. T | 45. T | 79. A |
| 12. T | 46. F | 80. A |
| 13. T | 47. T | 81. D |
| 14. T | 48. T | 82. B |
| 15. T | 49. T | 83. A |
| 16. T | 50. T | 84. B |
| 17. T | 51. B | 85. D |
| 18. T | 52. C | 86. D |
| 19. T | 53. D | 87. C |
| 20. T | 54. D | 88. C |
| 21. T | 55. C | 89. A |
| 22. F | 56. A | 90. B |
| 23. T | 57. B | 91. D |
| 24. T | 58. C | 92. C |
| 25. T | 59. B | 93. D |
| 26. T | 60. B | 94. D |
| 27. T | 61. A | 95. A |
| 28. T | 62. B | 96. A |
| 29. T | 63. C | 97. C |
| 30. T | 64. D | 98. D |
| 31. T | 65. A | 99. A |
| 32. F | 66. C | 100. D |
| 33. F | 67. B | |
| 34. T | 68. C | |

## Core Knowledge

- Ideally, a period of 2 to 3 weeks before radiation therapy should be allowed for primary healing of the sockets after dental extractions.

- The most frequent acute sequelae of head and neck radiation therapy are mucositis, dysgeusia, dysphagia, and ropy saliva.

- The most frequent chronic sequealae and complications of radiation therapy to the oral cavity are xerostomia, caries, periodontal disease, trismus, and osteoradionecrosis.

- Before ablative surgery of the hard and/or soft palate, a mold of the oral cavity should be made to fabricate a surgical obturator.

- After ablative surgery of the hard and/or soft palate, the patient may experience hypernasality making speech unintelligible, difficulty chewing, difficulty swallowing, nasal regurgitation, desiccation of nasal mucous membranes, difficulty controlling nasal and/or sinus secretions, and facial disfigurement.

- Approximately 7 to 10 days after maxillectomy, the surgical packing and obturator are removed and replaced with a removable interim obturator.

- The soft palate and lateral and posterior pharyngeal walls form the velopharyngeal sphincter.

- The soft palate elevates posterosuperiorly, the lateral walls move medially, and the posterior wall moves anteriorly. Failure of this sphincter to form is known as velopharyngeal inadequacy.

- The Passavant ridge assists in velopharyngeal competence in patients who have undergone soft palate resection.

- An anatomically intact but nonfunctional soft palate is known as velopharyngeal incompetence.

- A functional but anatomically deficient soft palate is known as velopharyngeal insufficiency.

- A resected mandible will deviate toward the side of the resection because of the unopposed pull of the contralateral pterygoid muscles.

- Facial prostheses are held in place by natural undercuts in the defect, water soluble adhesives, physical retainers (e.g., glasses, straps, or tape), or craniofacial implants with magnets or clips.

- Typically, a mold of the patient's facial defect is made, a sculpting is completed, tinting of the silicone prosthesis is finalized, and the prosthesis is delivered.

- Facial prostheses are usually made of medical-grade silicone that lasts between 2 and 5 years, depending on the environment in which the patient resides.

## SUGGESTED READING

Bohle 3rd G, Rieger J, Huryn J, Verbel D, Hwang F, Zlotolow I. Efficacy of speech aid prostheses for acquired defects of the soft palate and velopharyngeal inadequacy—clinical assessments and cephalometric analysis: a Memorial Sloan-Kettering study. Head Neck 2005;27(3):195–207.

Bohle GC, Mitcherling WW, Mitcherling JJ, Johnson RM, Bohle 3rd GC. Immediate obturator stabilization using mini dental implants. J Prosthodont 2008;17(6):482–6.

Chrcanovic BR, Reher P, Sousa AA, Harris M. Osteoradionecrosis of the jaws—a current overview—part 1: Physiopathology and risk and predisposing factors. Oral Maxillofac Surg 2010;14(1):3–16.

Cordeiro PG, Santamaria E. A classification system and algorithm for reconstruction of maxillectomy and midfacial defects. Plast Reconstr Surg 2000;105:2331–46.

Depprich R, Naujoks C, Lind D, Ommerborn M, Meyer U, Kübler NR, et al. Evaluation of the quality of life of patients with maxillofacial defects after prosthodontic therapy with obturator prostheses. Int J Oral Maxillofac Surg 2011;40(1):71–9.

Fritz GW, Gunsolley JC, Abubabker O, Laskin DM. Efficacy of pre- and postirradiation hyperbaric oxygen therapy in the prevention of post-extraction osteoradionecrosis: a systematic review. J Oral Maxillofac Surg 2010;68(11):2653–60.

Huryn JM, Piro JD. The maxillary immediate surgical obturator prosthesis. J Prosthet Dent 1989;61(3):343–7.

Kornblith AB, Zlotolow IM, Gooen J, Huryn JM, Lerner T, Strong EW, et al. Quality of life of maxillectomy patients using an obturator prosthesis. Head Neck 1996;18(4):323–34.

Kubicek GJ, Machtay M. New advances in high-technology radiotherapy for head and neck cancer. Hematol Oncol Clin North Am 2008;22(6):1165–80.

Okay DJ, Genden E, Buchbinder D, Urken M. Prosthodontic guidelines for surgical reconstruction of the maxilla: a classification system of defects. J Prosthet Dent 2001;86(4):352–63.

Rieger J, Bohle G, Huryn J, Tang JL, Harris J, Seikaly H. Surgical reconstruction versus prosthetic obturation of extensive soft palate defects: a comparison of speech outcomes. Int J Prosthodont 2009;22(6):566–72.

Spiro RH, Strong EW, Shah JP. Maxillectomy and its classification. Head Neck 1997;19(4):309–14.

Stubblefield MD, Manfield L, Riedel ER. A preliminary report on the efficacy of a dynamic jaw opening device (dynasplint trismus system) as part of the multimodal treatment of trismus in patients with head and neck cancer. Arch Phys Med Rehabil 2010;91(8):1278–82.

Vissink A, Mitchell JB, Baum BJ, Limesand KH, Jensen SB, Fox PC, et al. Clinical management of salivary gland hypofunction and xerostomia in head-and-neck cancer patients: successes and barriers. Int J Radiat Oncol Biol Phys 2010;78(4):983–91.

# 16 Radiation Oncology

## Questions

### TRUE/FALSE

1. Contouring in head and neck cancer typically involves outlining gross disease and areas at risk for microscopic disease on cross-sectional imaging. (T/F)

2. The accuracy of head and neck tumor contouring affects outcomes of radiation therapy. (T/F)

3. Simulation involves making sure patients are in the correct position before their first treatment session. (T/F)

4. Patients who receive external beam radiation therapy are very mildly radioactive and should not interact with small children. (T/F)

5. The term *Gray* (Gy) refers to joules per kilogram of tissue. (T/F)

6. Chemotherapy and radiation therapy do not interact, so they are often given together to save time. (T/F)

7. Regardless of treatment intent (i.e., definitive, adjuvant, or palliative), all patients receive the same dose of radiation therapy. (T/F)

8. The standard radiation therapy technique in head and neck cancer is two-dimensional radiation therapy, or conventional treatment. (T/F)

9. Intensity-modulated radiation therapy (IMRT) has been shown in randomized trials to provide a survival benefit compared with two-dimensional radiation therapy. (T/F)

10. In general, electrons penetrate tissue deeper than photons. (T/F)

11. A typical palliative radiation therapy dose is 10 Gy in five fractions. (T/F)

12. Stereotactic radiosurgery can only be performed with a Gamma Knife or a CyberKnife. (T/F)

13. Accelerated fractionation schemes have been shown to improve local control compared with standard fractionation. (T/F)

14. In the era of concurrent chemoradiation therapy, accelerated fractionation continues to demonstrate improved outcomes compared with standard fractionation. (T/F)

15. Split-course radiation therapy is associated with equivalent outcomes to conventional fractionated treatment. (T/F)

16. The depth at which the dose is maximum for a particular beam of energy (Dmax) for 6 MV is 1.5 cm. (T/F)

17. Penumbra is the radiation dose falloff from 80% to 20% isodose lines. (T/F)

18. T1 glottic cancers with anterior commissure involvement should not receive a bolus during radiation therapy. (T/F)

19. It is a standard procedure to obtain weekly portal images to verify field setup. (T/F)

20. Hypoxic cell sensitizers have been shown to clinically improve outcomes when given concurrently with radiation therapy. (T/F)

21. Adjuvant or neoadjuvant chemotherapy appears as effective in maintaining locoregional control as concurrent chemotherapy. (T/F)

22. Images like that shown in Figure 16-1 are useful for ensuring that the tumor is adequately being treated and critical structures are not receiving an excessive dose. (T/F)

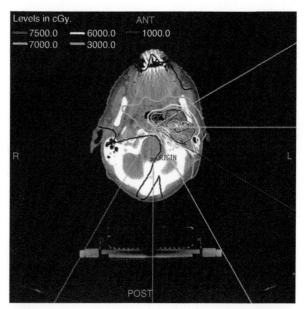

**Figure 16-1** (Courtesy of Memorial Sloan Kettering Cancer Center, New York.)

23. Every patient that receives radiation therapy for laryngopharyngeal cancer requires a percutaneous endoscopic gastrostomy (PEG). (T/F)

24. IMRT has been shown in randomized trials to reduce toxic effects compared with two-dimensional radiation therapy. (T/F)

25. Hypothyroidism is common after radiation therapy for squamous cell carcinoma (SCC) of the head and neck. (T/F)

26. Long-term rates of xerostomia have decreased with the advent of IMRT. (T/F)

27. Accelerated fractionated radiation therapy results in higher long-term toxic effects than conventionally fractionated radiation therapy. (T/F)

28. The spinal cord can safely receive 70 Gy of radiation therapy without significant concern for toxic effects. (T/F)

29. Hyperbaric oxygen is a reasonable treatment for mild osteoradionecrosis. (T/F)

30. Temporal lobe necrosis is a common late side effect after radiation therapy for nasopharyngeal carcinoma. (T/F)

31. A small increase in the risk of stroke may result from radiation therapy to the neck. (T/F)

32. Grade 2 or greater acute skin toxicity is uncommon (fewer than 5% of cases) after definitive chemoradiation therapy for oropharyngeal cancer. (T/F)

33. Patients who present with a single well-encapsulated lymph node less than 2 cm and an unknown primary site should be offered surgery over radiation therapy as initial definitive treatment because it is associated with a better survival outcome. (T/F)

34. Human papillomavirus (HPV)-positive tumors are more sensitive to radiation than HPV-negative tumors. (T/F)

35. HPV-positive tumors may be safely treated with lower doses of radiation therapy than HPV-negative tumors. (T/F)

36. A typical definitive radiation therapy dose used to treat unresectable oropharyngeal cancer is 60 Gy. (T/F)

37. The treatment of locoregionally advanced nasopharyngeal cancer consists of platinum-based chemoradiation therapy. (T/F)

38. T1 and T2 glottic larynx cancers receive the same dose of definitive radiation therapy. (T/F)

39. Lower doses of radiation are used to treat papillary thyroid cancer compared with anaplastic thyroid carcinoma. (T/F)

40. Adenoid cystic cancers respond well to neutron beam radiation therapy. (T/F)

41. T1N0 tonsil cancer requires irradiation to both sides of the neck. (T/F)

42. Definitive radiation therapy with high-energy sources is equivalent to surgery for salivary gland tumors. (T/F)

43. After definitive chemoradiation therapy for SCC of the head and neck, a neck dissection is mandatory for all patients with node-positive disease, staged N2b, regardless of the response. (T/F)

44. In the node-negative neck, level 2 contours should always extend to the base of the skull. (T/F)

45. In the node-negative neck, level 2 treatment can stop where the posterior belly of the digastric crosses the internal jugular vein (or the lateral process of C1). (T/F)

46. Reirradiation after salvage surgery has been demonstrated in randomized trials to improve the disease-free survival rate. (T/F)

47. Almost every patient that undergoes reirradiation will develop some type of grade 3 or greater late toxic effects. (T/F)

48. There are no long-term survivors of reirradiation. (T/F)

## MULTIPLE CHOICE

49. After a consultation with a radiation oncologist, patients must have the following tasks completed before they can receive their first fraction of treatment: contouring, simulation, treatment, port film, and treatment planning. Which of the following choices is in the correct order?
    A. Planning, contouring, simulation, port film, treatment
    B. Planning, simulation, contouring, port film, treatment
    C. Simulation, planning, contouring, port film, treatment
    D. Simulation, contouring, planning, port film, treatment

50. The primary mechanism by which radiation kills cancer cells is
    A. Damage to DNA.
    B. Inhibition of the cell cycle.
    C. Damage to the cell membrane.
    D. Induction of apoptosis.

51. Which of the following is not one of the four *R*s of radiobiology?
    A. Repair
    B. Restoration
    C. Reassortment
    D. Reoxygenation
    E. Repopulation

52. Which of the following may interfere with the effectiveness of radiation therapy?
    A. Antibiotics (especially macrolides)
    B. Antioxidants

C. Supplemental oxygen
D. Calcium channel blockers

53. In the postoperative setting, radiation therapy should typically begin within
    A. 6 weeks.
    B. 12 weeks.
    C. 18 weeks.
    D. 24 weeks.

54. Which of the following settings is generally not a preferred means of delivering radiation therapy in SCC of the head and neck?
    A. Definitive treatment
    B. Adjuvant treatment
    C. Salvage treatment
    D. Palliative treatment
    E. Preoperative treatment

55. Which of the following can be a contraindication to delivering radiation therapy?
    A. Scleroderma
    B. Psoriasis
    C. Acne
    D. Diabetes

56. Who is typically not a part of the team required to deliver radiation therapy?
    A. Medical physicists
    B. Radiation therapists
    C. Dosimetrists
    D. Radiation oncology nurses
    E. Anesthesiologists

57. Head and neck cancer patients are typically immobilized during delivery of radiation therapy with a(n)
    A. Alpha cradle.
    B. Face mask.
    C. Mold.
    D. Sedation.
    E. Bolus.

58. The purpose of immobilization in radiation therapy is to
    A. Make the patient comfortable.
    B. Help the radiation oncologist determine where the tumor is located.
    C. Make sure the patient is in the same position for treatment each day.
    D. Maintain sanitation.

59. Which of the following structures is not typically contoured on a routine head and neck treatment plan as an organ at risk?
    A. Parotid gland
    B. Cochlea
    C. C1 vertebral body
    D. Brachial plexus
    E. Pituitary gland

60. The clinical target volume (CTV) represents
    A. Gross disease.
    B. Gross disease and microscopic disease.
    C. Gross disease and a margin for setup uncertainty.
    D. Gross disease, microscopic disease, and a margin for setup uncertainty.

*In Questions 61 through 65, choose the best dose for the specified targets in SCC of the head and neck.*

61. Gross disease dose
    A. 80 Gy
    B. 70 Gy
    C. 60 Gy
    D. 54 Gy
    E. 50 Gy
    F. 40 Gy

62. Typical low anterior neck dose
    A. 80 Gy
    B. 70 Gy
    C. 60 Gy
    D. 54 Gy
    E. 50 Gy
    F. 40 Gy

63. Low-risk dose
    A. 80 Gy
    B. 70 Gy
    C. 60 Gy
    D. 54 Gy
    E. 50 Gy
    F. 40 Gy

64. Moderate-risk dose
    A. 80 Gy
    B. 70 Gy
    C. 60 Gy
    D. 54 Gy
    E. 50 Gy
    F. 40 Gy

65. Postoperative dose (low risk)
    A. 80 Gy
    B. 70 Gy
    C. 60 Gy
    D. 54 Gy
    E. 50 Gy
    F. 40 Gy

66. IMRT stands for
    A. Intensity-mandated radiation therapy.
    B. Intensely-marketed radiation therapy.
    C. Intensity-modulated radiation therapy.
    D. Imaging-modulated radiation therapy.

67. The typical daily fraction size in definitive treatment for head and neck cancer is
    A. 1 Gy.
    B. 2 Gy.
    C. 3 Gy.
    D. 4 Gy.

68. The most routinely used type of radiation therapy beam to treat head and neck cancers is:
    A. 6 MV photons
    B. 15 MV photons
    C. Cobalt radiation therapy
    D. Proton radiation therapy

69. Which tumor is most likely to have retropharyngeal lymph node metastasis?
    A. Nasopharynx
    B. Oral cavity

C. Glottic larynx
D. Parotid

70. Which of the following agents delivered concurrently with radiation therapy does not result in an improvement in overall survival?
    A. Cisplatin
    B. Cetuximab
    C. Tirapazamine
    D. Carboplatin/5-FU

*Questions 71 through 74 refer to Figure 16-2.*

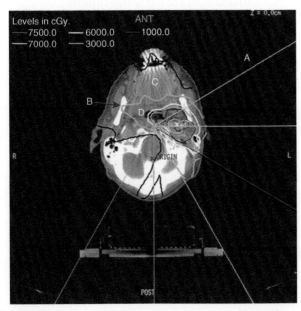

**Figure 16-2** (Courtesy of Memorial Sloan Kettering Cancer Center, New York.)

71. In Figure 16-2, *A* refers to
    A. An isodose line.
    B. A beam angle.
    C. An isometric line.
    D. All of the above.

72. In Figure 16-2, *B* refers to
    A. An isodose line.
    B. A beam angle.
    C. An isometric line.
    D. All of the above.

73. The dose delivered to *region C* in Figure 16-2 is
    A. 1000 cGy.
    B. 3000 cGy.
    C. 6000 cGy.
    D. 7000 cGy.

74. The dose delivered to *region D* in Figure 16-2 is
    A. 1000 cGy.
    B. 3000 cGy.
    C. 6000 cGy.
    D. 7000 cGy.

*Questions 75 and 76 refer to Figure 16-3.*

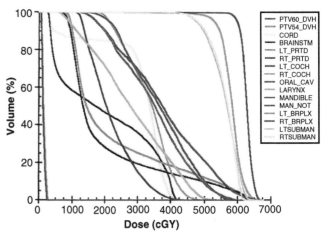

**Figure 16-3** (Courtesy of Memorial Sloan Kettering Cancer Center, New York.)

75. Figure 16-3 is an example of
    A. An isodose curve.
    B. A dose–volume histogram.
    C. Organ dose distribution curves.
    D. A contour of an organ at risk.

76. Figure 16-3 allows one to determine
    A. How to properly line up a patient at the time of treatment.
    B. How much of a dose that a certain organ at risk or target is receiving.
    C. Which part of the tumor is receiving most of the dose.
    D. All of the above.

77. The most common acute toxic effect from radiation therapy to the head and neck is
    A. Headache.
    B. Nausea.
    C. Mucositis.
    D. Visual changes.

78. Which of the following is the most common late toxic effect from radiation therapy to the head and neck?
    A. Xerostomia
    B. Osteoradionecrosis
    C. Feeding tube dependence
    D. Brachial plexopathy

79. Which of the following is the most common late sequela after radiation therapy to the head and neck?
    A. Osteoradionecrosis
    B. Feeding tube dependence
    C. Hypothyroidism
    D. Brachial plexopathy

80. In oropharyngeal cancer, the rate of PEG dependence 2 years after treatment with definitive chemoradiation therapy (IMRT-based) is
    A. 1%.
    B. 5%.
    C. 15%.
    D. 20%.

81. Rates of osteoradionecrosis are dependent on
    A. The amount of radiation delivered to the mandible.
    B. Dental extractions after radiation therapy.
    C. Poor oral hygiene.
    D. All of the above.

*For the postoperative clinical scenarios in Questions 82 through 88, identify the best adjuvant treatment.*

82. A 40-year-old man with T1N0 SCC of the oral tongue s/p hemiglossectomy has clear margins and negative nodes as determined from the neck dissection specimen. The depth of invasion of the primary tumor was 3 mm.
    A. Postoperative chemoradiation therapy
    B. Postoperative radiation therapy
    C. No adjuvant therapy

83. A 43-year-old man has T3N2 SCC of the floor of the mouth with a positive margin.
    A. Postoperative chemoradiation therapy
    B. Postoperative radiation therapy
    C. No adjuvant therapy

84. A 28-year-old man had T4aN0 SCC of the larynx s/p laryngectomy with negative margins.
    A. Postoperative chemoradiation therapy
    B. Postoperative radiation therapy
    C. No adjuvant therapy

85. A 60-year-old man has T1N2 SCC of the oral tongue with 4 of 30 ipsilateral nodes involved with extracapsular extension (ECE).
    A. Postoperative chemoradiation therapy
    B. Postoperative radiation therapy
    C. No adjuvant therapy

86. A 39-year-old woman has a T3N2 SCC of the floor of the mouth with a positive margin.
    A. Postoperative chemoradiation therapy
    B. Postoperative radiation therapy
    C. No adjuvant therapy

87. A 44-year-old man has a T1N0 SCC of the tonsil s/p tonsillectomy with negative margins.
    A. Postoperative chemoradiation therapy
    B. Postoperative radiation therapy
    C. No adjuvant therapy

88. A 1.5-cm low-grade mucoepidermoid carcinoma of the parotid has a close margin.
    A. Postoperative chemoradiation therapy
    B. Postoperative radiation therapy
    C. No adjuvant therapy

89. Which of the following is not true regarding the Radiation Therapy Oncology Group (RTOG) randomized larynx organ preservation trial (RTOG-91-11) comparing induction chemotherapy followed by radiation therapy versus concurrent chemoradiation therapy versus radiation alone?
    A. The majority of patients had locoregional failure.
    B. No overall survival difference was seen among the three treatment arms.
    C. Those who required surgical salvage had similar outcomes to those who did not require surgical salvage.
    D. Those treated with induction chemotherapy had better disease-free survival rates compared with those undergoing radiation therapy alone.

90. According to the Meta-analysis of Chemotherapy in Head and Neck Cancer (MACH-NC) study, which patients do not benefit from the addition of concurrent chemotherapy to definitive radiation therapy?
    A. Patients older than 70 years
    B. Patients with oropharynx cancers
    C. Patients with HPV-positive tumors
    D. Patients without ECE

91. In which of the following sites is surgery clearly superior to definitive chemoradiation therapy?
    A. Oropharynx
    B. Larynx
    C. Oral cavity
    D. Nasopharynx

92. After definitive chemoradiation therapy for SCC of the head and neck, when should the first posttreatment positron emission tomography/computed tomography (PET/CT) scan be performed?
    A. After 3 weeks
    B. After 12 weeks
    C. After 24 weeks
    D. After 36 weeks

93. Which of the following laboratory test results should be routinely checked in follow-up visits after a patient receives radiation therapy?
    A. CBC
    B. TSH
    C. Chem-7
    D. LDL

94. Which of the following is not an indication for neck dissection after definitive chemoradiation therapy?
    A. Gross/palpable residual node
    B. Initial N3 disease
    C. Fluorodeoxyglucose (FDG)-avid disease on a posttreatment scan
    D. Initial N2 disease

95. After radiation therapy, which of the following is not a suspicious feature of a persistent metastatic lymph node?
    A. Size greater than 1.5 cm
    B. Focal enhancement on CT
    C. Well-circumscribed node
    D. Calcification

96. Which cranial nerve is rarely involved in patients with nasopharyngeal cancer?
    A. VII
    B. V
    C. III
    D. XII

97. Which CT-based landmark differentiates level II from level III?
    A. Hyoid bone
    B. Thyroid cartilage

C. Cricoid cartilage
D. Posterior belly of the digastric

98. Which CT-based landmark differentiates level III from level IV?
    A. Hyoid bone
    B. Thyroid cartilage
    C. Cricoid cartilage
    D. Tendon of the omohyoid muscle

99. Which of the following is associated with worse outcomes when patients undergo reirradiation?
    A. Nasopharynx subsite
    B. Prior salvage surgery
    C. Oral cavity subsite
    D. Isolated nodal disease

100. The feasibility of reirradiation does not depend on the
    A. Time since the prior course of radiation therapy.
    B. Location of recurrence.
    C. Dose received by prior critical structures.
    D. Prior delivery of chemotherapy.

## Answers

| | | |
|---|---|---|
| 1. T | 27. T | 53. A |
| 2. T | 28. F | 54. E |
| 3. F | 29. T | 55. A |
| 4. F | 30. F | 56. E |
| 5. T | 31. T | 57. B |
| 6. F | 32. F | 58. C |
| 7. F | 33. T | 59. C |
| 8. F | 34. T | 60. B |
| 9. F | 35. F | 61. B |
| 10. F | 36. F | 62. E |
| 11. F | 37. F | 63. D |
| 12. F | 38. F | 64. C |
| 13. T | 39. F | 65. C |
| 14. F | 40. T | 66. C |
| 15. F | 41. F | 67. B |
| 16. T | 42. F | 68. A |
| 17. T | 43. F | 69. A |
| 18. F | 44. F | 70. C |
| 19. T | 45. T | 71. B |
| 20. F | 46. T | 72. A |
| 21. F | 47. F | 73. A |
| 22. T | 48. F | 74. B |
| 23. F | 49. D | 75. B |
| 24. T | 50. A | 76. B |
| 25. T | 51. B | 77. C |
| 26. T | 52. B | 78. A |

| | | |
|---|---|---|
| 79. C | 87. C | 95. C |
| 80. B | 88. C | 96. A |
| 81. D | 89. C | 97. A |
| 82. C | 90. A | 98. C |
| 83. A | 91. C | 99. C |
| 84. B | 92. B | 100. D |
| 85. A | 93. B | |
| 86. A | 94. D | |

## Core Knowledge

- Arranging for a patient's radiation treatment involves a number of steps before treatment can commence, of which the first is a dental evaluation and appropriate dental care. After consultation, a patient is simulated, which usually involves obtaining a computed tomographic (CT) scan while the patient is immobilized with a face mask. Afterward, the radiation oncologist outlines the disease on the scan (contouring). Then a medical physicist and dosimetrist devise a method to deliver the radiation safely to the patient while avoiding radiation to normal structures. At the time of treatment, the radiation therapists verify that the patient lines up appropriately before treatment can begin.

- Radiation therapy is thought to kill tumor cells via damage to their DNA. The amount of radiation is typically measured in the unit gray (Gy), which represents joules of energy per kilogram. The following gives the conversion between grays, radiation absorbed dose (rad), and centigrays: 1 Gy = 100 rad = 100 cGy.

- In the past decade, intensity-modulated radiation therapy (IMRT) has become the standard of care for treating patients with head and neck cancer. Unlike older forms of radiation therapy, IMRT is better able to focus the dose of radiation on the tumor while simultaneously minimizing the dose received by healthy tissue. This has led to a dramatic reduction in toxicity.

- IMRT requires that the radiation oncologist outline the tumor, the areas at risk for microscopic spreading, and the critical normal structures on every CT slice (contouring). Outlining the gross disease (gross tumor volume [GTV]) and areas at risk of microscopic spreading (clinical target volume [CTV]) requires a thorough understanding of the anatomy of the region and is significantly more labor-intensive than prior two-dimensional or conventional radiation therapy techniques.

- Often, radiation to the head and neck involves the selection of different doses depending on the amount of disease in that area. Typically, gross disease receives a dose of 70 Gy. Areas at high risk of microscopic disease often receive a dose of between 60 and 66 Gy. Areas at low risk of microscopic disease typically receive a dose of 50 to 54 Gy. The areas designated at high risk and low risk will depend on the site of presentation, the stage, and other pathological features. The most common fraction size is 2 Gy of radiation per day.

- Contouring and dose selection are operator-dependent variables, and wide discrepancies in contours have been reported between different radiation oncologists. A difference in survival outcomes was reported between poor quality radiation therapy and good quality radiation therapy in the Trans-Tasman Radiation Oncology Group (TROG) study on tirapazamine.

- Evaluating the quality of a radiation therapy plan involves reviewing the dose–volume histogram (DVH) and the isodose curves. The DVH summarizes how much of a particular structure is receiving the prescribed dose (i.e., what fraction of the tumor is receiving the full prescribed dose). The isodose curves display this visually and help determine whether a certain part of the tumor is being undertreated.

- The more common acute toxic effects from radiation therapy to the head and neck are mucositis, erythema, dermatitis, odynophagia, weight loss, pain, and fatigue. Acute toxic effects typically do not arise until the third week of treatment and usually resolve within 6 weeks after the end of treatment. The time needed to recover from acute toxic effects is longer when concurrent chemotherapy is administered. Aggressive management of acute toxic effects as they arise and prophylactic measures can help minimize treatment breaks.

- The role of prophylactic percutaneous endoscopic gastrostomy (PEG) tube placement is controversial: some authorities believe it may lead to PEG dependence and an increased rate of long-term dysphagia.

- The most common late toxic effect after head and neck radiation therapy is hypothyroidism. Thyroid-stimulating hormone (TSH) levels should be routinely monitored after treatment. Other common late toxic effects include xerostomia and trismus.

- Rare late toxic effects (occurring in fewer than 5% of cases) include osteoradionecrosis, dysphagia, and carotid stenosis. These are highly dependent on patient factors. Osteoradionecrosis rates depend on patients' oral hygiene and dental extractions after radiation therapy, as well as the dose received by the mandible.

- Acute and late toxic effects appear to increase with the use of altered fractionation or the addition of concurrent systemic therapy.

- When hypofractionation (high dose per fraction) is used, the amount of radiation received by the target is much higher than the numerical sum of radiation (Gy) delivered. This is called the biological effective dose.

- Radiation therapy is widely used for head and neck cancers and can be used as a definitive treatment with or without chemotherapy, in an adjuvant—usually postoperative—setting, or for palliative treatment.

- Radiation therapy is often used as a definitive modality for squamous cell carcinoma (SCC) of the larynx, hypopharynx, oropharynx, and nasopharynx. It can be used in the adjuvant or palliative setting for almost any malignancy in the head and neck.

- In the locally advanced setting, multiple studies have documented the benefit of concurrent chemotherapy. The Meta-analysis of Chemotherapy in Head and Neck Cancer (MACH-NC) study demonstrated that the addition of chemotherapy leads to an absolute increase in overall survival of 6.5%. Platinum-based regimens typically had the best results.

- To try and exploit the four Rs of radiobiology (repair of DNA damage, redistribution of cells in the cell cycle, repopulation, and reoxygenation of hypoxic tumor areas), investigators have looked at altered fractionation schemes. The most common scheme involves delivering two fractions of radiation therapy a day for the entire course of radiation or delivering two fractions of radiation therapy a day for the last one third of the course of treatment. These schemes have been shown to improve local control. In a metaanalysis, a small improvement was seen in overall survival rates. However, the combination of altered fractionation and concurrent chemotherapy does not appear to be superior to standard fractionation and concurrent chemotherapy.

- Human papillomavirus (HPV)-positive tumors have improved outcomes compared with HPV-negative tumors after definitive chemoradiation therapy. Deescalating treatment in these patients with lower risk is an active area of investigation; however, for now, they should be treated in a fashion similar to those with HPV-negative tumors.

- Radiation therapy with concurrent cetuximab, a monoclonal antibody to epidermal growth factor receptor (EGFR), has been shown to significantly improve overall survival rates compared with radiation therapy alone in the palliative setting. A direct randomized comparison of cetuximab versus platinum-based regimens is under way. At present, platinum-based regimens are preferred over other drugs, as long as patients can tolerate the regimen.

- In the adjuvant setting for SCC, the most commonly accepted indications for radiation therapy are T3-T4 disease or multiple metastatic lymph nodes. Other less definitive indications include nodal disease in levels IV or V, a depth of invasion greater than 4 mm, perineural invasion, and lymphovascular invasion.

- In the adjuvant setting, patients with positive margins or extracapsular extension should receive adjuvant chemoradiation therapy because two randomized trials have demonstrated an overall survival advantage compared with radiation therapy alone.

- After radiation therapy, the preferred method for assessment of tumor response, in addition to clinical and endoscopic examination, is a posttreatment positron emission tomographic (PET)/CT scan at 12 weeks. In most patients with a complete response to therapy and negative PET scan results, routine neck dissection is not recommended.

## SUGGESTED READING

Ang KK, Harris J, Wheeler R, Weber R, Rosenthal DI, Nguyen-Tân PF, et al. Human papillomavirus and survival of patients with oropharyngeal cancer. N Engl J Med 2010;363(1):24–35.

Bernier J, Cooper JS, Pajak TF, van Glabbeke M, Bourhis J, Forastiere A, et al. Defining risk levels in locally advanced head and neck cancers: a comparative analysis of concurrent postoperative radiation plus chemotherapy trials of the EORTC (#22931) and RTOG (# 9501). Head Neck 2005;27(10):843–50.

Bonner JA, Harari PM, Giralt J, Azarnia N, Shin DM, Cohen RB, et al. Radiotherapy plus cetuximab for squamous-cell carcinoma of the head and neck. N Engl J Med 2006;354(6):567–78.

Bourhis J, Overgaard J, Audry H, Ang KK, Saunders M, Bernier J, et al. Hyperfractionated or accelerated radiotherapy in head and neck cancer: a meta-analysis. Lancet 2006;368(9538):843–54.

Grégoire V, Levendag P, Ang KK, Bernier J, Braaksma M, Budach V, et al. CT-based delineation of lymph node levels and related CTVs in the node-negative neck: DAHANCA, EORTC, GORTEC, NCIC, RTOG consensus guidelines. Radiother Oncol 2003;69(3):227–36.

Lee NY, de Arruda FF, Puri DR, Wolden SL, Narayana A, Mechalakos J, et al. A comparison of intensity-modulated radiation therapy and concomitant boost radiotherapy in the setting of concurrent chemotherapy for locally advanced oropharyngeal carcinoma. Int J Radiat Oncol Biol Phys 2006;66(4):966–74.

Lee NY, O'Meara W, Chan K, Della-Bianca C, Mechalakos JG, Zhung J, et al. Concurrent chemotherapy and intensity-modulated radiotherapy for locoregionally advanced laryngeal and hypopharyngeal cancers. Int J Radiat Oncol Biol Phys 2007;69(2):459–68.

Lee NY, Zhang Q, Pfister DG, Kim J, Garden AS, Mechalakos J, et al. Addition of bevacizumab to standard chemoradiation for locoregionally advanced nasopharyngeal carcinoma (RTOG 0615): a phase 2 multi-institutional trial. Lancet Oncol 2012;13(2):172–80.

Liauw SL, Mancuso AA, Amdur RJ, Morris CG, Villaret DB, Werning JW, et al. Postradiotherapy neck dissection for lymph node-positive head and neck cancer: the use of computed tomography to manage the neck. J Clin Oncol 2006;24(9):1421–7.

Pignon JP, le Maître A, Maillard E, Bourhis J, MACH-NC Collaborative Group. Meta-analysis of chemotherapy in head and neck cancer (MACH-NC): an update on 93 randomised trials and 17,346 patients. Radiother Oncol 2009;92(1):4–14.

# 17 Chemotherapy

## Questions

**TRUE/FALSE**

1. Neoadjuvant (i.e., induction) TPF chemotherapy (docetaxel, cisplatin, and 5-fluorouracil [5-FU]) for patients with locally and/or regionally advanced disease shows a significant difference in survival outcomes compared with PF chemotherapy. (T/F)

2. In the GORTEC trial by Calais and colleagues comparing concurrent chemoradiation therapy with carboplatin plus infusional 5-FU versus radiation therapy alone for unresectable oropharynx cancer, chemoradiation therapy was shown to be superior to radiation therapy alone. (T/F)

3. The central finding of the Veterans Affairs Laryngeal Cancer Study Group randomized trial was that attempting organ preservation with induction chemotherapy and radiation therapy does not significantly compromise overall survival at 3 years compared with primary laryngectomy. (T/F)

4. Common adverse events associated with cetuximab include neuropathy, vomiting, alopecia, and myelosuppression. (T/F)

5. Paclitaxel acts by formation of DNA cross-links. (T/F)

6. In the study by Bonner and colleagues for patients with stage III/IV (M0) head and neck squamous cell carcinoma (HNSCC), the addition of cetuximab to definitive radiation therapy improved 3-year overall survival rates by approximately 10%. (T/F)

7. The results of RTOG 91-11 by Forastiere and colleagues did not address the management of patients with T1 disease or large-volume T4 disease. (T/F)

8. Cetuximab has the most data to support its use as a radiosensitizer for fit patients with stage III/IV(M0) HNSCC. (T/F)

9. Magnesium infusions to prevent methotrexate-associated mucositis represent a major advance that has occurred in supportive care to improve the tolerability of chemotherapy for HNSCC patients. (T/F)

10. In a study of patients with advanced head and neck cancer by Morton and colleagues, cisplatin was associated with an approximate 10-week improvement in overall survival time compared with best supportive care. (T/F)

11. Cetuximab is a fully humanized monoclonal antibody against the HER2 receptors. (T/F)

12. Regarding neoadjuvant chemotherapy, the Head and Neck Contracts Program demonstrated improved overall survival and improved locoregional control rates. (T/F)

13. A design feature of the Veterans Affairs Laryngeal Cancer Study Group randomized trial was that patients with less than a partial response after two cycles of induction chemotherapy (cisplatin plus 5-FU) were directed to undergo total laryngectomy. (T/F)

14. The cisplatin and 5-fluorouracil doses and schedules in TPF were identical in the TAX 323 study by Vermorken and colleagues and the TAX 324 study by Posner and colleagues. (T/F)

15. Carboplatin exerts its cytotoxic effect by binding to DNA. (T/F)

16. A 48-year-old man with newly diagnosed stage IVA SCC of the tonsil is referred to a medical oncologist for consideration of concurrent chemotherapy. He has never smoked. The patient's tumor and the patient's peripheral blood should both be tested for the presence of human papilloma virus (HPV) because the presence of virus in the tumor is not clinically meaningful unless it can be corroborated by a peripheral blood test indicating active virus in the circulation. (T/F)

17. The TAX 323 study and the TAX 324 study established that the addition of docetaxel to cisplatin plus 5-FU, as induction therapy followed by definitive radiation therapy, improves the overall survival rate in patients with locally/regionally advanced HNSCC. (T/F)

18. Regarding randomized phase III clinical trials comparing cytotoxic chemotherapy regimens for patients with metastatic HNSCC, the use of cisplatin plus 5-FU is superior to cisplatin plus paclitaxel. (T/F)

19. At the doses and schedules commonly used in the treatment of patients with metastatic HNSCC, cisplatin is more likely to cause kidney damage than other chemotherapeutic agents typically used for this disease. (T/F)

20. The peripheral neuropathy associated with taxane chemotherapy is generally permanent, whereas the neuropathy associated with cisplatin chemotherapy is almost always reversible with discontinuation of the drug. (T/F)

21. In a randomized trial comparing PF chemotherapy before locoregional therapy versus locoregional therapy alone, Paccagnella and colleagues found a modest improvement in overall survival for the PF induction chemotherapy arm, but only for patients with resectable disease. (T/F)

22. Regarding overall survival rates, the TAX 323 and TAX 324 studies established that TPF followed by locoregional therapy was superior to locoregional therapy alone. (T/F)

23. The study by Bonner and colleagues that led to the approval of cetuximab given with radiation therapy for patients with locally/regionally advanced disease found that, with the exception of acneiform rash and infusion reactions, the addition of cetuximab was not associated with an increased risk of grade 3 or 4 toxic effects. (T/F)

24. In the Intergroup Study for patients with locally advanced (M0) head and neck cancer conducted by Adelstein and colleagues, the treatment group with the best overall survival rate was with radiation plus concurrent cisplatin. (T/F)

25. The MACH-NC metaanalysis reported an absolute benefit of 8% at 5 years associated with chemotherapy administered concurrently with radiation therapy. (T/F)

26. Level I evidence from mature, large, randomized clinical trials conclusively establishes that HPV-associated head and neck cancer should be treated with cetuximab plus radiation therapy, not cisplatin plus radiation therapy. (T/F)

27. For patients with recurrent HNSCC, the major response rate typically achieved with single-agent chemotherapy is typically 10% to 30%. (T/F)

28. An important factor for the better survival outcomes seen with TPF in TAX 324 compared with TPF in TAX 323 is that TAX 324 included patients with both resectable and unresectable disease but TAX 323 included only patients with unresectable disease. (T/F)

29. Cisplatin is excreted almost entirely in the urine. (T/F)

30. Regarding palliative chemotherapy for patients with metastatic HNSCC, all patients, regardless of performance status, should receive first-line therapy with cisplatin plus 5-FU plus cetuximab. (T/F)

31. High-dose isotretinoin reverses oral leukoplakia but has not been demonstrated to reduce the risk of invasive SCC. (T/F)

32. Regarding patients in whom surgical pathological analysis demonstrates extracapsular extension and/or microscopically involved surgical margins who

received chemoradiation therapy versus those who received radiation therapy alone, the combined analysis of EORTC 22931 and RTOG 9501 did not demonstrate an improved overall survival rate for the patients receiving chemoradiation therapy. (T/F)

33. In the trial by Bonner and colleagues, radiation therapy with concurrent weekly cetuximab was associated with a superior overall survival rate. (T/F)

34. For patients with previously untreated HNSCC that is locally and/or regionally advanced, the major response rate achieved with cisplatin-based combination chemotherapy is typically in the range of 10% to 20%. (T/F)

35. Long-term complications of chemoradiation therapy can include hypothyroidism, stricture requiring pharyngoesophageal dilation (especially among patients with tumors arising in the hypopharynx or larynx), and xerostomia. (T/F)

36. Using the T-A-M End Results System (short-term toxicity, adverse long-term effects, and mortality risk from treatment [TAME]), RTOG 91-11 showed that sequential (or induction) therapy is associated with an extreme acute toxicity risk. (T/F)

37. Combined modality trials for patients with oropharynx SCC should at least stratify patients by HPV status. (T/F)

38. Combined modality trials for patients with larynx SCC should at least stratify patients by Epstein–Barr virus status. (T/F)

39. The TAME system was developed to demonstrate that the acute toxic effects of combined modality therapy are generally much lower than commonly believed. (T/F)

40. In RTOG 91-11, neck dissection after completion of radiation/chemoradiation therapy was planned if clinical imaging showed multiple lymph nodes or a single lymph node 3 cm or larger. (T/F)

41. The GORTEC study found that radiation therapy plus concurrent carboplatin plus 5-FU chemotherapy compared with radiation therapy alone was associated with an improved overall survival rate among patients with stage III or IV oropharynx SCC without distant metastases. (T/F)

42. The Veterans Affairs trial demonstrated that induction chemotherapy followed by radiation therapy resulted in superior overall survival rates compared with primary surgery (total laryngectomy) and larynx preservation in 66% of survivors. (T/F)

43. In the Intergroup Study for patients with unresectable HNSCC, radiation therapy alone was associated with the highest incidence of ≥grade 3 toxic effects. (T/F)

44. For patients with recurrent and/or metastatic HNSCC, a 1985 study by Vogl and colleagues demonstrated that the objective response rate was

the same for both the methotrexate arm and for the methotrexate plus cisplatin plus bleomycin group. (T/F)

45. For patients with metastatic HNSCC, the addition of cetuximab to the cisplatin plus 5-FU doublet should only be contemplated in patients with epidermal growth factor receptor (EGFR) amplification. (T/F)

46. In a randomized study of adjuvant therapy for patients with resected HNSCC in whom the surgical pathological results were notable for extracapsular extension, the treatment arm with the highest overall survival rate at 5 years was radiation therapy plus concurrent weekly cisplatin. (T/F)

47. Perineural invasion and two or more involved lymph nodes were identified as poor risk features found on surgical pathological examination in both RTOG 9501 and EORTC 22931 that mandate the concurrent administration of cisplatin with postoperative radiation therapy. (T/F)

48. In a randomized clinical trial for patients with recurrent and/or metastatic HNSCC, the addition of cetuximab to the platinum plus 5-FU doublet improved overall survival rates. (T/F)

49. In EORTC 22931 comparing postoperative radiation therapy alone versus postoperative radiation therapy plus concurrent cisplatin, the combined treatment arm was notable for improved progression-free survival and 5-year overall survival rates. (T/F)

50. For patients receiving first-line therapy with cetuximab plus cisplatin plus 5-FU for recurrent and/or metastatic HNSCC, the EXTREME trial found that the median overall survival time was approximately 7 months. (T/F)

## MULTIPLE CHOICE

51. Which of the following toxic effects is not typically associated with the indicated therapy for head and neck cancer?
    A. Renal toxicity, cisplatin
    B. Acneiform rash, paclitaxel
    C. Mucositis, 5-FU
    D. Xerostomia, radiation therapy

52. Which of the following toxic effects is commonly associated with cisplatin?
    A. Renal toxicity
    B. Ototoxicity
    C. Myelosuppression
    D. All of the above

53. The EORTC trial of larynx preservation in hypopharyngeal SCC found that
    A. Induction chemotherapy was associated with significantly worse locoregional control.
    B. The larynx preservation rate at 5 years was 65%.
    C. Primary surgery is associated with a superior overall survival rate in this patient population.

D. At 5 years, overall survival and disease-free survival rates were comparable between the primary surgery group and the primary induction chemotherapy group.

54. Which of the following chemotherapeutic agents used in the treatment of HNSCC inhibits dihydrofolate reductase?
    A. Cisplatin
    B. Methotrexate
    C. Paclitaxel
    D. Cetuximab

55. An 83-year-old man is given a diagnosis of stage IVA oropharyngeal cancer. Which of the following medical comorbidities would make cetuximab preferable to cisplatin, from a safety and tolerability standpoint, in this patient?
    A. Renal insufficiency
    B. Tinnitus
    C. Peripheral neuropathy
    D. All of the above

56. The 83-year-old man from Question 55 has a grade 4 hypersensitivity reaction during the first cetuximab infusion. He recovers fully, but no further cetuximab is planned. The oncologist discusses options including radiation therapy alone or radiation therapy with different chemotherapy. Which of the following concurrent chemotherapy regimens has been shown to improve the overall survival rate when added to radiation therapy for locally/regionally advanced oropharynx cancer?
    A. Carboplatin plus infusional 5-FU
    B. Bolus paclitaxel plus weekly methotrexate
    C. Weekly paclitaxel plus gemcitabine
    D. Weekly methotrexate plus gemcitabine

57. Which of the following describes the main mechanism of action of platinum chemotherapy?
    A. Formation of DNA cross-links
    B. Stabilization of microtubules to block M phase
    C. Inhibition of dihydrofolate reductase during S phase
    D. Inhibition of thymidylate synthase during S phase

58. A 56-year-old woman with metastatic hypopharynx cancer presents for her first cycle with palliative paclitaxel. During the infusion, she develops a severe hypersensitivity reaction, with hypotension and wheezing. The reaction resolves, and the patient stabilizes after discontinuation of the infusion and administration of epinephrine, steroids, and antihistamines. Which of the following statements is not correct?
    A. She probably reacted to the lipid solvent rather than the paclitaxel itself.
    B. It is important to review the timing and dosing of her steroid premedications to determine whether improper premedication may have been a causal factor for the hypersensitivity reaction.

C. If she took the steroid premedications properly, the risk of rechallenge with paclitaxel is prohibitively high because she would probably have a more severe reaction if rechallenged.

D. She should never receive cetuximab because hypersensitivity to taxol is highly predictive of hypersensitivity to cetuximab.

59. Which of the following is a preclinical observation that provided a biological rationale for the clinical development of cetuximab in HNSCC?
    A. Almost all HNSCCs express EGFR on the cell membrane.
    B. Activating somatic mutations in the tyrosine kinase domain of EGFR are found in approximately 30% of all HNSCCs.
    C. EGFR/EGFR homodimers only are found in HNSCCs, but EGFR does not dimerize with other HER 2 family members in these cells.
    D. EGFR is expressed in only about 10% of HNSCCs, but binding of cetuximab triggers rapid cell death in any EGFR-expressing HNSCC.

60. In RTOG 91-11 study by Forastiere and colleagues, the concurrent chemoradiation group (arm B) was associated with
    A. Similar rates of grade 3 and 4 toxic effects as in arms A and C.
    B. A 2% increase in the incidence of death that may have been treatment related.
    C. A larynx preservation rate that was better than that of arm A but worse than that of arm C.
    D. A superior overall survival rate compared with arm A and arm C.

61. In the GORTEC trial by Calais and colleagues comparing concurrent chemoradiation therapy versus radiation therapy alone, concurrent chemoradiation therapy was associated with
    A. An improved overall survival rate but not improved locoregional control.
    B. Improved locoregional control but not an improved overall survival rate.
    C. Higher rates of mucositis, the need for a feeding tube, and late complications.
    D. Higher rates of mucositis and the need for a feeding tube but not higher rates of late complications.

62. Which of the following chemotherapeutic agents is not typically associated with neuropathy?
    A. Methotrexate
    B. Paclitaxel
    C. Docetaxel
    D. Cisplatin

63. Which of the following is true for the TAX 323 study by Vermorken and colleagues but not for the TAX 324 study by Posner and colleagues?
    A. Only patients with unresectable disease were allowed to participate.
    B. The study compared TPF with PF.
    C. The study called for antibiotic prophylaxis to decrease the risk of neutropenic sepsis.

D. The study compared cetuximab plus PF versus PF alone.

64. A 58-year-old man with metastatic laryngeal cancer is admitted to the hospital with profound diarrhea and mucositis during his first cycle with cisplatin plus 5-FU and cetuximab. What is the most likely cause of these symptoms?
    A. Cisplatin
    B. 5-FU
    C. Cetuximab
    D. *Clostridium difficile*

65. A 67-year-old man with metastatic oral cavity SCC has completed six cycles of cisplatin plus 5-FU plus cetuximab, as per the EXTREME regimen. The metastatic disease has undergone a radiographic partial response, but cycles 5 and 6 were complicated by neuropathy, diarrhea, and neutropenia. According to the EXTREME study, what would be the next step in treatment?
    A. Stop all treatment and refer to hospice.
    B. Continue cisplatin plus 5-FU plus cetuximab, but reduce the dose of cisplatin, until disease progression or worsening toxic effects.
    C. Continue 5-FU plus cetuximab, but substitute carboplatin for cisplatin, until disease progression or worsening toxic effects.
    D. Continue cetuximab as monotherapy until disease progression.

66. Examples of drugs from the four main classes of active cytotoxic chemotherapy regimens for the treatment of HNSCC are
    A. Cisplatin, docetaxel, methotrexate, and 5-FU.
    B. Cisplatin, fludarabine, methotrexate, and cetuximab.
    C. Bleomycin, gemcitabine, doxorubicin (Adriamycin), and cisplatin.
    D. Carboplatin, mitoxantrone, 5-FU, and cetuximab.

67. Which of the following is not true of the toxicity profile of TPF in the TAX 324 study?
    A. Approximately 83% of patients experienced grade 3 or 4 neutropenia.
    B. Approximately 12% of patients experienced febrile neutropenia.
    C. The rate of grade 3 or 4 mucositis was higher with TPF compared with PF.
    D. The rate of grade 3 or 4 neutropenia was higher with TPF compared with PF.

68. A fit 67-year-old woman with metastatic SCC of the oral tongue presents to the clinic for consideration of palliative chemotherapy options. She states that it is very important for her quality of life to avoid any treatments that cause alopecia or skin rashes. With this in mind, which regimen would most likely be acceptable to her?
    A. Cisplatin plus paclitaxel
    B. Cisplatin plus 5-FU
    C. Cisplatin plus 5-FU plus cetuximab
    D. Docetaxel

69. Which of the following chemotherapeutic agents used in the treatment of HNSCC is commonly administered as a continuous intravenous infusion over 4 or 5 days?
    A. Methotrexate
    B. 5-FU
    C. Paclitaxel
    D. Cisplatin

70. In studies that have compared combination cytotoxic chemotherapy regimens versus monotherapy with a cytotoxic agent, which of the following is generally true?
    A. The combination regimen is associated with more toxicity.
    B. The combination regimen is associated with more nonhematological toxicity but not higher response rates.
    C. The combination chemotherapy regimen is associated with longer overall survival rates.
    D. All of the above are true.

71. A 58-year-old man with metastatic head and neck cancer who is receiving palliative chemotherapy presents to a local emergency department with inability to eat due to oral mucositis pain. He does not recall the name of the chemotherapy drug that he is being treated with, but he said he has received other chemotherapy drugs over the last year for his head and neck cancer. He started this new drug 3 weeks ago and receives one infusion per week. With which drug is he most likely being treated?
    A. Docetaxel
    B. Gemcitabine
    C. Methotrexate
    D. Bleomycin

72. The study by Bonner and colleagues that led to the approval of cetuximab given with radiation therapy for patients with locally/regionally advanced disease found that
    A. Cetuximab plus radiation therapy yielded a superior overall survival rate compared with radiation therapy alone.
    B. Cetuximab plus radiation therapy yielded a superior overall survival rate compared with cisplatin plus radiation therapy.
    C. Cetuximab plus radiation therapy was superior to radiation therapy alone in terms of the larynx preservation rate, although overall survival rates did not differ between the two arms.
    D. Cetuximab plus radiation therapy was superior to cisplatin plus radiation therapy in terms of the larynx preservation rate, although overall survival rates did not differ between the two arms.

73. Patients with low levels of dihydropyrimidine dehydrogenase are at increased risk of severe toxicity when treated with
    A. 5-FU.
    B. Cisplatin.
    C. Cetuximab.
    D. Any of the above.

74. In the Intergroup Study for patients with locally advanced (M0) head and neck cancer conducted by Adelstein and colleagues, treatment with concurrent radiation plus cisplatin was associated with
    A. A superior overall survival rate compared with the other treatment groups.
    B. An increased incidence of acute toxic effects (including mucositis and nausea/vomiting).
    C. A toxic death rate of approximately 4%.
    D. All of the above.

75. Which of the following targeted agents has received regulatory approval by the Food and Drug Administration of the United States for the treatment of head and neck cancer?
    A. Gefitinib
    B. Cetuximab
    C. Erlotinib
    D. Both cetuximab and erlotinib

76. Data from randomized prospective phase III clinical trials support the use of cisplatin plus concurrent chemoradiation therapy in which of the following settings?
    A. A 58-year-old man has locally/regionally advanced larynx SCC, and it will be used as an organ preservation strategy.
    B. A 31-year-old woman has undergone resection of an adenoid cystic carcinoma of the submandibular salivary gland.
    C. A 52-year-old man has anaplastic thyroid cancer.
    D. A 42-year-old man will be undergoing reirradiation; he has already undergone resection of recurrent SCC of the oral tongue.

77. In the EORTC study on larynx preservation in hypopharyngeal cancer by Lefebvre and colleagues, patients randomly assigned to induction chemotherapy underwent a response assessment at the primary site after each cycle of induction chemotherapy. After cycle 3, patients were directed to proceed
    A. To radiation therapy if there was at least a partial response.
    B. To laryngectomy if there was a partial response.
    C. To laryngectomy if there was a complete response.
    D. With two more cycles of induction chemotherapy if there was less than a complete response, and then to repeat the response assessment to guide subsequent locoregional therapy.

78. In RTOG 91-11, the group with the worst larynx preservation rate was
    A. Radiation therapy alone.
    B. Radiation therapy with concurrent carboplatin.
    C. Chemotherapy followed by radiation therapy.
    D. Radiation therapy with concurrent cisplatin.

79. Docetaxel
    A. Is a semisynthetic taxane.
    B. Was first isolated from the bark of the Pacific yew tree.

C. Is formulated as a lipid emulsion of polyeth-oxylated castor oil (Cremophor).

D. Is highly emetogenic.

80. In a phase III study by Burtness and colleagues for patients with recurrent or metastatic HNSCC that was previously untreated, cisplatin plus cetuximab was compared with cisplatin plus placebo. Which of the following was observed in the cisplatin plus cetuximab group?

A. A higher radiographic response rate and a longer overall survival rate

B. A higher radiographic response rate but not a longer overall survival rate

C. A lower response rate in patients who developed skin rashes

D. Both B and C

81. Which class of chemotherapy drug stabilizes microtubules to block the M phase?

A. Platinum

B. Taxane

C. Antifolate

D. Fluoropyrimidine

82. Which of the following strategies has been shown to reduce the risk of second primary tumors in patients with head and neck cancer?

A. Oral retinoids

B. Antioxidant vitamins

C. Smoking cessation

D. All of the above

83. The available data from randomized prospective clinical trials of standard cisplatin-based chemoradiation therapy for head and neck cancer indicates that the incidence of early treatment-related death is approximately

A. Less than 1%.

B. 4%.

C. 15%.

D. 25%.

84. Which statement regarding the mechanism of action of cetuximab is correct?

A. Cetuximab binds to the extracellular domain of VEGFR.

B. Cetuximab binds to the intracellular tyrosine kinase domain of EGFR.

C. Cetuximab binds to the extracellular domain of EGFR and other erbB-B/HER family members.

D. Cetuximab binds to the extracellular domain of EGFR.

85. Which of the following was not a finding of the Head and Neck Contracts Program Trial?

A. A significantly improved disease-free survival rate was seen in the neoadjuvant therapy arm.

B. Overall survival times were comparable in the three arms.

C. Poor compliance was seen with the adjuvant phase of the neoadjuvant/adjuvant arm.

D. On subset analysis, adjuvant therapy was of greatest benefit in N2 disease.

86. Which of the following is a reasonable possible explanation for the longer survival times for patients treated with TPF in TAX 324 compared with the survival times for patients treated with TPF in TAX 323?

A. TAX 323 was restricted to patients with unresectable disease, whereas TAX 324 included both patients with resectable disease and patients with unresectable disease.

B. After induction TPF, patients in TAX 324 received radiation therapy with concurrent weekly carboplatin, whereas patients in TAX 323 received radiation therapy only after TPF.

C. In TAX 324, the cisplatin dose was higher than the cisplatin dose used in TAX 323.

D. All of the above are true.

87. Which of the following are findings regarding TPF in the TAX 323 study?

A. A higher objective response rate but no significant difference in the median overall survival rate

B. An improved median overall survival rate but increased treatment-related mortality

C. A higher objective response rate and significantly improved median overall survival and improved median progression-free survival rates

D. An improved median progression-free survival rate but no significant improvement in the overall survival rate

88. Which of the following toxic effects are most typically associated with cetuximab monotherapy?

A. Xerostomia and acneiform rash

B. Hypomagnesemia and acneiform rash

C. Alopecia and acneiform rash

D. Mucositis and acneiform rash

89. In the randomized study by Burtness and colleagues that compared cisplatin plus cetuximab versus cisplatin plus placebo for patients with recurrent or metastatic HNSCC, which of the following was observed?

A. In a subset analysis of patients who had received at least one prior cytotoxic regimen for recurrent or metastatic disease, the objective response rate was higher in the cisplatin plus cetuximab arm.

B. In a subset analysis of patients who had received at least one prior cytotoxic regimen for recurrent or metastatic disease, the overall survival rate was higher in the cisplatin plus cetuximab arm.

C. In the cetuximab plus cisplatin group, the objective response rate was higher among patients who experienced skin toxic effects.

D. Unexpectedly, the response rate was higher in the cisplatin plus placebo group.

90. You are evaluating a 53-year-old man with newly diagnosed bulky transglottic T4N2c laryngeal SCC with thyroid cartilage invasion. He has a 30-year history of alcohol abuse and a creatinine level of

2.5 mg/dL. His Eastern Cooperative Oncology Group (ECOG) performance status is 2. He has been offered primary laryngectomy but has refused. Which of the following is the appropriate management strategy for this patient?

A. Individualized management based on the consensus clinical judgment of the treating physicians is appropriate because this patient would not have met eligibility criteria for the large randomized clinical trials that compared combined modality strategies for patients with HNSCC.

B. Cetuximab plus radiation therapy is appropriate because the study by Bonner and colleagues showed improved outcomes for patients with renal insufficiency with this regimen.

C. Cisplatin plus radiation is appropriate because RTOG 91-11 established this as the organ preservation strategy for patients in his situation.

D. Induction TPF is appropriate because TAX 323 and TAX 324 showed improved long-term survival rates with the use of TPF for patients in his situation.

91. In the phase III "Studio" study for patients with locally/regionally advanced HNSCC comparing PF induction chemotherapy before locoregional therapy versus locoregional therapy alone, Paccagnella and colleagues found that

A. PF induction chemotherapy was associated with a modest survival advantage in a subgroup analysis restricted to patients with operable disease.

B. PF induction chemotherapy was associated with a modest survival advantage in a subgroup analysis restricted to patients with inoperable disease.

C. PF induction chemotherapy was not associated with a modest survival advantage among patients with either operable disease or inoperable disease.

D. PF induction chemotherapy was associated with a modest survival advantage among all patients, regardless of whether they had operable or inoperable disease.

92. In the study of radiation therapy plus concurrent cetuximab by Bonner and colleagues, cetuximab adverse events included a

A. Severe infusion reaction in 10% of patients.

B. Statistically significant intensification of mucositis in the radiation field.

C. Statistically significant increase in dysphagia requiring percutaneous endoscopic gastrostomy (PEG) tube placement.

D. Severe acneiform rash in 17% of patients.

93. RTOG 8503 (Intergroup 0034), which evaluated the addition of concurrent chemotherapy to adjuvant radiation therapy for patients with resected head and neck cancer,

A. Failed to show significant differences in survival between the treatment groups.

B. Identified patients with high-risk features in surgical pathological specimens in a retrospective analysis.

C. Found that the most effective concurrent regimen was cisplatin plus paclitaxel.

D. Found that the most effective concurrent regimen was hydroxyurea.

94. A 65-year-old man with metastatic oral tongue SCC has received one cycle of cetuximab plus cisplatin plus 5-FU. Treatment was complicated by diarrhea and mucositis that required hospitalization but now have resolved. In planning a second cycle, dose modification in which of the following drugs would be most appropriate?

A. 5-FU

B. Cisplatin and cetuximab

C. Cisplatin

D. Cetuximab

95. In the EORTC study on larynx preservation in hypopharyngeal carcinoma, induction chemotherapy plus radiation therapy compared with primary surgery resulted in

A. A statistically significant improvement in local control.

B. No difference in 5-year overall survival or disease-free survival rates.

C. Larynx preservation in 35% at 5 years.

D. All of the above.

96. In the Southwest Oncology Group study by Forastiere and colleagues that randomly assigned 277 patients with advanced head and neck cancer to three different treatment regimens,

A. Cisplatin plus 5-FU yielded the same response rate as carboplatin plus 5-FU.

B. Cisplatin plus 5-FU was associated with a significantly longer median survival time than methotrexate.

C. Median survival times for the cisplatin plus 5-FU arm and the carboplatin plus 5-FU arm were significantly longer than for the methotrexate arm.

D. Median survival times were similar in all three treatment groups in the study.

97. In RTOG 9501 comparing postoperative radiation therapy alone versus postoperative radiation therapy plus concurrent cisplatin, the combined treatment arm was notable for

A. A significantly improved overall survival rate but only a trend toward improved 2-year locoregional control.

B. Improved 2-year locoregional control and an improved disease-free survival rate.

C. Improved 2-year locoregional control and a significantly improved overall survival rate.

D. A trend toward an improved survival rate but no increase in incidence of ≥grade 3 toxic effects.

98. Premedication with steroids before infusion is required to reduce the risk of an anaphylactic reaction with which of the following chemotherapeutic agents?

A. Paclitaxel
B. Cetuximab
C. Methotrexate
D. 5-FU

99. A 50-year-old male former smoker presents for a medical oncology consultation. He has undergone resection of T3N2 SCC of the supraglottic larynx, and the surgical pathological results are notable for extracapsular extension in the resected cervical lymph nodes. He has no significant medical co-morbidities and wishes to be maximally aggressive to improve his chance of durable disease-free survival. Postoperative radiation therapy is planned. For his situation, which of the following concurrent chemotherapy regimens is best supported by data from prospective randomized clinical trials?
A. Cetuximab
B. Cetuximab plus cisplatin
C. Cisplatin
D. Cisplatin plus 5-FU

100. In a phase II study conducted by Vermorken and colleagues for patients with recurrent and/or metastatic HNSCC with clinical progression after prior platinum-based therapy, cetuximab
A. Yielded a median time to progression of 70 days.
B. Was not associated with any objective responses.
C. Was associated with radiation recall in 15% of patients.
D. Was associated with uncomplicated grade 3 neutropenia in 15% of patients.

## Answers

| | | | | | |
|---|---|---|---|---|---|
| 1. T | 20. F | 39. F | 58. D | 73. A | 88. B |
| 2. T | 21. F | 40. T | 59. A | 74. D | 89. C |
| 3. T | 22. F | 41. T | 60. B | 75. B | 90. A |
| 4. F | 23. T | 42. F | 61. C | 76. A | 91. B |
| 5. F | 24. T | 43. F | 62. A | 77. B | 92. D |
| 6. T | 25. T | 44. F | 63. A | 78. A | 93. B |
| 7. T | 26. F | 45. F | 64. B | 79. A | 94. A |
| 8. F | 27. T | 46. T | 65. D | 80. B | 95. D |
| 9. F | 28. T | 47. F | 66. A | 81. B | 96. D |
| 10. T | 29. T | 48. T | 67. C | 82. C | 97. B |
| 11. F | 30. F | 49. T | 68. B | 83. B | 98. A |
| 12. F | 31. T | 50. F | 69. B | 84. D | 99. C |
| 13. T | 32. F | 51. B | 70. A | 85. A | 100. A |
| 14. F | 33. T | 52. D | 71. C | 86. D | |
| 15. T | 34. F | 53. D | 72. A | 87. C | |
| 16. F | 35. T | 54. B | | | |
| 17. T | 36. F | 55. D | | | |
| 18. F | 37. T | 56. A | | | |
| 19. T | 38. F | 57. A | | | |

## Core Knowledge

• Chemotherapy may be given before definitive radiation therapy (induction chemotherapy), during radiation therapy (concurrent chemoradiation therapy), or after radiation therapy (adjuvant chemoradiation therapy) in selected patients.

• The main classes of cytotoxic agents used in head and neck squamous cell carcinoma (HNSCC) are platinums, taxanes, and antimetabolites. Cetuximab, a novel chimeric antibody directed against the epidermal growth factor receptor, is the only molecularly targeted agent that is currently approved for the treatment of head and neck cancer.

• Adverse effects of cisplatin include bone marrow suppression (which can lead to infection), hearing loss (particularly in the high-frequency range), peripheral neuropathy, and severe emesis (which usually can be prevented or controlled by antinausea medications).

• Adverse effects of taxanes include fatigue, alopecia, myelosuppression, and peripheral neuropathy. Taxanes are metabolized by the liver and not administered in patients with significant liver dysfunction.

• Cisplatin is the drug with the most data to support its use as a radiosensitizer in patients with head and neck cancer and is associated with increased mucositis in the radiation field.

• The antimetabolites methotrexate and 5-fluorouracil (5-FU) are associated with myelosuppression, fatigue, and mucositis. 5-FU can also cause diarrhea.

• Cetuximab binds the extracellular domain of the epidermal growth factor receptor and acts as a radiosensitizer. The most common adverse effect is an acneiform rash. A small risk of a severe allergic-type hypersensitivity reaction also exists during the first exposure to cetuximab.

- In the Veterans Affairs Laryngeal Cancer Study Group, standard treatment (primary laryngectomy followed by radiation therapy) versus organ preservation therapy (induction chemotherapy with cisplatin plus 5-FU followed by radiation therapy) showed no significant difference in median and overall survival rates at 2 years, but larynx preservation was reported in 66% of the cases in the organ preservation group.

- The addition of docetaxel to cisplatin plus 5-FU (TPF) in stage III or IV disease with no distant metastasis (M0) has demonstrated superiority over the platinum plus 5-FU (PF) regimen in the TAX 323 and TAX 324 studies. There was a higher objective response rate, improved median overall survival rate, and improved progression-free survival rate.

- For patients with locally and/or regionally advanced unresectable HNSCCs, the Intergroup study by Adelstein and colleagues demonstrated that concurrent chemoradiation therapy (100 mg/m$^2$ cisplatin every 3 weeks for three cycles) was superior to radiation therapy alone or split-course radiation therapy and chemotherapy.

- RTOG 91-11 established chemoradiation therapy (100 mg/m$^2$ cisplatin every 3 weeks for three cycles) as a standard regimen for larynx preservation.

- The GORTEC trial showed that concurrent chemoradiation therapy (carboplatin plus infusional 5-FU) was associated with improved locoregional control and overall 5-year survival rates compared with radiation therapy alone. Chemoradiation therapy was associated with an increased incidence of mucositis, percutaneous endoscopic gastrostomy (PEG) tube requirement, and long-term complications.

- In the study by Bonner et al, weekly concurrent cetuximab with radiation therapy improved overall survival rates and progression-free survival rates compared with radiation therapy alone. Cetuximab was associated with an increased incidence of acneiform rash.

- HNSCC patients who have undergone primary surgery and who have high-risk surgical pathological features (e.g., extracapsular extension or positive surgical margins) appear to derive a modest survival benefit from chemoradiation therapy (cisplatin 100 mg/m$^2$ every 3 weeks for three cycles) compared with radiation therapy alone. However, the application of concurrent cisplatin with postoperative radiation therapy intensifies acute toxic effects.

- Single-agent palliative chemotherapy achieves partial responses of approximately 10% to 30%; no single agent has shown conclusive evidence of superiority over another. The drugs most commonly used for palliative chemotherapy include cisplatin, taxanes, methotrexate, 5-FU, and cetuximab.

- One randomized study of recurrent or metastatic HNSCC has shown palliative cisplatin to be associated with an improved survival duration (approximately 10 weeks longer) compared with best supportive care (BSC). Subsequent studies have generally not included a BSC arm.

- In studies before the introduction of cetuximab, combination cytotoxic chemotherapy was associated with higher response rates and more acute toxic effects compared with single-agent chemotherapy but without an increase in overall survival rates.

- For patients with recurrent or metastatic disease, the regimen reported in the EXTREME study (i.e., platinum, 5-FU, and cetuximab) yielded higher response rates with increased overall survival rates compared with standard treatment (platinum and 5-FU).

- The treatment-related mortality rate for chemoradiation therapy for head and neck cancers in randomized clinical trials was approximately 3% to 4%.

- Long-term complications of chemoradiation therapy may include xerostomia, taste disturbances, hypothyroidism, pharyngeal stricture, and osteoradionecrosis.

- Extensively evaluated compounds for chemoprevention in head and neck cancer include vitamin A and its derivatives. Although high-dose isotretinoin reverses oral leukoplakia, it does not prevent or reverse invasive SCC.

## SUGGESTED READING

Adelstein DJ, Li Y, Adams GL, Wagner Jr H, Kish JA, Ensley JF, et al. An intergroup phase III comparison of standard radiation therapy and two schedules of concurrent chemoradiotherapy in patients with unresectable squamous cell head and neck cancer. J Clin Oncol 2003;21(1):92–8.

Adjuvant chemotherapy for advanced head and neck squamous carcinoma. Final report of the Head and Neck Contracts Program. Cancer 1987;60(3):301–11.

Bachaud JM, Cohen-Jonathan E, Alzieu C, David JM, Serrano E, Daly-Schveitzer N. Combined postoperative radiotherapy and weekly cisplatin infusion for locally advanced head and neck carcinoma: final report of a randomized trial. Int J Radiat Oncol Biol Phys 1996;36(5):999–1004.

Bernier J, Cooper JS, Lefèbvre JL. Defining risk levels in locally advanced head and neck cancers: a comparative analysis of concurrent postoperative radiation plus chemotherapy trials of the EORTC (#22931) and RTOG (# 9501). Head Neck 2005;27(10):843–50.

Bernier J, Cooper JS. Chemoradiation after surgery for high-risk head and neck cancer patients: how strong is the evidence? Oncologist 2005;10(3):215–24.

Bonner JA, Harari PM, Giralt J, Azarnia N, Shin DM, Cohen RB, et al. Radiotherapy plus cetuximab for squamous-cell carcinoma of the head and neck. N Engl J Med 2006;354(6):567–78.

Burtness B, Goldwasser MA, Flood W, Mattar B, Forastiere AA. Eastern Cooperative Oncology Group. Phase III randomized trial of cisplatin plus placebo compared with cisplatin plus cetuximab in metastatic/recurrent head and neck cancer: an Eastern Cooperative Oncology Group study. J Clin Oncol 2005;23(34):8646–54.

Calais G, Alfonsi M, Bardet E, Sire C, Germain T, Bergerot P, et al. Randomized trial of radiation therapy versus concomitant chemotherapy and radiation therapy for advanced-stage oropharynx carcinoma. J Natl Cancer Inst 1999;91(24):2081–6.

Denis F, Garaud P, Bardet E, Alfonsi M, Sire C, Germain T, et al. Final results of the 94–01 French Head and Neck Oncology and Radiotherapy Group randomized trial comparing radiotherapy alone with concomitant radiochemotherapy in advanced-stage oropharynx carcinoma. J Clin Oncol 2004;22:69–76.

Forastiere AA, Goepfert H, Maor M, Pajak TF, Weber R, Morrison W, et al. Concurrent chemotherapy and radiotherapy for organ preservation in advanced laryngeal cancer. N Engl J Med 2003;349(22):2091–8.

Induction chemotherapy plus radiation compared with surgery plus radiation in patients with advanced laryngeal cancer. The Department of Veterans Affairs Laryngeal Cancer Study Group. N Engl J Med 1991;324(24):1685–90.

Lefebvre JL, Chevalier D, Luboinski B, Kirkpatrick A, Collette L, Sahmoud T. Larynx preservation in pyriform sinus cancer: preliminary results of a European Organization for Research and Treatment of Cancer phase III trial. EORTC Head and Neck Cancer Cooperative Group. J Natl Cancer Inst 1996;88(13):890–9.

Morton RP, Rugman F, Dorman EB, Stoney PJ, Wilson JA, McCormick M, et al. Cisplatinum and bleomycin for advanced or recurrent squamous cell carcinoma of the head and neck: a randomised factorial phase III controlled trial. Cancer Chemother Pharmacol 1985;15(3):283–9.

Paccagnella A, Orlando A, Marchiori C, Zorat PL, Cavaniglia G, Sileni VC, et al. Phase III trial of initial chemotherapy in stage III or IV head and neck cancers: a study by the Gruppo di Studio sui Tumori della Testa e del Collo. J Natl Cancer Inst 1994;86(4):265–72.

Pignon JP, le Maître A, Maillard E, Bourhis J, MACH-NC Collaborative Group. Meta-analysis of chemotherapy in head and neck cancer (MACH-NC): an update on 93 randomised trials and 17,346 patients. Radiother Oncol 2009;92(1):4–14.

Posner MR, Hershock DM, Blajman CR, Mickiewicz E, Winquist E, Gorbounova V, et al. Cisplatin and fluorouracil alone or with docetaxel in head and neck cancer. TAX 324 Study Group. N Engl J Med 2007;357(17):1705–15.

Rivera F, García-Castaño A, Vega N, Vega-Villegas ME, Gutiérrez-Sanz L. Cetuximab in metastatic or recurrent head and neck cancer: the EX-TREME trial. Expert Rev Anticancer Ther 2009;9(10):1421–8.

Vermorken JB, Mesia R, Rivera F, Remenar E, Kawecki A, Rottey S, et al. Platinum-based chemotherapy plus cetuximab in head and neck cancer. N Engl J Med 2008;359(11):1116–27.

Vermorken JB, Trigo J, Hitt R, Koralewski P, Diaz-Rubio E, Rolland F, et al. Open-label, uncontrolled, multicenter phase II study to evaluate the efficacy and toxicity of cetuximab as a single agent in patients with recurrent and/or metastatic squamous cell carcinoma of the head and neck who failed to respond to platinum-based therapy. J Clin Oncol 2007;25(16):2171–7.

Vogl SE, Schoenfeld DA, Kaplan BH, Lerner HJ, Engstrom PF, Horton J. A randomized prospective comparison of methotrexate with a combination of methotrexate, bleomycin, and cisplatin in head and neck cancer. Cancer 1985;56(3):432–42.

# 18 Radiology

## Questions

### TRUE/FALSE

1. Imaging is a useful adjunct for accurate mapping of the superficial extent of mucosal cancer in the upper aerodigestive tract. (T/F)

2. Perineural spread (PNS) of cancer can be detected on magnetic resonance imaging (MRI) in an asymptomatic patient. (T/F)

3. Computed tomography (CT) and MRI often complement each other in the workup of head and neck cancer. (T/F)

4. The major advantage of MRI over CT is sagittal and coronal views. (T/F)

5. CT scans show medullary bone involvement in adults more accurately than MRI. (T/F)

6. CT is able to identify early extracapsular spread from nodal metastasis better than MRI. (T/F)

7. MRI is less susceptible to artifacts from dental amalgam compared with CT. (T/F)

8. Imaging features of many clinical entities such as neurogenic and vascular tumors are typical enough to allow accurate diagnosis without examination of tissue. (T/F)

9. CT-guided biopsy is a safe and effective option for diagnosis of carotid space (poststyloid parapharyngeal space) lesions. (T/F)

10. MRI is useful for assessment of hard palate tumors. (T/F)

11. CT of the sinuses is an adequate investigation for estimating the local extent of paranasal sinus cancer. (T/F)

12. CT of the oropharynx may provide more anatomical information on the extent of a large tumor at the base of the tongue than would MRI. (T/F)

13. Imaging provides little additional benefit in pretreatment assessment of the clinically negative neck if surgical treatment is planned. (T/F)

14. Ultrasonography is more sensitive than CT, MRI, and positron emission tomography (PET) for identifying early lymph node metastasis in well-differentiated papillary thyroid cancer. (T/F)

15. A PET scan is a cost-effective modality for the initial workup of squamous cell carcinoma of the oral cavity. (T/F)

16. A PET scan may not be able to identify a clinically occult oropharyngeal primary tumor in a patient with a human papillomavirus (HPV)-positive metastatic neck node. (T/F)

17. A CT scan of the chest is preferred over a PET scan for imaging of suspected pulmonary metastases in adenoid cystic carcinoma. (T/F)

18. A PET scan is the most effective and widely used modality for posttreatment assessment after chemoradiation therapy of head and neck squamous cell carcinoma. (T/F)

19. The optimal time for a PET scan after completion of chemoradiation therapy is 6 to 8 weeks. (T/F)

20. Osteoradionecrosis of the mandible (ORNM) is easily differentiated from a recurrent tumor on a PET scan. (T/F)

21. Unilateral middle ear fluid on MRI in an adult patient should trigger a search for nasopharyngeal carcinoma. (T/F)

22. Prominent soft tissue of the nasopharynx is a normal feature in children and adolescents. (T/F)

23. Skull base invasion from nasopharyngeal carcinoma can be detected earlier with MRI than with CT. (T/F)

24. Retropharyngeal nodes are normally located in the infrahyoid neck between the scalene muscles and common carotid artery. (T/F)

25. Retropharyngeal nodal metastasis can occur from cancer of the hard palate. (T/F)

26. Primary tonsil cancers rarely extend to the masticator space. (T/F)

27. Tonsil cancers can spread to the buccal space by tracking along the pharyngobasilar fascia. (T/F)

28. Subtle invasion of the prevertebral fascia from posterior pharyngeal wall carcinoma is difficult to detect on imaging. (T/F)

29. Tumors of the base of the tongue commonly extend to the preepiglottic space. (T/F)

30. Imaging is of limited value in evaluation of submucosal skip areas of involvement in hypopharyngeal carcinoma. (T/F)

31. Carotid artery encasement is likely if a tumor is noted to encircle at least 180 degrees of the carotid. (T/F)

32. Imaging can help assess the extent of planned surgical resection in early stage supraglottic squamous cell carcinoma. (T/F)

33. The majority of patients with early stage glottic squamous cell carcinoma do not need imaging before endoscopic resection. (T/F)

34. The hyoepiglottic ligament separates the preepiglottic from the paraglottic spaces. (T/F)

35. The plane of imaging for an optimal CT or MRI larynx study should be parallel to the C4-5 and C5-6 vertebral disk spaces. (T/F)

36. The supraglottic portion of the paraglottic space predominantly contains muscle, which can be differentiated from the glottic portion on a CT scan. (T/F)

37. MRI is more helpful than CT for imaging cartilage invasion in the adult larynx. (T/F)

38. The hyoepiglottic ligament is an effective barrier to tumor spread from the preepiglottic space to the base of the tongue. (T/F)

39. Involvement of the preepiglottic space is more common with tumors of the suprahyoid epiglottis than with those of its infrahyoid portion. (T/F)

40. Cartilage involvement and extralaryngeal spread is more frequent with glottic than with supraglottic squamous cell carcinoma. (T/F)

41. CT findings can upstage a T1 glottic squamous cell carcinoma to T2. (T/F)

42. Cartilage invasion should be suspected in all glottic T1 lesions that involve the anterior commissure. (T/F)

43. Radiographic imaging is unreliable in detecting early invasion of the laryngeal cartilage framework. (T/F)

44. Imaging adds limited information to the clinical examination in evaluation of floor-of-the-mouth squamous cell carcinoma with palpable nodal metastasis at level IB. (T/F)

45. Imaging of the mandible is not necessary for surgical planning of a posteriorly based cancer of the oral tongue. (T/F)

46. Clinical examination is the most sensitive modality for detection of early cortical invasion of the mandible from a primary tumor of the floor of the mouth. (T/F)

47. PNS along major nerves can be seen on imaging before development of symptoms or clinical signs. (T/F)

48. PNS can occur in skip areas or in an antegrade direction. (T/F)

49. CT has no value in imaging PNS. (T/F)

50. Precontrast T1-weighted (T1W) MRI is best for imaging extracranial PNS whereas postcontrast T1W MRI is best for imaging intracranial PNS. (T/F)

## MULTIPLE CHOICE

51. Which of the following is not true about CT imaging of head and neck tumors?
    A. Modern multidetector 64-slice scanners allow imaging in axial, coronal, and sagittal planes.
    B. Long examination time
    C. Excellent resolution of fine cortical bone detail
    D. Detects extracapsular nodal spread of disease earlier than MRI
    E. Not limited by incompatible implants in the patient's body

52. The limitations of MRI for head and neck imaging include the following, except
    A. Body habitus.
    B. Long examination time.
    C. Motion artifacts from swallowing and vascular pulsation.
    D. Limited ability to differentiate tumors from obstructive sinus disease.
    E. Lack of detail when cortical bone is imaged.

53. MRI of a 35-year-old patient shown in Figure 18-1 shows features that should prompt a workup for

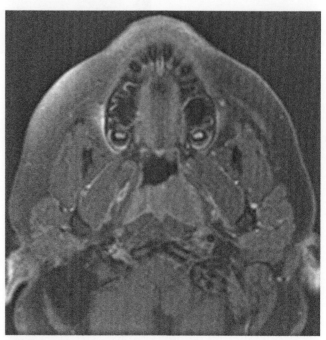

**Figure 18-1** Postcontrast T1-weighted magnetic resonance imaging. (Courtesy of Memorial Sloan Kettering Cancer Center, New York.)

    A. Benign adenoidal hypertrophy.
    B. Chronic mastoiditis.
    C. Carcinoma of the nasopharynx.
    D. Benign tonsillar hypertrophy.
    E. Carcinoma of the palatine tonsil.

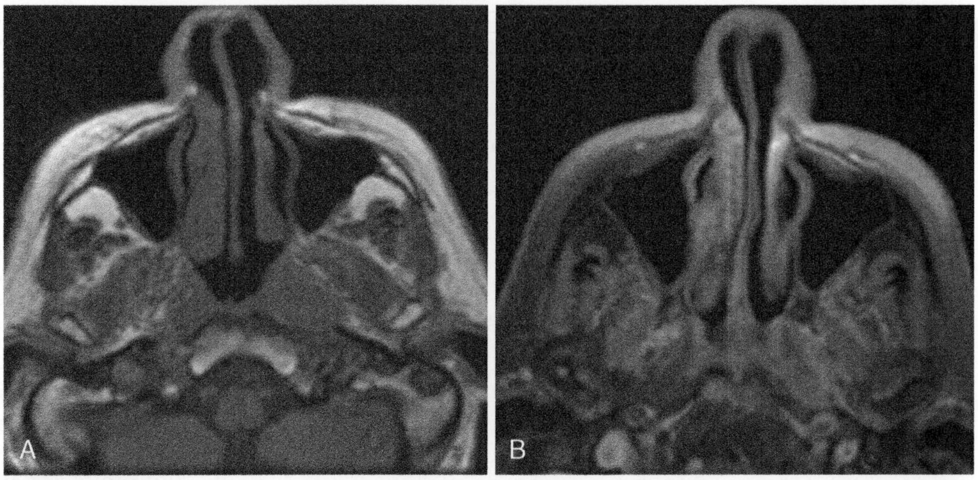

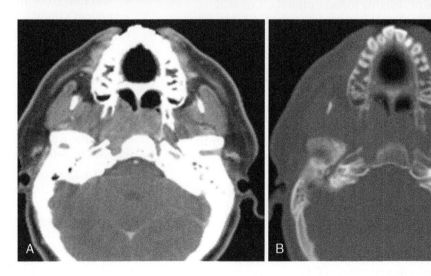

**Figure 18-2 A,** Precontrast T1-weighted magnetic resonance imaging (T1W MRI). **B,** Postcontrast T1W fat-saturated MRI. (Courtesy of Memorial Sloan Kettering Cancer Center, New York.)

**Figure 18-3** (Courtesy of Memorial Sloan Kettering Cancer Center, New York.)

54. T1W MRI of the nasopharynx shown in Figure 18-2 demonstrates
    A. PNS along $V_3$.
    B. Petroclival fissure involvement.
    C. Skull base invasion.
    D. Retropharyngeal node involvement.
    E. Pterygopalatine fossa involvement.

55. The CT scan in Figure 18-3 shows
    A. Invasion of the pterygoid plate.
    B. Widening of the petroclival fissure.
    C. Invasion of the clivus.
    D. Erosion of the hard palate.
    E. Retropharyngeal node involvement.

56. The presence of peripheral cysts around the intracranial component of a sinonasal lesion is generally associated with which of the following tumors?
    A. Sinonasal undifferentiated carcinoma
    B. Melanoma
    C. Esthesioneuroblastoma
    D. Squamous cell carcinoma
    E. Adenoid cystic carcinoma

57. Based on the imaging features shown in this postcontrast T1W fat-saturated MRI (Figure 18-4), the following can be expected in this patient with nasopharyngeal carcinoma:

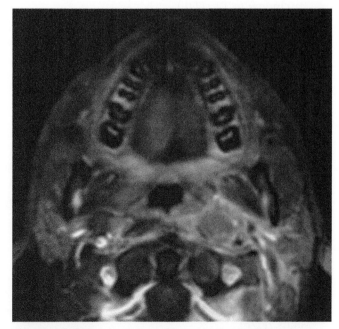

**Figure 18-4** Postcontrast axial T1-weighted magnetic resonance imaging (T1W MRI) with fat saturation. (Courtesy of Memorial Sloan Kettering Cancer Center, New York.)

A.  Carotid artery insufficiency.
B.  Carotid artery blowout.
C.  Cranial neuropathy.
D.  Trismus.
E.  Middle ear effusion.

58.  Which of the following is seen in the scans of the patient shown in Figure 18-5?
A.  Hypertrophied palatine tonsils
B.  Hypertrophic lingual tonsillar tissue
C.  Lingual thyroid
D.  Squamous cell carcinoma of the base of the tongue
E.  Minor salivary gland carcinoma of the base of the tongue

59.  The following are true for the patient whose CT scan is shown in Figure 18-6, except
A.  Right-sided otalgia may be a symptom.
B.  The tumor is invading the right mandible.
C.  The patient is at risk of retropharyngeal nodal metastasis.

D.  The internal carotid artery is at risk of encasement with progression of right level II adenopathy.
E.  The tumor can spread to the buccal space via the pterygomandibular raphe.

60.  The CT scan in Figure 18-7 shows a
A.  Right branchial cleft cyst.
B.  Metastatic right level II lymph node.
C.  Metastatic right retropharyngeal lymph node.
D.  Right vagal schwannoma.
E.  Right lateral nasopharyngeal cyst.

61.  The lateral retropharyngeal nodes are
A.  Lateral to the internal carotid artery.
B.  Not accessible to the surgeon during conventional neck dissection.
C.  Between the internal carotid artery and vertebral artery.
D.  Between scalene muscles and the common carotid artery.
E.  Between the sympathetic chain and the internal carotid artery.

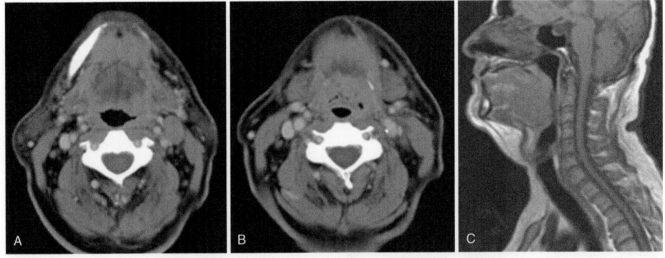

**Figure 18-5** (Courtesy of Memorial Sloan Kettering Cancer Center, New York.)

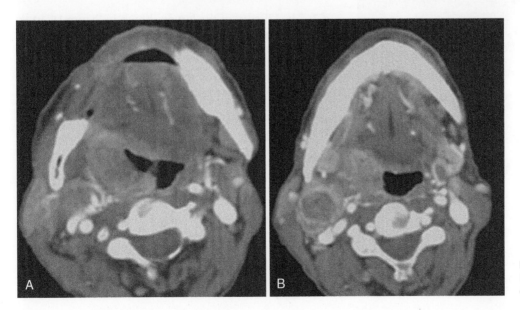

**Figure 18-6** (Courtesy of Memorial Sloan Kettering Cancer Center, New York.)

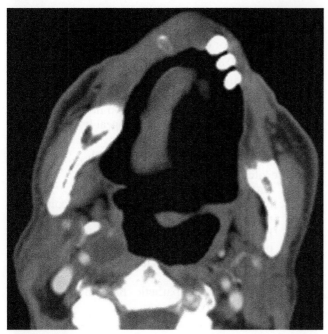

**Figure 18-7** (Courtesy of Memorial Sloan Kettering Cancer Center, New York.)

62. Which of the following tumors is not commonly associated with lateral retropharyngeal lymphadenopathy?
    A. Nasopharyngeal carcinoma
    B. Paranasal sinus carcinoma
    C. Tonsil carcinoma
    D. Papillary carcinoma of the thyroid
    E. Pyriform sinus carcinoma

63. The most significant finding in the CT scan in Figure 18-8 is

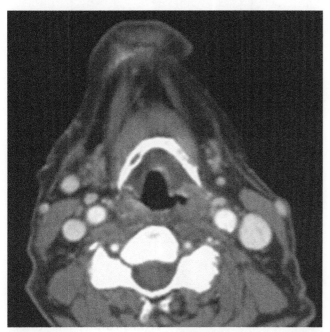

**Figure 18-8** (Courtesy of Memorial Sloan Kettering Cancer Center, New York.)

A. Asymmetrical internal jugular veins.
B. Thickening and enhancement of the left pyriform sinus mucosa.
C. Left cervical lymphadenopathy.
D. Invasion of preepiglottic space.
E. Involvement of the hyoid bone.

64. The most likely cause of left vocal fold paralysis in the patient shown in Figure 18-9 with a left pyriform sinus cancer is
    A. Retropharyngeal lymphadenopathy.
    B. Extralaryngeal spread and involvement of the left recurrent laryngeal nerve.
    C. Direct extension of the tumor into the left paraglottic space.
    D. Idiopathic.
    E. Involvement of the left recurrent laryngeal nerve by tracheoesophageal groove nodal metastases.

65. Hypopharyngeal cancers can cause paralysis of the ipsilateral vocal cord by all of the following mechanisms except
    A. Direct invasion of the paraglottic space.
    B. Direct invasion of the cricoarytenoid joint.
    C. Perineural involvement of the recurrent laryngeal nerve.
    D. Direct invasion of the recurrent laryngeal nerve.
    E. Involvement of the recurrent laryngeal nerve by paratracheal lymphadenopathy.

66. Which of the following statements about laryngeal cartilages is false?
    A. The cricoid is the only complete cartilaginous ring in the airway.
    B. The thyroid cartilage encloses the supraglottic and glottic larynx.
    C. The thyroid cartilage has natural fenestrations within the cartilage.
    D. The arytenoid cartilages span the supraglottis and glottis.
    E. The vocal ligaments attach to the arytenoid cartilages.

67. The CT scan of the larynx shown in Figure 18-10, performed on a patient with a submucosal bulge on the midline of the infrahyoid epiglottis, illustrates the following findings except
    A. Involvement of the preepiglottic space.
    B. Pushing borders of the invasive component of the tumor.
    C. Infiltration of the hyoid bone.
    D. Submucosal involvement of the bilateral aryepiglottic folds.
    E. A normal posterior pharyngeal wall.

68. Which of the following is not true of the conus elasticus (CE)?
    A. The CE is an intralaryngeal membrane that is an important landmark on MRI.
    B. The CE spans from the vocal ligament to the superior edge of the cricoid cartilage.
    C. The CE funnels a tumor from the paraglottic space toward the cricothyroid membrane.

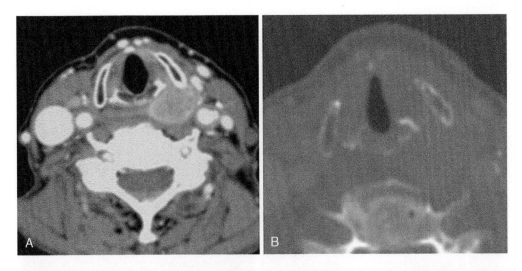

**Figure 18-9** (Courtesy of Memorial Sloan Kettering Cancer Center, New York.)

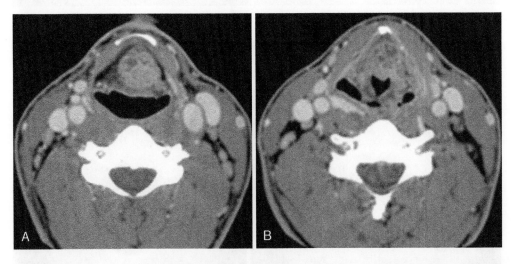

**Figure 18-10** (Courtesy of Memorial Sloan Kettering Cancer Center, New York.)

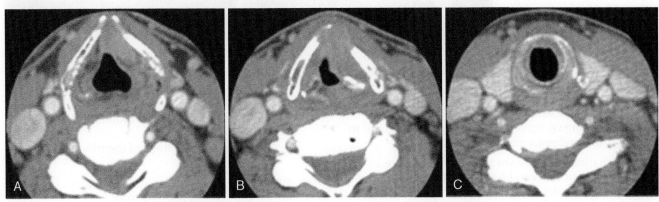

**Figure 18-11** (Courtesy of Memorial Sloan Kettering Cancer Center, New York.)

D. The cricothyroid membrane is a pathway for extralaryngeal spread of a tumor.
E. Areas of ossified cricoid and thyroid cartilage bordering the inferior attachment of the CE are at higher risk of tumor invasion.

69. Which of the following features is not seen in the CT images shown in Figure 18-11?
A. Extralaryngeal extension of the tumor
B. Invasion of the ala of the thyroid cartilage

C. Invasion of the paraglottic space
D. Invasion of the right arytenoid cartilage
E. Subglottic extension

70. Which of the following statements is not true about the imaging studies shown in Figure 18-12?
A. The *white open arrows* point to the genioglossus muscles.
B. The *white closed arrow* points to the hyoglossus muscle.

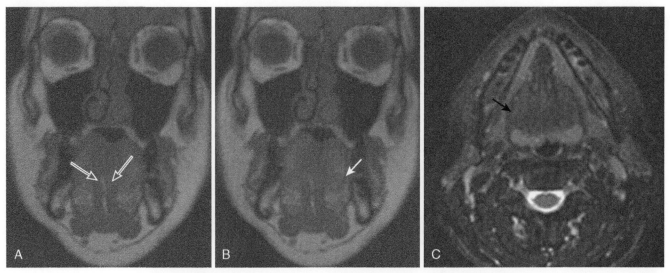

**Figure 18-12** (Courtesy of Memorial Sloan Kettering Cancer Center, New York.)

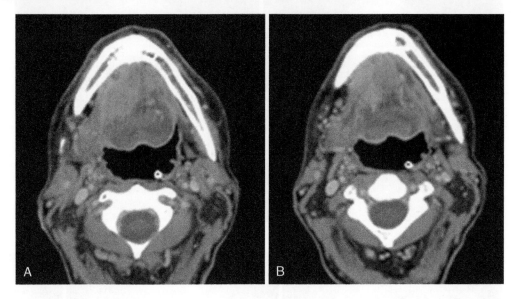

**Figure 18-13** (Courtesy of Memorial Sloan Kettering Cancer Center, New York.)

C. The *black arrow* points to the submandibular salivary duct.
D. The lingual artery and IXn are located medial to the hyoglossus muscle.
E. The lingual nerve and XIIn are located lateral to the hyoglossus muscle.

71. The patient whose scans are shown in Figure 18-13 has a tumor that can be adequately treated with a
    A. Right partial glossectomy without reconstruction.
    B. Right partial glossectomy and reconstruction.
    C. Right partial glossectomy and right segmental mandibulectomy.
    D. Subtotal anterior glossectomy and reconstruction.
    E. Total glossectomy and laryngectomy.

72. The patient whose scan is shown in Figure 18-14 has
    A. Carcinoma of the floor of the mouth with no nodal metastasis.
    B. Carcinoma of the floor of the mouth with level IB nodal metastasis.

C. Carcinoma of the floor of the mouth with an obstructed submandibular salivary gland.
D. Direct extension of carcinoma of the floor of the mouth into the submandibular triangle.
E. Carcinoma of the floor of the mouth invading the mandible.

73. Which of the following statements about the pterygomandibular raphe is not true?
    A. It has a fibrous aponeurosis that extends from the hamulus of the medial pterygoid plate to the mylohyoid line on the lingual aspect of the mandible.
    B. It provides attachment to the buccinator and superior pharyngeal constrictor muscles.
    C. The inferior alveolar nerve passes under it in the retromolar trigone.
    D. It is an effective barrier to tumor spread from the oropharynx to the buccal space.
    E. It is separated from the ramus of the mandible by adipose tissue.

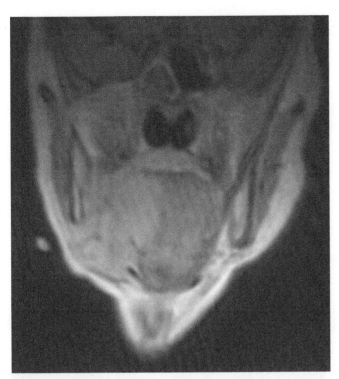

**Figure 18-14** (Courtesy of Memorial Sloan Kettering Cancer Center, New York.)

74. The most appropriate management for the patient whose scans are shown in Figure 18-15 would include a
    A. Right partial glossectomy without mandible resection.
    B. Right partial glossectomy with a marginal mandibulectomy.
    C. Right partial glossectomy, a marginal mandibulectomy, and free flap reconstruction.
    D. Right partial glossectomy with a segmental mandibulectomy.
    E. Right partial glossectomy, a segmental mandibulectomy, and free flap reconstruction.

75. A patient has a remote history of right partial glossectomy for squamous cell carcinoma. She underwent excisional biopsy of another lesion in the right retromolar trigone by an oral surgeon and underwent extraction of the posterior mandibular and maxillary molar teeth. Pathological examination revealed squamous cell carcinoma, which prompted a referral to the head and neck surgeon, who saw no findings suggestive of cancer in the oral cavity. The diagnosis of cancer prompted MRI and CT scans for evaluation of the extent of the disease. Which of the following statements is true about the series of scans shown in Figure 18-16?
    A. A tumor is tracking along the pterygomandibular raphe to invade the maxilla and mandible.
    B. Postdental extraction changes are visible in the mandible and maxilla.
    C. Postdental extraction changes are visible in the mandible and maxilla with tumor extension to the superior constrictor muscle.
    D. There is PNS along $V_3$.
    E. There is invasion of the right buccinator muscle.

76. The most likely diagnosis in the patient whose MRI scans are shown in Figure 18-17 is
    A. Benign maxillary sinus polyp.
    B. Nasal cavity tumor with extension into the maxillary antrum.
    C. Minor salivary gland neoplasm of the hard palate.
    D. Squamous cell carcinoma of the maxillary antrum.
    E. Squamous cell carcinoma of the hard palate.

77. Risk factors for development of the condition shown in the CT scan shown in Figure 18-18 include all except
    A. Poor dental hygiene.
    B. Chemoradiation therapy for carcinoma of the retromolar trigone.
    C. Marginal mandibulectomy and neck dissection with postoperative radiation therapy for a pT1N2b carcinoma of the floor of the mouth.
    D. Postoperative intensity-modulated radiation therapy to a total dose of 55 cGy for a T2N1 HPV+ carcinoma of the tonsil after transoral robotic resection.

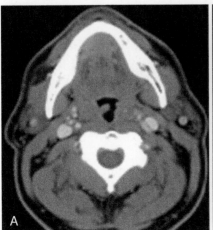
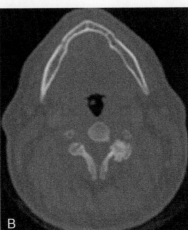
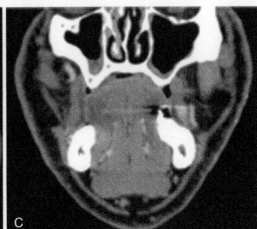

**Figure 18-15** (Courtesy of Memorial Sloan Kettering Cancer Center, New York.)

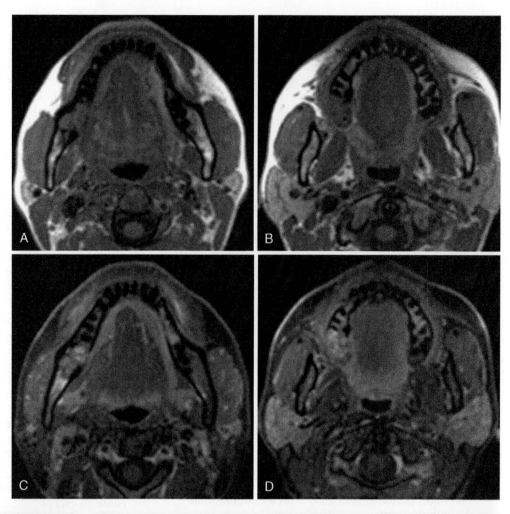

**Figure 18-16 A** and **B,** Precontrast axial T1-weighted magnetic resonance imaging (T1W MRI). **C** and **D,** Postcontrast axial T1W MRI with fat suppression. (Courtesy of Memorial Sloan Kettering Cancer Center, New York.)

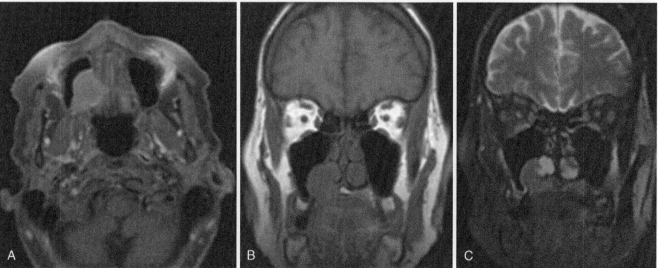

**Figure 18-17 A,** Postcontrast T1-weighted magnetic resonance imaging (T1W MRI) with fat saturation. **B,** Precontrast T1W MRI. **C,** T2W MRI with fat saturation. (Courtesy of Memorial Sloan Kettering Cancer Center, New York.)

    E. Conventional two-dimensional postoperative radiation therapy after a partial glossectomy and neck dissection for T2N2b carcinoma of the oral tongue.

78. The patients whose imaging studies are shown in Figure 18-19 are candidates for surgical resection

and reconstruction of the mandible for treatment of osteoradionecrosis. Which of the following features is not seen on the imaging studies?

    A. Pathological fracture of the mandible

    B. Trabecular changes in the marrow of the mandible

    C. Orocutaneous fistula

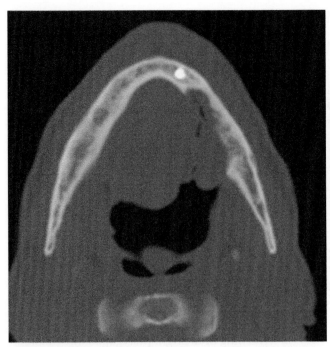

**Figure 18-18** (Courtesy of Memorial Sloan Kettering Cancer Center, New York.)

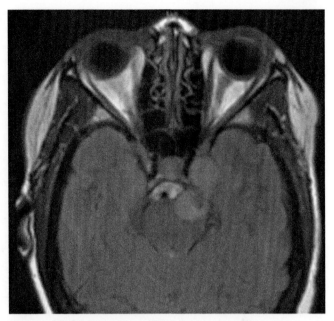

**Figure 18-20** T2-weighted (T2W) fluid attenuated inversion recovery (FLAIR) axial magnetic resonance imaging (MRI). (Courtesy of Memorial Sloan Kettering Cancer Center, New York.)

D. Soft tissue changes around necrotic bone
E. Unicortical dehiscence of mandibular bone

79. PNS of a tumor is a frequent feature of which of the following tumors?
A. Lymphoma
B. Acinic cell carcinoma of the parotid gland
C. Squamous cell carcinoma of the hard palate
D. Mucosal melanoma of the supraglottic larynx
E. Malignant peripheral nerve sheath tumor

80. Which of the following statements best describes the findings in the scan shown in Figure 18-20?
A. There is involvement of the left cavernous sinus by PNS of the tumor.
B. The patient has an internal carotid artery aneurysm in the left cavernous sinus.

C. The patient has a meningioma of the left cavernous sinus.
D. The patient has thrombosis of the left cavernous sinus.
E. The patient has a schwannoma of the left cavernous sinus.

81. A 74-year-old male patient developed lancing pain in the right half of his face 5 years before the scans shown in Figure 18-21. He had a history of excision of multiple skin lesions from the face and scalp, all of which were reportedly benign. A year later he developed numbness of the face, which was followed by diplopia, drooling from the right side of the mouth, and difficulty chewing food. The imaging studies show perineural invasion involving the

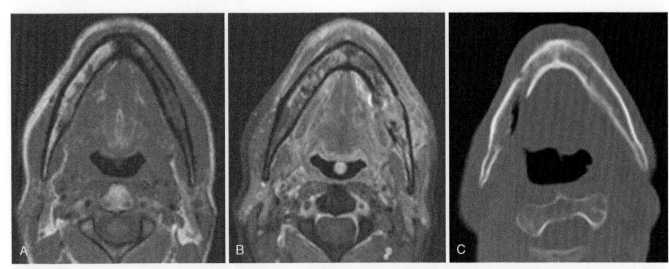

**Figure 18-19 A,** Precontrast axial T1-weighted magnetic resonance imaging (T1W MRI). **B,** Postcontrast T1W MRI with fat saturation. **C,** Axial computed tomographic (CT) bone window. (Courtesy of Memorial Sloan Kettering Cancer Center, New York.)

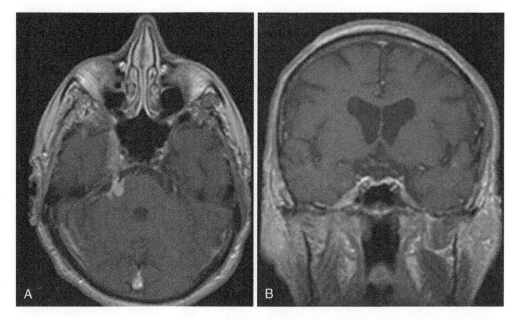

**Figure 18-21 A,** Postcontrast axial T1-weighted magnetic resonance imaging (T1W MRI). **B,** Postcontrast coronal T1W MRI. (Courtesy of Memorial Sloan Kettering Cancer Center, New York.)

A. Infraorbital nerve up to the orbital apex.
B. Infraorbital nerve and intracranial V₂.
C. Infraorbital nerve, intracranial V₂, and gasserian ganglion.
D. Infraorbital nerve, intracranial V₂, gasserian ganglion, and main trunk of cranial nerve V.
E. Infraorbital nerve skipping intracranial V₂ but involving the gasserian ganglion.

82. The most likely diagnosis of the tumor seen on the MRI scans shown in Figure 18-22 is
    A. Adenoid cystic carcinoma of the hard palate.
    B. Squamous cell carcinoma of the hard palate.
    C. Mucosal melanoma of the hard palate.
    D. Adenocarcinoma of the maxillary sinus.
    E. Squamous cell carcinoma of the maxillary sinus.

83. The radiographic findings seen on the MRI scans shown in Figure 18-23 include all of the following except
    A. PNS along the right infraorbital nerve.

B. Widening of the right pterygopalatine canal.
C. Erosion of the right mandibular cortex.
D. An asymmetrically enlarged right foramen ovale.
E. Involvement of the right inferior alveolar nerve.

84. The patient whose scans are shown in Figure 18-24 presented with hoarseness of recent onset in the setting of a known thyroid mass. Which of the following findings is not seen in these scans?
    A. Extrathyroid extension of the tumor
    B. Encasement of the common carotid artery
    C. Right vocal fold paralysis
    D. Intralaryngeal extension of the tumor
    E. Retropharyngeal lymphadenopathy

85. The most likely diagnosis in the patient whose scans are shown in Figure 18-25 is
    A. Chondrosarcoma of the cricoid cartilage.
    B. Papillary carcinoma of the thyroid with cricoid cartilage destruction.

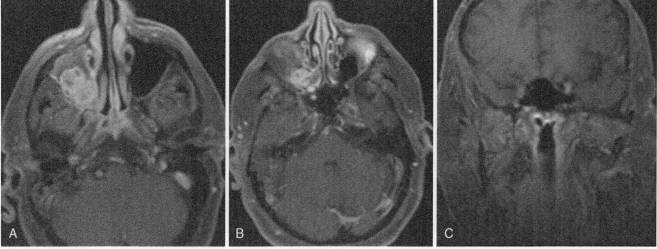

**Figure 18-22** (Courtesy of Memorial Sloan Kettering Cancer Center, New York.)

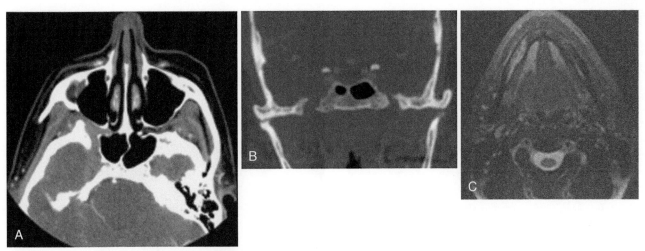

**Figure 18-23** (Courtesy of Memorial Sloan Kettering Cancer Center, New York.)

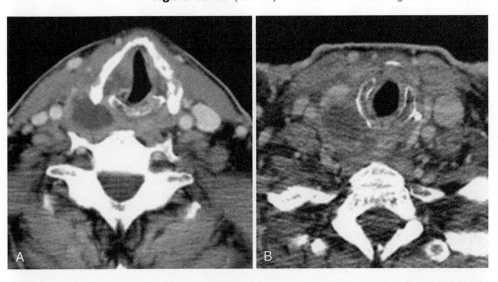

**Figure 18-24** (Courtesy of Memorial Sloan Kettering Cancer Center, New York.)

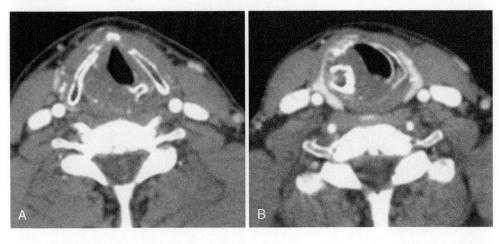

**Figure 18-25** (Courtesy of Memorial Sloan Kettering Cancer Center, New York.)

C. Adenoid cystic carcinoma of the subglottic larynx.
D. Squamous cell carcinoma of the subglottic larynx.
E. Chondroradionecrosis after radiation therapy for squamous cell carcinoma of the larynx.

86. A 45-year-old nonsmoking woman presented with a firm, nontender, mobile mass in the right preauricular region. What is the most likely diagnosis based on the scan shown in Figure 18-26?
A. Normal intraparotid lymph node
B. Lymphoepithelial cyst
C. Benign or malignant parotid tumor
D. Level II lymph node
E. Parotid abscess

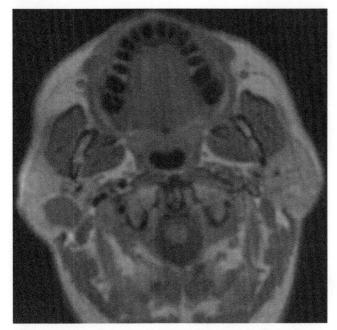

**Figure 18-26** (Courtesy of Memorial Sloan Kettering Cancer Center, New York.)

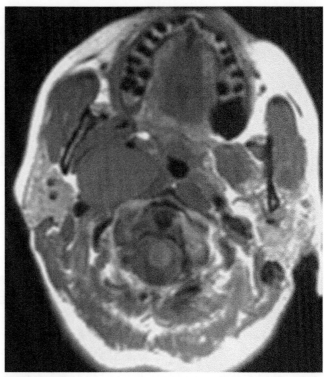

**Figure 18-28** (Courtesy of Memorial Sloan Kettering Cancer Center, New York.)

87. Which of the following imaging studies is most likely to be helpful in the diagnosis for the patient in Question 86?
    A. Postcontrast T1W MRI
    B. Contrast-enhanced CT scan
    C. PET-CT scan
    D. T2W MRI
    E. Postcontrast T1W MRI with fat suppression

88. The T2W MRI scans shown in Figure 18-27 most likely represent which of the following conditions?
    A. Carcinoma ex pleomorphic adenoma
    B. Recurrent pleomorphic adenoma
    C. Sjögren syndrome
    D. Intraparotid lymph node metastases
    E. Lymphoepithelial cysts

89. A 62-year-old woman presents for evaluation of difficulty swallowing. Clinical examination revealed a smooth submucosal bulge on the right lateral oropharyngeal wall. The imaging study shown in Figure 18-28 shows a mass located in which space?
    A. Parapharyngeal space
    B. Carotid space
    C. Masticator space
    D. Parotid space
    E. Retropharyngeal space

90. The T2W axial MRI scan in Figure 18-29 shows features most consistent with the diagnosis of
    A. Paraganglioma.
    B. Retropharyngeal lymphadenopathy.
    C. Schwannoma.
    D. Neurofibroma.
    E. Benign mixed tumor of the deep lobe of the parotid gland.

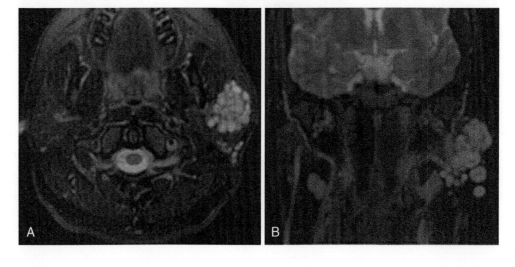

**Figure 18-27** (Courtesy of Memorial Sloan Kettering Cancer Center, New York.)

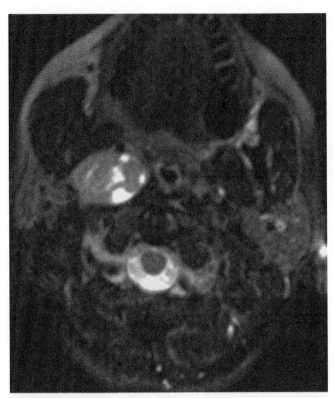

**Figure 18-29** (Courtesy of Memorial Sloan Kettering Cancer Center, New York.)

A. Lymphoma of the base of the tongue
B. Paraganglioma of the base of the tongue
C. Schwannoma of the base of the tongue
D. Lingual thyroid
E. Minor salivary gland tumor of the base of the tongue

93. The patient whose scan is shown in Figure 18-32 presented with an otherwise asymptomatic lump in the neck. What is the most likely diagnosis?
    A. Inflamed thyroglossal duct cyst
    B. Squamous cell carcinoma of the larynx
    C. Metastatic Delphian lymph node
    D. Tumor within thyroglossal duct remnant or metastatic Delphian lymph node
    E. None of the above

94. Which of the following conditions is most likely in the patient whose CT scan is shown in Figure 18-33?
    A. Squamous cell carcinoma of the larynx with anterior commissure invasion
    B. Cartilage invasion from a poorly differentiated thyroid carcinoma
    C. Chondronecrosis of the larynx after radiation therapy
    D. Foreign body in the larynx
    E. Chondrosarcoma of the larynx

95. Which of the statements for the patient whose scan is shown in Figure 18-34 is true?
    A. The patient has right true vocal fold paralysis.
    B. The patient has papillary carcinoma of the right thyroid lobe invading the thyroid cartilage.
    C. The patient has laryngeal edema and chondronecrosis of the larynx after chemoradiation therapy.
    D. The patient has a hemangioma of the right paraglottic space.
    E. The patient has a paraganglioma of the right paraglottic space.

96. Which of the following radiographic changes should raise suspicion for a recurrent tumor in the larynx after chemoradiation therapy?

91. Which is the most likely diagnosis in the patient whose scans are shown in Figure 18-30?
    A. Paraganglioma
    B. Retropharyngeal lymphadenopathy
    C. Schwannoma
    D. Neurofibroma
    E. Benign mixed tumor of the deep lobe of the parotid gland

92. A 61-year-old woman presented with a 2-year history of globus sensation and laryngopharyngeal reflux without otalgia or any other significant symptoms. The physical examination of the head and neck was unremarkable. Based on the CT images shown in Figure 18-31, what is the most likely diagnosis?

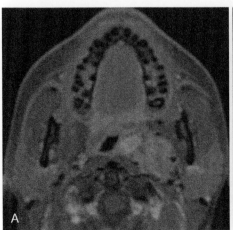
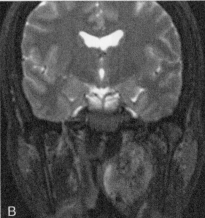
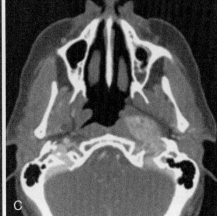

**Figure 18-30 A,** Postcontrast axial T1-weighted magnetic resonance imaging (T1W MRI). **B,** Coronal T2W MRI. **C,** Contrast-enhanced axial computed tomography (CT). (Courtesy of Memorial Sloan Kettering Cancer Center, New York.)

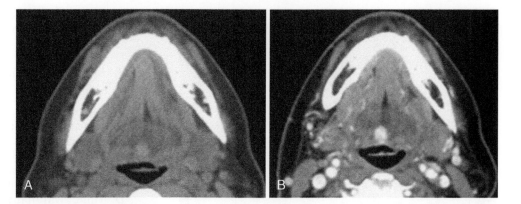

**Figure 18-31 A,** Precontrast axial computed tomography (CT). **B,** Postcontrast axial CT. (Courtesy of Memorial Sloan Kettering Cancer Center, New York.)

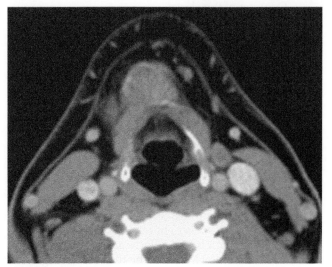

**Figure 18-32** Postcontrast axial computed tomography (CT). (Courtesy of Memorial Sloan Kettering Cancer Center, New York.)

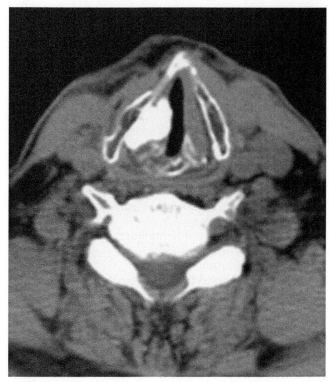

**Figure 18-34** (Courtesy of Memorial Sloan Kettering Cancer Center, New York.)

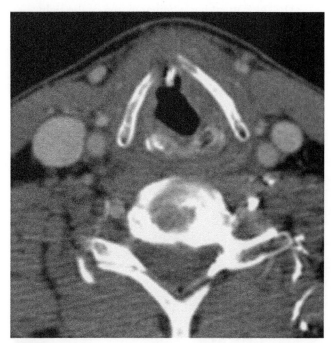

**Figure 18-33** (Courtesy of Memorial Sloan Kettering Cancer Center, New York.)

   A. Thickened omega-shaped epiglottis
   B. Edematous aryepiglottic folds
   C. Obliteration of paraglottic fat
   D. Enhancing mucosal surface
   E. New onset cartilage sclerosis

97. Reasons for a false-positive PET scan after treatment of a T2N1M0 squamous cell carcinoma of the tonsil include all the following except
   A. Mucositis
   B. Paralyzed vocal fold
   C. Osteoradionecrosis
   D. Laryngeal muscular activity
   E. Necrotic tumor

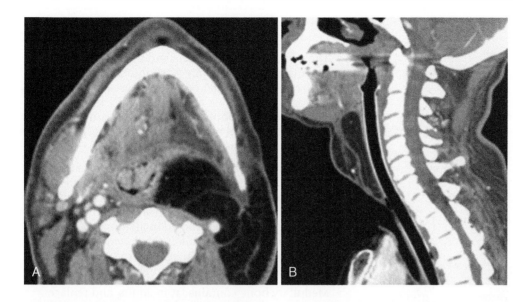

**Figure 18-35** (Courtesy of Memorial Sloan Kettering Cancer Center, New York.)

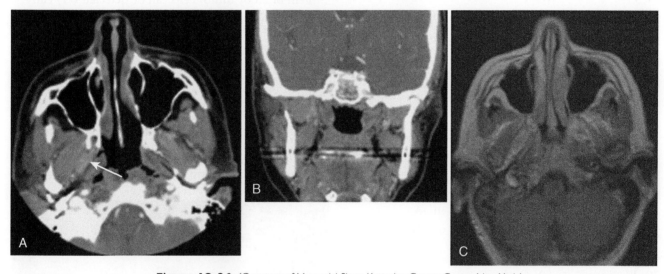

**Figure 18-36** (Courtesy of Memorial Sloan Kettering Cancer Center, New York.)

98. The patient whose CT scans are shown in Figure 18-35 was treated with a total laryngectomy and partial pharyngectomy with reconstruction for locally advanced hypopharyngeal cancer. Which of the following options is true for the type of reconstructive surgery used to restore the continuity of the pharynx and esophagus?
    A. The patient has had jejunal free flap reconstruction.
    B. The patient has had a pharyngeal tube without any reconstruction.
    C. The patient has had rectus abdominis free flap reconstruction.
    D. The patient has a recurrent tumor after rectus abdominis free flap reconstruction and pharyngeal tube placement.
    E. The patient has a pharyngocutaneous fistula after rectus abdominis free flap reconstruction and pharyngeal tube placement.

99. Which of the following statements is not true for CT-guided biopsy?
    A. It is often the least invasive approach for obtaining a diagnosis.
    B. It can help a patient avoid general anesthesia and a more complicated open surgical procedure for diagnosis.
    C. It can help a patient avoid unnecessary surgery for disease that can be treated nonsurgically.
    D. It requires inpatient admission.
    E. It is a low-risk procedure in experienced hands.

100. Which of the following approaches would be optimal for biopsy of the lesion in the scans shown in Figure 18-36 using CT guidance?
    A. Suprazygomatic
    B. Infrazygomatic (condylar notch)
    C. Retromandibular (transparotid)
    D. Transfacial paramaxillary (buccal)
    E. Transoral

## Answers

| | | |
|---|---|---|
| 1. F | 35. T | 69. D |
| 2. T | 36. F | 70. C |
| 3. T | 37. T | 71. D |
| 4. F | 38. T | 72. D |
| 5. F | 39. F | 73. D |
| 6. T | 40. T | 74. C |
| 7. T | 41. T | 75. B |
| 8. T | 42. F | 76. C |
| 9. T | 43. T | 77. D |
| 10. T | 44. F | 78. A |
| 11. F | 45. F | 79. A |
| 12. T | 46. F | 80. E |
| 13. F | 47. T | 81. D |
| 14. T | 48. T | 82. A |
| 15. F | 49. F | 83. C |
| 16. T | 50. T | 84. E |
| 17. T | 51. B | 85. A |
| 18. T | 52. D | 86. C |
| 19. F | 53. C | 87. D |
| 20. F | 54. C | 88. B |
| 21. T | 55. B | 89. B |
| 22. T | 56. C | 90. C |
| 23. T | 57. C | 91. A |
| 24. F | 58. D | 92. D |
| 25. F | 59. B | 93. D |
| 26. F | 60. C | 94. C |
| 27. F | 61. B | 95. A |
| 28. T | 62. B | 96. E |
| 29. F | 63. B | 97. B |
| 30. F | 64. C | 98. D |
| 31. F | 65. C | 99. D |
| 32. T | 66. C | 100. B |
| 33. F | 67. C | |
| 34. F | 68. A | |

## Core Knowledge

- Superficial mucosal lesions are best assessed by detailed clinical examination. Imaging studies are most helpful in estimating deep extension that may not be evident clinically.

- Perineural spread (PNS) of a tumor is seen as an enlarged and enhancing nerve on postcontrast imaging. Magnetic resonance imaging (MRI) is often very helpful in detecting PNS in asymptomatic patients;

however, disease is most often advanced by the time radiographic changes become evident.

- The clinician should understand the pros and cons of computed tomography (CT) and MRI to be able to utilize their individual benefits in answering clinically relevant questions. As a general rule, CT is better at imaging cortical bone and certain soft tissue features such as extranodal extension, whereas MRI provides superior soft tissue resolution.

- Modern multidetector CT scanners can be used to rapidly scan patients within a few minutes compared with the much longer scan times of MRI, which can take 30 to 45 minutes for each anatomical area to be studied. CT data can then be displayed in all three planes: axial, sagittal, and coronal. In addition, the raw data can be used to perform three-dimensional reconstructions that may be useful in surgical planning (see Question 51).

- Medullary bone contains fat in adults, and replacement of fat by tumor cells can be detected very early on the T1-weighted (T1W) sequence of an MR image (see Question 76).

- Early extracapsular spread (ECS) of metastatic disease around an involved lymph node is best imaged on a contrast-enhanced CT scan, especially in small lymph nodes.

- The CT scan in Figure 18-37 shows a metastatic lymph node at right level III. The node has irregular borders with reticulation of the surrounding soft tissue indicative of ECS in this patient who had not previously received any treatment.

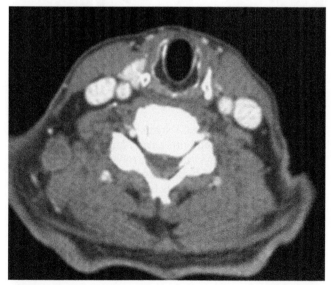

**Figure 18-37** (Courtesy of Memorial Sloan Kettering Cancer Center, New York.)

- Dental amalgam can cause significant deterioration in the quality of CT imaging, and this can be partially overcome by reangling the scan around the teeth to minimize loss of information. MRI is less susceptible to artifacts, but dental amalgam can cause a black "blooming" artifact that can obscure evaluation of

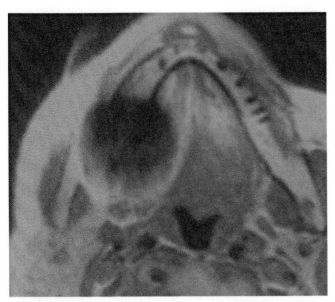

**Figure 18-38** (Courtesy of Memorial Sloan Kettering Cancer Center, New York.)

the adjoining oral cavity, as seen in the MRI scan in Figure 18-38.

- Imaging characteristics of many neurovascular tumors including hemangiomas, lymphangiomas, paragangliomas, and schwannomas are typical enough to allow a reliable diagnosis to be made. Needle biopsy in these situations, especially for vascular tumors, is not informative, and, in fact, may cause complications related to hemorrhaging (see Questions 89 through 91).

- CT-guided biopsy with a fine needle or core biopsy is an accurate and reliable option for diagnosis of many head and neck tumors, including those of the carotid space (poststyloid parapharyngeal space [PPS]). However, as discussed in Questions 8 and 89 through 91, the radiographic characteristics of many tumors are typical enough to allow treatment decisions without tissue diagnosis.

- Early bone involvement of the hard palate is easy to identify on T1W MRI because adult marrow is fatty and provides natural contrast to grayish tumor (see Questions 5 and 76). In addition, tumors of the hard palate are also susceptible to PNS, which can easily be seen on MRI (see Questions 82 and 83).

- Contrast-enhanced CT in axial and coronal planes is an excellent initial study for evaluation of sinus malignancy because bone destruction is more easily seen on CT. Early stage tumors present as unilateral masses that generally do not densely enhance on CT. Bony destruction is a common feature of squamous cell carcinoma, whereas regressive remodeling of adjacent bone occurs more frequently in minor salivary gland carcinomas and sinonasal sarcomas. Most tumors have low to intermediate signals on T1W MRI. Because they generally are highly cellular with little water content, they have intermediate signal on T2W images and are therefore easy to differentiate from postobstructive sinus secretions, which are hyperintense on T2W MRI. Some minor salivary gland tumors, schwannomas, and inverted papillomas have

sufficient water content and can be bright on T2W MRI. Postcontrast T1W MRI is particularly important in identifying dural/intracranial extension of tumors.

- Motion artifacts on MRI from swallowing are a major problem in patients who have bulky tumors of the oropharynx or tongue (Figure 18-39). These patients usually have pooling of saliva in the oropharynx, especially when they lay flat, and this requires them to swallow frequently, which, in turn, degrades the quality of images on an MRI exam, which may take 30 to 45 minutes to complete. A CT scan with coronal and sagittal reformation is an excellent substitute in these situations because it can be accomplished in a few minutes.

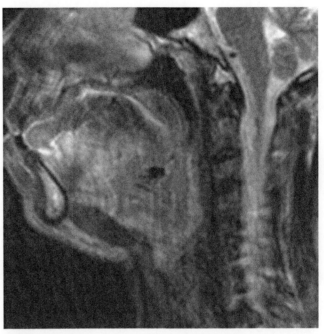

**Figure 18-39** (Courtesy of Memorial Sloan Kettering Cancer Center, New York.)

- The accuracy of clinical examination in identifying metastatic disease is appreciably lower compared with imaging modalities such as CT and ultrasound. Adequate staging of the neck should therefore include a baseline imaging study. Certain nodal basins, such as the lateral retropharyngeal nodes, are not amenable to clinical examination (see Questions 24 and 25) but can be easily detected on imaging. Other advantages of imaging studies include the ability to detect normal-sized metastatic nodes and early extracapsular nodal spread (see Question 6) and better assessment of the "difficult" neck (e.g., the neck of a patient with a muscular/stocky habitus or the posttreatment neck).

- The most accurate modality for assessment of lymphadenopathy in differentiated thyroid carcinoma is ultrasound examination. The lymph nodes at highest risk are the central compartment nodes, which are easily and accurately assessed by ultrasound. Features such as loss of the normal fatty hilum, increased internal vascularity, and microcalcification are indicative of metastatic lymphadenopathy. Fluorodeoxyglucose

(FDG) avidity is generally inversely proportional to the degree of differentiation of a tumor, and well-differentiated thyroid carcinoma is therefore not particularly FDG avid.

- The risk of occult nodal metastasis is used to determine the need for elective treatment of the clinically negative neck in oral cavity carcinoma. A positron emission tomographic (PET) scan is susceptible to false-positive results from reactive lymphadenopathy secondary to inflammation in the oral cavity or superinfection of the primary tumor. Although there are proponents of the PET scan as an initial staging modality for oral cavity carcinoma, the most cost-effective modality remains CT.

- The normal lymphoid tissue of the Waldeyer ring is FDG avid on a PET scan and can easily mask a clinically occult primary tumor in the oropharynx.

- Most malignant neoplasms of salivary gland origin, including adenoid cystic carcinoma, are not particularly avid on a PET scan. In addition, a dedicated CT scan of the chest has finer anatomical resolution than a PET-CT scan and is therefore more accurate at identifying pulmonary metastases.

- The normal anatomy of the head and neck becomes distorted by treatment-related changes after surgery and/or chemoradiation therapy. Distinguishing residual or recurrent tumors from treatment-related change is therefore often impossible on anatomical imaging studies such as CT and MRI. A PET scan relies on FDG activity for identification of a viable tumor and is therefore the first-line modality in monitoring patients after therapy. The negative predictive value of a PET scan is very high in this situation, but false-positive results can occur because of infection, inflammation, and early treatment-related changes that take up to 3 months to resolve.

- The baseline posttreatment PET study should be performed no earlier than approximately 3 months after completion of treatment to minimize false-positive results that can occur from inflammation or infection (see Question 18).

- Osteoradionecrosis of the mandible (ORNM) is usually complicated by some degree of inflammation and even infection, which makes differentiation from the tumor extremely difficult on a PET scan (see Question 20).

- Middle ear effusion is common in children and can often be unilateral. However, unilateral middle ear effusion in an adult signifies blockage of eustachian tube drainage and should trigger a search for a mass in the nasopharnx, the most ominous of which is nasopharyngeal carcinoma.

- Prominent soft tissue in the nasopharynx from adenoidal hypertrophy is not uncommon in children and adolescents. Gross asymmetric soft tissue on the other hand, especially in the adult patient, should be investigated carefully to rule out nasopharyngeal carcinoma. Although rare, nasopharyngeal carcinoma can be seen in adolescents.

- The bone marrow in the adult clivus is replaced by fat, which provides excellent contrast against which a tumor can be easily distinguished on T1W MRI (see Question 54).

- The lateral retropharyngeal lymph nodes are located in the suprahyoid part of the neck between the longus colli/longus capitis muscles and the internal carotid artery.

- Retropharyngeal lymph nodes are not typically at risk of involvement from primary tumors of the oral cavity. Metastases occur more commonly from anatomical sites such as the nasopharynx and tonsils. However, these nodes are also at risk from remotely located tumors such as the hypopharynx and thyroid (see Questions 60 through 62).

- The masticator space containing the lateral and medial pterygoid muscles is in close anatomical proximity and is immediately deep to the pharyngeal constrictor muscle on the lateral wall of the oropharynx and parapharyngeal fat. Primary tumors of the tonsil have ready access to this space after they have invaded through the pharyngeal constrictor, and invasion of the muscles of mastication is manifest clinically as trismus, which is a poor prognostic indicator.

- Tumors of the tonsil and lateral oropharyngeal wall can extend anteriorly toward the oral cavity. Deep extension into the retromolar trigone allows these tumors access to the pterygomandibular raphe and therefore to the buccal space (see Questions 59 and 73).

- The prevertebral fascia is not a discretely definable anatomical structure on radiographic imaging. Early infiltration of the fascia by a tumor is therefore not easy to identify and is most often not evident until the surgeon is able to examine the area directly on the operating table.

- The hyoepiglottic ligament provides early resistance to tumor spread from the base of the tongue to the preglottic space (see Questions 34 and 38).

- Hypopharyngeal carcinomas can spread caudad to the cervical esophagus along submucosal lymphatics. This submucosal spread is often discontiguous from the primary tumor and can appear as "skip areas" of tumor involvement along the esophagus. Imaging is useful for evaluating the distal extent of hypopharyngeal tumors, especially if an endoscope cannot be negotiated beyond a circumferential constricted tumor.

- The most commonly accepted definition of a surgically unresectable tumor from carotid artery "encasement" is a tumor that is in relation to 270 degrees of the arterial circumference. Tumors with lesser degrees of involvement are more likely to be amenable to total resection without leaving gross residual disease.

- Involvement of the preepiglottic space (PES) from a supraglottic tumor is impossible to detect on clinical examination. Evaluation of the PES is easy on radiographic imaging because the normal space contains fat (see Question 38). Extension of the tumor into the fat-filled PES can be detected early on CT or MRI, and this finding has implications in staging and treatment. Patients with early supraglottic cancer are also at higher risk of occult nodal metastases compared with those with glottic cancer. Imaging is therefore indicated for a baseline assessment of the neck in these patients.

- Imaging has traditionally not been advocated in patients undergoing treatment for early glottic cancer because clinical examination is superior to imaging in assessing the mucosal extent of the disease. However, the submucosal extent of the tumor cannot only upstage glottic lesions but also have implications in terms of treatment selection, especially if endoscopic resection is being planned (see Questions 41 and 42). More importantly, a pretreatment baseline study is a useful frame of reference for interpreting posttreatment imaging studies because treatment-related changes can be difficult to differentiate from recurrent tumors.

- The hyoepiglottic ligament is a natural barrier to tumor spread from the oropharynx to the larynx but does not prevent tumor spread within the larynx (see Questions 29 and 38).The PES is contiguous with the paired paraglottic spaces.

- The unequal anterior and posterior laminae of the cricoid cartilage result in an angulation of the normal true and false vocal folds so that the anterior commissure is situated at a plane more caudad to the posterior commissure. This angular plane of the vocal folds corresponds to a plane parallel to the disk spaces between C4-5 and C5-6. If this angle is not maintained on a laryngeal imaging study, interpretation of tumor spread becomes very difficult and inaccurate.

- The thyroarytenoid muscle occupies the paraglottic space at the level of the true vocal folds (glottic larynx). This portion of the paraglottic space is therefore of muscle density on CT and MRI. In contrast, the supraglottic portion of the paraglottic space is largely occupied by fat, which is easily distinguishable from muscle and tumor on imaging.

- The adult human laryngeal cartilages contain fatty marrow if they are ossified. Infiltration or replacement of the normal fatty signal in these ossified areas of cartilage denotes involvement by tumor that may not be readily evident on CT (see Questions 40, 42, and 43). MRI of the larynx is generally reserved for directed examination of cartilage in question or early extralaryngeal spread if the CT findings are ambiguous.

- The hyoepiglottic ligament located under the mucosa of the vallecular fossae is a tough natural barrier to the spread of tumors from the base of the tongue to the PES of the larynx.

- Sagittal reconstruction of a CT scan (Figure 18-40) shows a tumor of the base of the tongue *(T)* confined to the oropharynx. Note the fat-filled PES *(arrow)* in immediate proximity to the tumor, which is prevented from spreading caudad by the hyoepiglottic ligament (see Questions 29 and 34).

- The infrahyoid epiglottic cartilage has more natural fenestrations that allow tumors on its mucosal surface easier access to the PES compared with suprahyoid epiglottic tumors. Tumors of the infrahyoid epiglottis

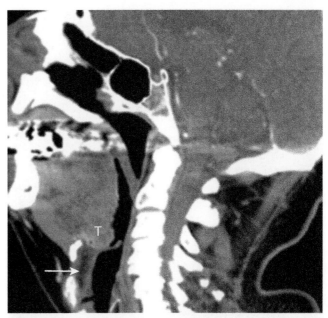

**Figure 18-40** (Courtesy of Memorial Sloan Kettering Cancer Center, New York.)

are therefore more prone to extend into the PES (see Question 66).

- Laryngeal anatomy places glottic tumors in closer proximity to the cartilaginous framework of the larynx compared with supraglottic tumors. Cartilage invasion occurs most commonly in areas of early ossification, including the lower border of the thyroid cartilage and the upper border of the cricoid cartilage, around the attachments of the cricothyroid membrane (CTM). Glottic tumors that infiltrate the paraglottic space encounter the conus elasticus (CE), which also plays an important role in directing tumors to these areas that are at high risk of cartilage involvement (see Question 68).

- Although radiographic imaging is generally not indicated for T1 glottic lesions, radiographically evident submucosal extension of a T1 glottic cancer to the supraglottis or subglottis can upstage it to T2.

- The anterior commissure is in close proximity to the perichondrium of the thyroid cartilage. However, most patients with mobile vocal cords do not have cartilage invasion, even with extension across the anterior commissure (T1b). If radiographic imaging is performed in these patients, minor cartilage demineralization is likely a normal anatomical variation. Tumors that are more likely to invade the cartilage at the anterior commissure include a bulky anteriorly located tumor with vocal cord fixation or more than 10 mm of caudad spread into the anterior subglottic region. An exception to this rule is the rare situation in which an aggressive small-volume anterior commissure lesion can extend cephalad to invade the insertion of the petiole of the epiglottis to the thyroid cartilage (Figure 18-41) and even extend into the PES.

- The normal adult larynx shows variable patterns and degrees of cartilage sclerosis and ossification, which make radiographic assessment of early cartilage involvement extremely difficult (see Questions 40 and 42).

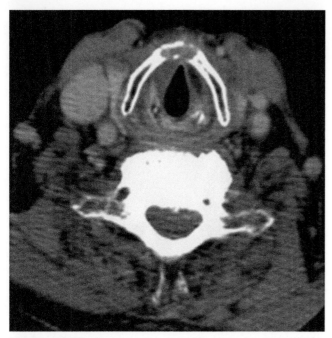

**Figure 18-41** (Courtesy of Memorial Sloan Kettering Cancer Center, New York.)

- A mass at level IB in a patient with carcinoma of the floor of the mouth can result from nodal metastasis, a blocked submandibular salivary gland from involvement of its duct in the floor of the mouth, or from direct extension of the floor-of-the-mouth tumor into the neck across the mylohyoid muscle (see Question 72). Although physical findings may direct the clinician to the appropriate scenario, imaging can readily assess the extent of the tumor, which is important not only for surgical resection with adequate margins but also for planning reconstruction of the surgical defect.

- The mandible should always be radiographically evaluated if mandibulotomy is a possibility. Adequate presurgical evaluation of these patients should include imaging to rule out the presence of any pathology at the site of the proposed mandibulotomy, such as cysts that may preclude secure placement of fixation plates and screws or hamper bony healing.

- Early cortical bone erosion from a carcinoma on the floor of the mouth is difficult to detect. If clinical examination reveals a tumor that is in close relation to the lingual aspect of the mandible, a fine-resolution CT scan, including a bone algorithm, can provide exquisite cortical detail of the mandible. However, the utility of imaging in these situations does not come from the ability to detect early cortical involvement but rather from the ability to rule out gross bony invasion: a marginal mandibulectomy constitutes adequate surgery for management of microscopic cortical bone involvement, but a segmental mandibulectomy is needed if gross, radiographically or clinically evident invasion of the mandible is present.

- PNS that is radiographically evident can predate symptoms of nerve involvement or signs of nerve dysfunction. The lack of symptoms or signs should therefore not be taken into account when patients who have tumors that are known to have a propensity for PNS are evaluated (see Questions 79 through 82).

- PNS generally occurs in a retrograde fashion (toward the central nervous system, starting from the smaller peripheral nerve). The involved nerve is most often contiguous to the end organ of innervation and appears enlarged and enhances on a postcontrast CT or MRI study. Occasionally, however, areas of PNS may be separated by patches of normal-appearing nerve, giving rise to the so-called skip areas of involvement along the course of the nerve. Antegrade spread of the tumor along an involved nerve is not infrequent and should always be anticipated when imaging studies of patients with PNS are evaluated. An example of antegrade PNS is shown in Figure 18-42. This patient had recurrent cutaneous squamous cell carcinoma of the right cheek with PNS along cranial nerve (CN) $V_2$ (i.e., infraorbital nerve, pterygopalatine fossa [PPF], cavernous sinus, Meckel cave, and the main trunk of CN V) denoted by the *arrowheads*. The tumor then spread antegrade from the main trunk of CN V along CN $V_1$ *(arrow)*.

- The soft tissue resolution of MRI is superior to CT for PNS, but PNS can also be reliably detected on CT

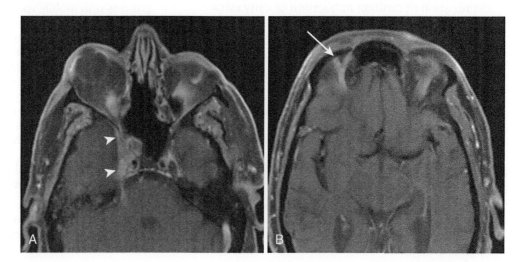

**Figure 18-42** (Courtesy of Memorial Sloan Kettering Cancer Center, New York.)

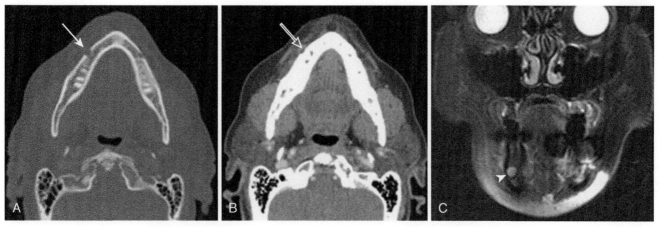

**Figure 18-43** (Courtesy of Memorial Sloan Kettering Cancer Center, New York.)

based on certain indirect signs such as widening of bony canals and foramina that transmit the CNs and their branches. The patient whose scans are shown in Figure 18-43 developed new-onset numbness of the right lower gum and teeth after previous surgical excision of a cutaneous melanoma of the chin. Note the widened right mental foramen *(white arrow)* on the bone window and the enlarged and enhancing right mental nerve *(open arrow)* on contrast-enhanced CT. The enlarged and enhancing right mental nerve *(white arrowhead)* is clearly seen within the alveolar canal on coronal T2W MRI.

- Precontrast T1W MRI is best suited for imaging PNS along the extracranial course of the involved CN because of the natural contrast of surrounding fat in the subcutaneous tissue or bone marrow. The involved nerve enhances with administration of contrast and blends with surrounding fat, making it less apparent. The intracranial enhancing component of an involved nerve is readily imaged on postcontrast T1W because there is no fat along the path of the nerve. The patient whose scans are shown in Figure 18-44 had a cutaneous melanoma of the left cheek with PNS along the left infraorbital nerve. The precontrast T1W MRI shows the grayish tumor *(T)* against adjacent subcutaneous fat and PNS along CN $V_2$ extending into the PPF

*(white arrow)*. Administration of contrast obscures the extracranial PNS, but now the extent of intracranial PNS along $V_2$ becomes very evident *(open arrow)*. Fat suppressed postcontrast T1W imaging nicely shows extracranial PNS; however, a susceptibility artifact from adjacent bone or air in the sinuses can cause incomplete fat suppression, and thus subtle PNS can be missed.

- Modern multidetector CT scanners are so quick that an entire study can be completed within a few minutes (see Question 4).

- T2W MRI is excellent at differentiating a tumor from postobstructive sinus disease and inspissated secretions. The patient whose scans are shown in Figure 18-45 had a locally advanced adenoid cystic carcinoma of the right maxillary sinus. T1W MRI shows an isointense tumor *(T)* that fills the right maxillary sinus; a rim and a patch of higher intensity signal in the anterior sinus *(white arrow)* appear different from the tumor. T2W MRI confirms that this difference in appearance is because of inspissated secretions in the maxillary sinus, which appear hyperintense compared with the tumor.

- Radiographic features that should raise suspicion for nasopharyngeal carcinoma include asymmetry in the

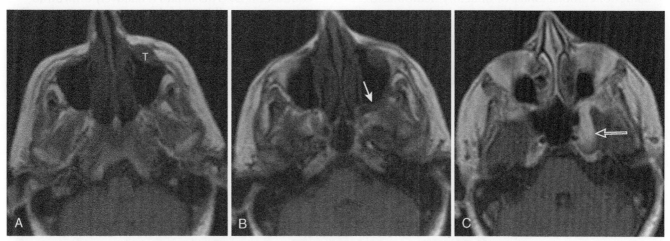

**Figure 18-44** (Courtesy of Memorial Sloan Kettering Cancer Center, New York.)

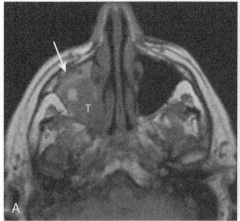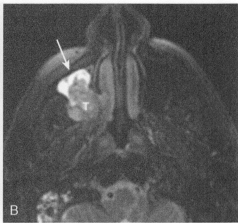

**Figure 18-45 A,** Precontrast T1-weighted magnetic resonance imaging (T1W MRI). **B,** T2W MRI. (Courtesy of Memorial Sloan Kettering Cancer Center, New York.)

nasopharyngeal wall, unilateral middle ear effusion, unexplained neuropathy of CN IX through XII, and level V and retropharyngeal lymph node metastases (see Questions 21 through 23).

• Invasion of the clivus by nasopharyngeal carcinoma is clearly seen on precontrast T1W MRI because the normal fatty marrow provides excellent contrast to the tumor. However, subtle bone involvement can be easily missed on postcontrast T1W imaging because the enhancing tumor blends with fatty marrow. Fat-saturated postcontrast T1W imaging confirms clival invasion because normal fat suppresses, whereas the enhancing tumor remains clearly visible and white. Clival involvement is even better imaged on sagittal sequences of the same patient, as shown in Figure 18-46. The gray tumor *(white arrow)* in the ventral clivus contrasts nicely with the uninvolved fat of the dorsal portion. This delineation between tumor and fat is lost on the postcontrast T1W sequence, and early clival involvement can be easily missed.

• Widening of the right petroclival fissure should raise suspicion of a malignant nasopharyngeal neoplasm in the patient whose CT scan shows prominent soft tissue in the nasopharynx (see Figure 18-3). Benign adenoidal hypertrophy would not cause regressive remodeling of bone in this area.

• Esthesioneuroblastomas or olfactory neuroblastomas are tumors of neural crest origin that arise from

the olfactory mucosa in the superior nasal cavity near the cribriform plate. Intracranial extension of these tumors occurs in about 25% of cases. A CT scan typically shows a homogeneous, enhancing mass that primarily remodels bone, and extension into the ethmoid and maxillary sinuses is common (Figure 18-47). Erosion of the cribriform plate *(A, arrow)* is frequent because of the location of the tumor. The tumor may occasionally have calcification *(B, arrow)*.

• These tumors generally have an intermediate signal on all precontrast MRI sequences. The presence of intracranial extension is often accompanied by cyst formation (Figure 18-48A, *white arrow*). Edema of the brain parenchyma on T2W MRI (Figure 18-48B, *black arrows*) is an ominous feature because it represents parenchymal invasion by the tumor.

• Figure 18-4 shows metastatic lateral retropharyngeal adenopathy with radiographic features of extracapsular nodal spread including invasion of the left prevertebral musculature (see Questions 6, 24, and 25). Infiltration of metastatic disease in this area at the skull base poses risk of invasion of the lower CNs IX to XII.

• Squamous cell carcinomas of the head and neck do not enhance significantly after administration of contrast on CT. This makes it relatively difficult to distinguish small base-of-the-tongue squamous cell

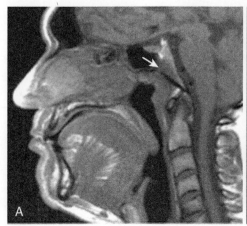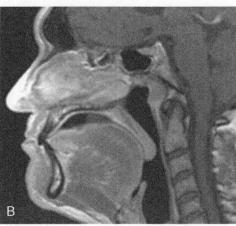

**Figure 18-46 A,** Precontrast T1-weighted magnetic resonance imaging (T1W MRI). **B,** Postcontrast T1W MRI without fat suppression. (Courtesy of Memorial Sloan Kettering Cancer Center, New York.)

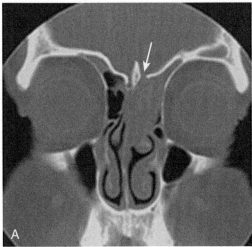 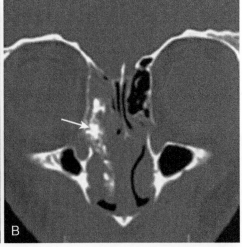

**Figure 18-47** (Courtesy of Memorial Sloan Kettering Cancer Center, New York.)

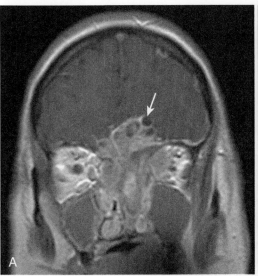 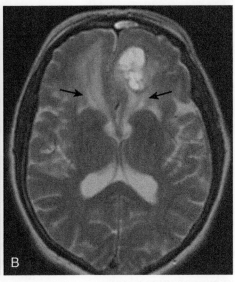

**Figure 18-48 A,** Postcontrast T1-weighted magnetic resonance imaging (T1W MRI). **B,** T2W MRI. (Courtesy of Memorial Sloan Kettering Cancer Center, New York.)

carcinoma from normal lingual tonsillar tissue. Asymmetry of lingual tonsillar tissue and local infiltration into the musculature of the base of the tongue and pharynx are signs of malignancy as seen in Figure 18-5 (see Question 92).

- The patient in Figure 18-6 had a squamous cell carcinoma of the right tonsil. The tumor extended posteriorly along the superior constrictor of the posterior pharyngeal wall up to the midline. Anteriorly, the tumor extended to the retromolar trigone without invading the underlying mandible. The pterygomandibular raphe is located in the vicinity, and its invasion allows oropharyngeal tumors access to the buccal space, posing significant challenges in management (see Questions 27 and 73).

- The patient in Figure 18-7 has a typical metastatic right lateral retropharyngeal lymph node (see Questions 24, 25, 57, 61, 62, and 84).

- The anatomical location of the lateral retropharyngeal lymph nodes medial to the internal carotid artery makes it difficult for the surgeon to access these nodes via the conventional transcervical approach to

neck dissection. The lack of anatomical access also precludes any systematic dissection of these nodes, although some surgeons advocate excision via a transoral approach (see Questions 24, 25, 62, and 84).

- The lateral retropharyngeal nodes receive lymphatic drainage from the nasopharynx, oropharynx, hypopharynx, and thyroid along the prevertebral plexus. Tumors at these anatomical sites are likely to cause metastatic lateral retropharyngeal lymphadenopathy.

- Tumors of the pyriform sinus most often do not become symptomatic until they become locally advanced. Early stage tumors are rare and are generally diagnosed incidentally on clinical examination or on imaging performed for investigation of other entities. The normal pyriform sinus mucosa is thin and enhances uniformly after contrast administration, as is seen on the right side in Figure 18-8. Thickening and enhancement of the left pyriform sinus is suggestive of a malignant lesion and should be investigated appropriately with endoscopy and biopsy.

- The paraglottic space is separated from the hypopharynx only by thin mucosa and the posterior arytenoid fat pad overlying the thyroarytenoid space. Tumors of the hypopharynx have access to the paraglottic space between the cricoarytenoid joint and the thyroid cartilage in this area. Widening of this space and sclerosis of the arytenoid cartilage as seen in the scan of the patient in Figure 18-49 are indicators of tumor involvement. Postcontrast axial T1W MRI clearly shows the tumor insinuating itself into the paraglottic space.

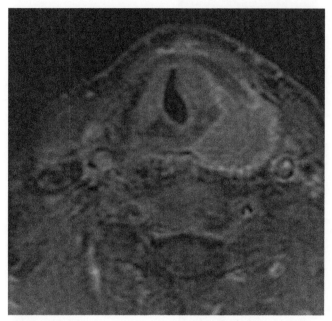

**Figure 18-49** (Courtesy of Memorial Sloan Kettering Cancer Center, New York.)

• The apex of the pyriform sinus is situated at the level of the cricoarytenoid joint, and the recurrent laryngeal nerve is in close proximity in the tracheoesophageal groove. Vocal cord paralysis in hypopharyngeal cancers can therefore result from direct invasion of the recurrent laryngeal nerve and fixation of the cricoarytenoid joint. Indirect involvement of the recurrent laryngeal nerve by metastatic lymphadenopathy in the tracheoesophageal groove can also occur but is relatively rare.

• The laryngeal cartilaginous framework is based on the cricoid cartilage, which is the only complete ring in the upper airway. The cricoid cartilage articulates with the thyroid, which encloses the supraglottis and glottis. The epiglottic cartilage attaches to the thyroid cartilage anteriorly at the level of the anterior commissure of the glottis. Natural fenestrations are present in the infrahyoid portion of the epiglottic cartilage (see Question 39). The paired arytenoid cartilages also articulate with the cricoid cartilage. They span the supraglottic and glottic larynx, and the vocal process of the arytenoid cartilage provides attachment to the vocal ligament.

• The PES is a fat-filled C-shaped space enclosed between the hyoid bone anteriorly and the epiglottic cartilage posteriorly. The thyrohyoid membrane wraps around to form the lateral boundary of the

PES. Its roof is covered by the vallecular mucosa and the hyoepiglottic ligament, which lies immediately under the mucosa and divides the PES into halves (see Questions 29, 34, and 38). It is bounded inferiorly by the petiole of the epiglottis, which attaches to the thyroid cartilage by the thyroepiglottic ligament. The pattern of invasion of the PES can indicate the nature of a tumor: squamous cell carcinoma invades with an infiltrative and destructive pattern, whereas tumors of minor salivary gland origin generally have a well-defined pushing border as seen in Figure 18-10. Involvement of the PES does place the hyoid bone at risk if the patient has an infiltrative squamous cell carcinoma but not if the patient has a minor salivary gland carcinoma with pushing borders. Infiltrative and destructive tumors can extend across the thyrohyoid membrane, but this is a feature of very advanced disease.

• There are two major intralaryngeal membranes: the quadrangular membrane (QM) and the CE. Neither membrane can be seen on MRI. The QM spans from the lateral margin of the epiglottis and aryepiglottic fold to the upper arytenoid and corniculate cartilages. Its upper margin supports the aryepiglottic fold while the condensed lower margin forms the ventricular ligament. It forms the medial boundary of the supraglottic paraglottic space. The CE spans from the vocal ligament to the superior edge of the cricoid cartilage. When a glottic tumor involves the paraglottic space, it is located cranial to the CE, which directs tumor spread laterally toward the CTM. This is where areas of ossified cricoid and thyroid cartilage border the inferior attachment of the CE, and these portions of the cartilage are therefore at higher risk of tumor invasion. The CTM provides some resistance to tumor invasion but is ultimately a pathway for extralaryngeal spread of the tumor. The lymphatics of the subglottic larynx also exit the larynx through the CT membrane.

• Invasion of the arytenoid cartilage is often seen as sclerosis, which is asymmetrical compared with the opposite normal side, as in the patient with a locally advanced squamous cell carcinoma of the left glottic larynx (see Figure 18-11). The tumor extends into the left paraglottic space, crosses the midline, destroys the thyroid cartilage ala anteriorly, and invades the adjacent sternothyroid muscle, which is thickened. Inferior extension into the anterior subglottis is manifest by thickening of the soft tissue underlying the mucosa and irregular enhancement on the postcontrast study. Sclerosis of thyroid cartilage can indicate invasion by a tumor or reactive changes, making the diagnosis of cartilage invasion by a tumor difficult.

• The paired genioglossus muscles flank the midline raphe of the tongue, which is occupied by fat. The hyoglossus muscle is an important radiographic landmark because the lingual artery and IXn are located medial to it while the lingual nerve and XIIn are located lateral to the muscle.

• The extent of involvement of the tongue by an infiltrative tumor is almost always underestimated

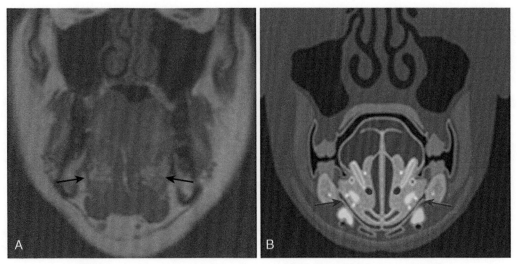

**Figure 18-50** (Courtesy of Memorial Sloan Kettering Cancer Center, New York.)

by both clinical examination and imaging studies. One of the key considerations in deciding on the extent of glossectomy is the relationship of the tumor to the neurovascular pedicles of the tongue. The surgeon usually aims to resect normal tissue to a distance of 1 to 1.5 cm from the visible and palpable borders of the tumor. In doing so for the patient, the surgeon will also have to sacrifice the left neurovascular bundle, which will result in an anterior subtotal glossectomy.

- The mylohyoid muscle forms a muscular diaphragm that separates the oral cavity from the neck. The muscle (Figure 18-50, *arrows*) spans from the mylohyoid line on the lingual aspect of the mandible to the hyoid bone on each side, and the submandibular salivary gland is wrapped around its posterior border.

- Tumors of the floor of the mouth can be associated with a palpable mass at level IB because of lymph node metastasis, an obstructed submandibular salivary gland from involvement of its duct in the floor of the mouth, or direct extension through the mylohyoid muscle. The treatment implications of each of these three scenarios is different; therefore it is important to determine the exact relation of a palpable level IB mass to a primary tumor of the floor of the mouth before surgical resection (see Question 44). The patient shown in Figure 18-14 will need an en bloc resection of the primary tumor with at least a marginal mandibulectomy and neck dissection. Reconstruction of the resultant defect in the floor of the mouth will require a microvascular free radial forearm flap. If direct extension of the tumor into the neck from the primary of the floor of the mouth were mistaken for an obstructed submandibular gland or a metastatic level IB lymph node, the patient's surgical plan would be for resection of the floor of the mouth with skin graft reconstruction and neck dissection; the misdiagnosis would have required major revision of the surgical plan on the operating table.

- The pterygomandibular raphe is a fibrous aponeurosis that extends from the hamulus of the medial ptery-

goid plate to the mylohyoid line on the lingual aspect of the mandible. The raphe is separated from the ramus of the mandible by adipose tissue, and the inferior alveolar nerve passes under it in the retromolar trigone. The fibers of the buccinator and the superior pharyngeal constrictor muscles interdigitate along this raphe so that involvement by a tumor facilitates tumor spread anteriorly to the buccal space and posteriorly to the pharynx. The patient whose scans are shown in Figure 18-51 has a right retromolar trigone tumor *(T)*. The tumor has extended on to the right pterygomandibular raphe and then anteriorly to the right buccinator muscle, which appears thickened *(white arrow)* compared with the opposite normal buccinator muscle *(black arrow)*.

- The patient in Figure 18-15 has a tumor of the right lateral border of the tongue with involvement of the floor of the mouth. The tumor is in close proximity to the lingual surface of the mandible, but there is no cortical erosion of the bone window on the CT scan. The patient has a good mandibular height, and the tumor will therefore be amenable to partial glossectomy with marginal mandibulectomy and free flap reconstruction.

- Dental extraction and manipulation of the gingiva can produce bony and soft tissue changes that can very easily be mistaken for tumor invasion on MRI scans. As seen on the precontrast T1W images in Figure 18-52, the fatty marrow of the mandible and maxilla is replaced by grayish signal that could be an invasive tumor. These areas of the bone also enhance on the postcontrast T1W MRI. In addition, note the extensive soft tissue changes in the retromolar trigone continuing anteriorly along the lateral aspect of the mandible and posteriorly along the superior constrictor muscle. A CT scan confirmed the bony changes noted on the MRI scan.

- In the context of a histologically proven squamous cell carcinoma of the retromolar trigone, the aforementioned radiographic findings appear consistent with invasion of the pterygomandibular raphe and spread

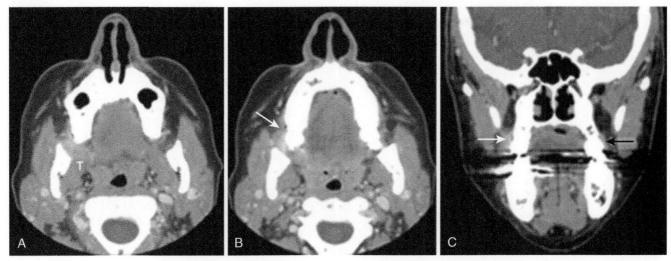

**Figure 18-51** (Courtesy of Memorial Sloan Kettering Cancer Center, New York.)

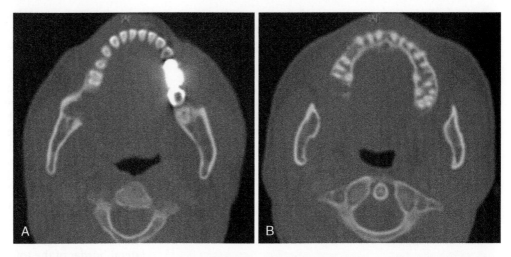

**Figure 18-52** (Courtesy of Memorial Sloan Kettering Cancer Center, New York.)

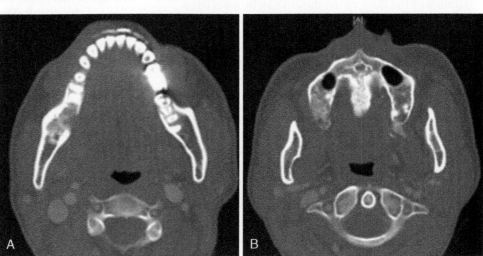

**Figure 18-53** (Courtesy of Memorial Sloan Kettering Cancer Center, New York.)

along the pharyngeal constrictor (see Question 73). However, the discrepancy between radiographic findings and the clinical examination, which did not reveal any obvious mucosal tumor in the oral cavity, was striking, and the radiographic findings were thought to be related to dental extraction and surgical manipulation.

This prompted the decision for short interval repeated imaging in 6 weeks, and a CT scan shown in Figure 18-53 confirms healing of the abnormal bone of the mandible as well as maxilla and resolution of the soft tissue changes noted on the previous MRI. The previously "lytic" dental sockets now show sclerotic new bone.

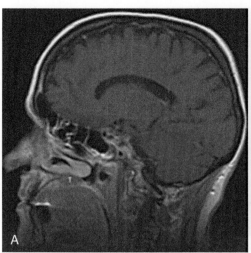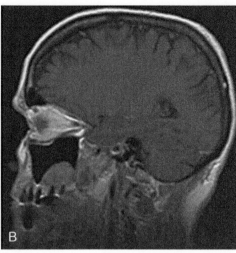

**Figure 18-54** (Courtesy of Memorial Sloan Kettering Cancer Center, New York.)

- Tumors of minor salivary gland origin generally have a pushing growth pattern in contrast to squamous cell carcinoma and poorly differentiated tumors that are infiltrative and destructive. Regressive remodeling of adjacent bone is a radiographic feature of a slow-growing neoplasm. The patient in Figure 18-17 had an adenoid cystic carcinoma arising from and expanding the hard palate, extending into the right nasal cavity and maxillary sinus. The precontrast T1W MRI clearly shows replacement of the fatty marrow of the right half of the hard palate by grayish tumor (T) as does the sagittal T1W postcontrast MRI shown in Figure 18-54. The floor of the maxillary antrum is intact on the sagittal T1W postcontrast MRI and the overlying mucosa appears normal on coronal T2W MRI.

- Osteoradionecrosis (ORN) is a devastating complication of radiation therapy that can be more difficult to treat than the original tumor. It is defined as devitalized, irradiated bone that is exposed through overlying mucosa or skin persisting for 6 months or longer. The etiopathogenesis of ORN is multifactorial and includes patient-, tumor-, and treatment-related factors. Patient factors include smoking and alcohol use, especially continued use during treatment, poor dental hygiene, dental extraction after radiation therapy, poor nutritional status, and severe mucositis and trismus. Tumor-related factors include a locally advanced infiltrative ulcerated lesion in close proximity or a lesion invading bone. Treatment-related factors include surgery, which requires manipulation of the mandibular bone (e.g., marginal mandibulectomy or mandibulotomy), and prior radiation therapy. Bone that receives radiation doses greater than 5500 cGy are at a higher risk of ORN. In the past, parallel opposed portals were used for delivering radiation therapy to the oral cavity and oropharynx; therefore the body of mandible was most susceptible to ORN. The mean time from completion of radiation therapy to development of ORN was approximately 3 years (range, 24 to 48 months). With the advent of intensity-modulated radiation therapy (IMRT), the mandible is routinely contoured as an avoidance structure in planning. However, tumor anatomy may not permit adequate

sparing of the mandible. For instance, delivery of adequate radiation to T3-4 tumors of the oropharynx expose even the anterior mandibular teeth to an average of more than 6000 cGy, which places these areas of the mandible at risk of ORN.

- Stage I or superficial ORN presents as a small necrotic ulcer with exposed cortical bone and appears as an irregularity of cortical bone (Figure 18-55, A, arrow) or early loss of integrity on imaging. Stage II ORN involves medullary bone with or without soft tissue changes. The imaging findings include loss of medullary trabeculation and fat on T1W MRI along with soft tissue changes on T2W MRI (B, arrow) that may be difficult to differentiate from the tumor. Progression to stage III ORN results from development of an orocutaneous fistula or sinus or from a pathological fracture (C, arrow).

- PNS of a tumor is defined as extension of the primary tumor along tissues of the neural sheath (epineurium and perineurium) of a named nerve. The term PNS has been used interchangeably with perineural invasion (PNI) in the literature. PNI is a histopathological feature of the tumor indicating involvement of microscopic or small nerves within the tumor and cannot be seen on radiographic imaging. PNS, on the other hand, denotes macroscopic or gross extension of a tumor along a large nerve that is distinct from and distant to the primary tumor. The presence of PNI on histological examination does not automatically portend PNS. The risk of PNS is influenced by the histological type of the tumor and its anatomical location. Certain tumors such as adenoid cystic carcinoma and desmoplastic melanoma have a propensity for PNS compared with other histological types such as squamous cell carcinoma. Lymphomas of the head and neck also have an affinity for nerves, and an accurate histological diagnosis is especially crucial in avoiding mistreatment. Tumors in anatomical locations such as the salivary glands (e.g., the parotid and hard palate) and skin in the distribution of CN V are therefore at higher risk. However, squamous cell carcinoma is the histological type found in the overwhelming major-

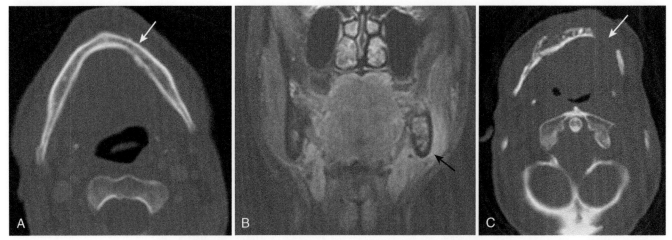

**Figure 18-55** (Courtesy of Memorial Sloan Kettering Cancer Center, New York.)

ity of patients with head and neck cancer; therefore the possibility of PNS should always be considered in these patients.

- The patient in Figure 18-56A has a well-circumscribed bilobed lesion in the left cavernous sinus with no evidence of extension along the nerves in the area. The tumor has features consistent with a schwannoma (see Questions 11 and 90). Unlike the typical bright tumor that is a feature of schwannoma on T2W MRI, this tumor was not as bright on T2W MRI or the T2W fluid attenuated inversion recovery (FLAIR) sequence (neither image is pictured here), which also suppresses the normal fluid in the brain and globes. The postcontrast T1W sequence shows a heterogeneously enhancing tumor that is located within the cavernous sinus and is not based on the dura. Meningiomas, on the other hand, tend to be densely homogeneous on postcontrast MRI, are dural based, and have a dural tail (Figure 18-56B, *white arrows*).

- Elderly patients with skin cancer often present with symptoms or clinical signs of PNS involving CN V and/ or CN VII. The patient shown in Figure 18-21 had a

long history of removal of skin lesions from the scalp and face that were reportedly all benign. Over time, he developed facial numbness and then diplopia, for which he was referred to a neurologist for a presumed cavernous sinus primary tumor. Postcontrast axial T1W MRI shows the classic appearance of PNS along the infraorbital nerve retrograde to $V_2$, through the foramen rotundum into the cavernous sinus and the Meckel cave, to the main trunk of CN V and into the CN V nucleus in the brainstem with involvement of the adjacent dura. CT and MRI are complementary in assessing patients for PNS, but each has its advantages. A PET scan is generally insensitive for detection of PNS but can occasionally give positive results. Imaging criteria used to diagnose PNS along a nerve include the following:

- Asymmetric enlargement
- Asymmetric enhancement
- Obliteration of perineural fat planes
- Denervation changes in end organs (e.g., muscles of facial expression and mastication)
- Widening of the foramina transmitting the nerve

- Adenoid cystic carcinoma has a particular affinity for nerves and is a common cause of PNS in tumors of

**Figure 18-56 A,** Postcontrast axial T1-weighted magnetic resonance imaging (T1W MRI). **B,** Postcontrast axial T1W MRI with fat saturation. (Courtesy of Memorial Sloan Kettering Cancer Center, New York.)

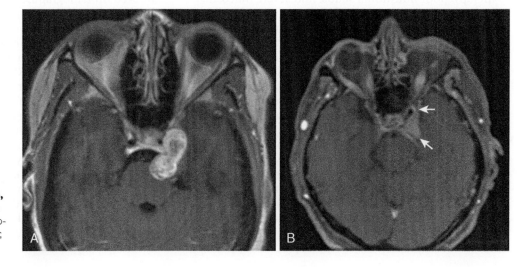

the maxillary sinus and hard palate. These tumors are generally treated with primary surgical resection, and accurate assessment for PNS is of critical importance in achieving complete resection of the tumor. Tumors of the hard palate gain access to the greater and lesser palatine nerves, which traverse the corresponding foramina and enter the PPF and then involve CN V$_2$ toward the central nervous system. As seen in this CT scan of another patient (Figure 18-57), widening of the PPF (*white arrow*) is an indirect sign of PNS. Note the normal opposite PPF.

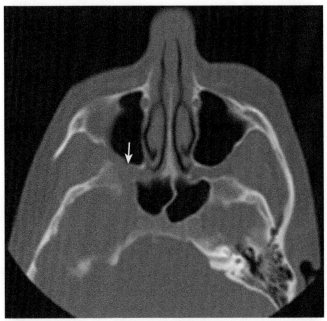

**Figure 18-57** (Courtesy of Memorial Sloan Kettering Cancer Center, New York.)

- Lymphoma is often ignored in the differential diagnosis of PNS. In the absence of other primary tumors that are known to cause PNS, lymphoma should be considered in the differential diagnosis because of the obvious implications in terms of treatment. Lymphoma is not treated surgically, and CT-guided biopsy is an excellent modality for obtaining tissue for diagnosis so that the patient can expeditiously proceed to appropriate treatment. The scans shown in Figure 18-23 demonstrate PNS along CN V$_2$ and antegrade PNS along V$_3$ and the inferior alveolar nerve. The asymmetrically widened right PPF and right foramen ovale without bone destruction are indicators of PNS along CN V$_2$, which also enhances on the postcontrast CT scan. Note the asymmetrically enlarged and enhancing right inferior alveolar nerve within the alveolar canal of the mandible.

- Soft tissue infiltration and invasion of the central compartment viscera is a feature of poorly differentiated locally aggressive thyroid cancer. The tumor shown in Figure 18-24 has ill-defined borders and infiltrates the right hemilarynx through the cricoarytenoid space. The course of the right recurrent laryngeal nerve is also occupied by infiltrative tumor signifying invasion, which has caused vocal fold paralysis denoted by

medial rotation of the right arytenoid and paramedian position of the right vocal fold. The hypodense mass represents tumor necrosis in a locally aggressive fast-growing tumor and is not consistent with the expected location of a lateral retropharyngeal lymph node (see Questions 24, 25, 57, 61, and 62).

- Chondromas and chondrosarcomas of the cricoid cartilage are the most common cartilaginous tumors of the laryngeal framework. The imaging features are consistent with an expansile lesion arising from and centered on the involved cartilage, which remains largely intact. These tumors are classically bright on T2W MRI and have chondroid calcifications on CT scan. The cricoid cartilage can be involved by other more common disease processes, such as squamous cell carcinoma of the larynx or papillary carcinoma of the thyroid, but the radiographic features in these entities would be consistent with soft tissue infiltration and cartilage destruction. Papillary carcinoma of the thyroid can also result in calcification, but this is typically present in the well-differentiated long-standing component of the thyroid tumor, not in the invasive intralaryngeal component. Adenoid cystic carcinoma is the most common minor salivary gland tumor of the subglottic larynx and cervical trachea. It is generally seen as a submucosal mass without destruction of cartilage. Chondroradionecrosis after radiation therapy can also be seen with destructive cartilage changes and is often difficult to differentiate from recurrent cancer. However, the imaging studies would also have other stigmata of radiation therapy, including edema of the airway and soft tissue stranding to indicate previous treatment.

- Pleomorphic adenoma or benign mixed tumor is the most common neoplasm of the parotid glands. This T2W MRI (Figure 18-58) shows a well-circumscribed

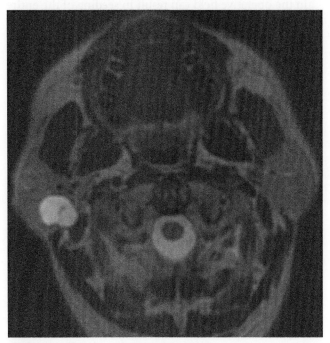

**Figure 18-58** (Courtesy of Memorial Sloan Kettering Cancer Center, New York.)

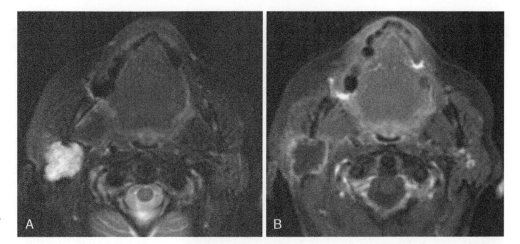

**Figure 18-59 A,** Axial T2-weighted magnetic resonance imaging (T2W MRI) with fat saturation. **B,** Postcontrast T1W MRI with fat saturation. (Courtesy of Memorial Sloan Kettering Cancer Center, New York.)

isointense lesion arising from the parotid gland. This appearance is not helpful in differentiating benign from malignant parotid tumors because malignant tumors of the parotid gland are commonly well-circumscribed. Infiltrative, irregular borders are the only consistent feature that allows radiographic diagnosis of a malignant tumor. This lesion is too large and too round to represent a normal intraparotid lymph node and shows no fatty hilum. This is not a lymphoepithelial cyst because the lesion is solid and is solitary.

- Benign mixed tumors are typically bright on T2W MRI, whereas most other parotid tumors are isointense on T2W MRI. This is an extremely useful sequence for assessing the extent of the lesion in relation to the parotid parenchyma.

- Local recurrence after surgical resection of pleomorphic adenoma is uncommon, especially after adequate resection. However, rupture of the tumor and spillage in the operative field can result in seeding of the entire surgical bed. Local recurrence in this situation appears as numerous discrete nodules like a cluster of grapes that is bright on T2W MRI. Malignant parotid tumors do not have any special features, except for possible irregular borders and an infiltrative appearance on imaging; however, many are well-defined. The T2W MRI shown in Figure 18-59 is of a patient who had a mucoepidermoid carcinoma. The T2 bright tumor is similar to the appearance of a benign mixed tumor, but note the thickened, irregular, and enhancing border of the tumor on T1W postcontrast MRI, which is consistent with a malignant process.

- The prestyloid space (i.e., parapharyngeal space or PPS) is separated from the poststyloid space (i.e., carotid space) by the fascia overlying the tensor veli palatini muscle (*white line* on Figure 18-60). The PPS is surrounded by other "spaces" as shown in Figure 18-61. The origin of tumors in this region can be deduced by the pattern of displacement of the fat-filled PPS and the contents of the carotid space relative to the tumor. For instance, tumors of the parotid space displace the fat-filled PPS medially and anteriorly, whereas tumors of the pharyngeal mucosal space displace it laterally and posteriorly. Tumors arising from

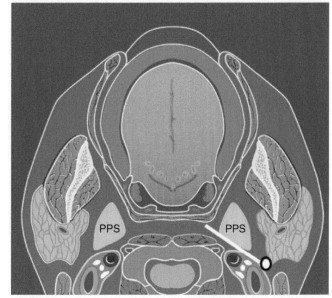

**Figure 18-60** (Courtesy of Memorial Sloan Kettering Cancer Center, New York.)

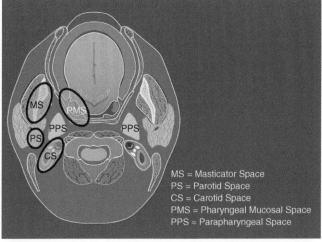

MS = Masticator Space
PS = Parotid Space
CS = Carotid Space
PMS = Pharyngeal Mucosal Space
PPS = Parapharyngeal Space

**Figure 18-61** (Courtesy of Memorial Sloan Kettering Cancer Center, New York.)

the masticator space displace the PPS medially and posteriorly.

- The PPS contains fat, branches of CN $V_3$, internal maxillary artery, ascending pharyngeal artery, pharyngeal venous plexus, and minor salivary gland rests (see Figure 18-61). Primary tumors of this space are uncommon, and this space is most commonly involved by extension of a deep lobe parotid tumor. The carotid space contains the common and internal carotid arteries, internal jugular vein, CNs IX through XII, and the sympathetic plexus. Tumors of this space are therefore largely of neurovascular origin, and they displace the PPS anteriorly. This "spatial approach" is very reliable for diagnosing tumors in this region.

- Schwannomas are benign tumors of Schwann cells and are generally asymptomatic; thus they are usually large at presentation unless they are discovered incidentally on an imaging study performed for unrelated reasons. Schwannomas appear as well-defined, ovoid masses that may be heterogeneous on imaging. They are typically bright on T2W MRI. Unlike paragangliomas (see Question 91), they do not show flow voids and do not vigorously enhance on a CT scan after administration of contrast, as shown in Figure 18-62.

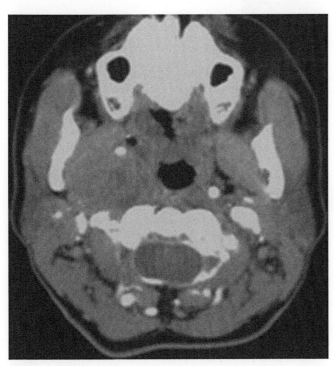

**Figure 18-62** (Courtesy of Memorial Sloan Kettering Cancer Center, New York.)

- Paragangliomas are benign tumors of neural crest origin. They are generally asymptomatic and are therefore most often large at presentation. Like other benign tumors of this area, they are well-defined and ovoid, but their distinguishing characteristic is the presence of prominent flow voids, which give the typical "salt and pepper" appearance on MRI. These tumors enhance densely on CT and MRI after administration of contrast

and can cause permeative changes in the osseous structures of the skull base as opposed to regressive remodeling seen with schwannomas and hyperostosis with meningiomas.

- Ectopic thyroid tissue can be found in any location along the thyroglossal duct (see Question 93). Lingual thyroid represents ectopic thyroid tissue at the opening of the thyroglossal duct in the base of the tongue (foramen cecum). The imaging appearance is that of a well-circumscribed median or paramedian tongue mass that is hyperdense compared with adjoining muscle on a CT scan and clearly enhances after contrast administration. Malignant transformation is rare, and no intervention is necessary unless there is suspicion of pathology, especially because the lingual thyroid may be the only functioning thyroid tissue in the patient. Ectopic thyroid tissue concentrates activity on an iodine-123 scan, as shown in Figure 18-63.

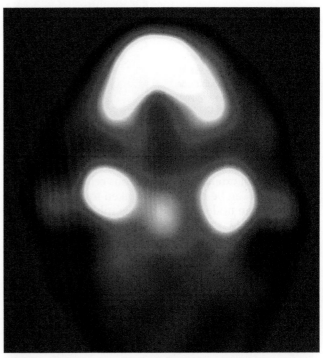

**Figure 18-63** (Courtesy of Memorial Sloan Kettering Cancer Center, New York.)

- The thyroid anlage descends from the foramen cecum on the base of the tongue to the infrahyoid neck. The normal thyroglossal duct (TGD) involutes at 5 to 6 weeks of gestation. However, pathology of the duct along the route of descent of the thyroid can result in ectopic thyroid tissue, including lingual thyroid, TGD cysts, and rarely, tumors of thyroid tissue origin (Figure 18-64). A TGD cyst results from secretions collecting in a persistent epithelial-lined TGD. It is the most common congenital neck lesion and is usually clinically silent unless it is infected or inflamed. Thyroid carcinoma within a TGD cyst is rare. An inflamed TGD cyst will show surrounding soft tissue changes including stranding. Most metastatic Delphian nodes are solid and enhancing, but cystic nodal metastases

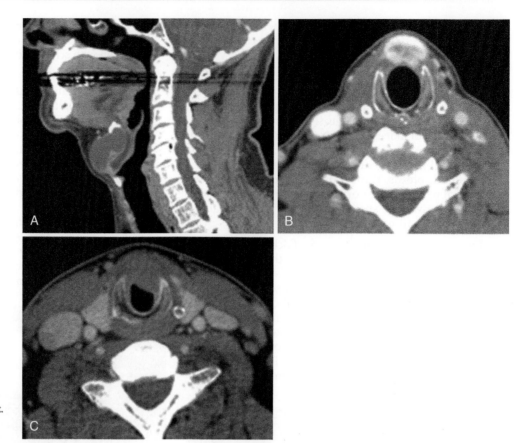

**Figure 18-64 A,** Inflamed thyroglossal duct (TGD) cyst. **B,** Metastatic Delphian lymph node. **C,** Extralaryngeal spread of squamous cell carcinoma of the larynx. (Courtesy of Memorial Sloan Kettering Cancer Center, New York.)

can be difficult to differentiate from a TGD cyst. Extralaryngeal extension of squamous cell carcinoma of the larynx can be clinically mistaken for a TGD tumor or Delphian node, but the radiographic appearance is unmistakable.

- Chondronecrosis of the larynx is a dreaded complication of radiation therapy of the larynx that very frequently results in the need for total laryngectomy to protect the airway from aspiration due to a dysfunctional larynx. Patients with locally advanced, bulky tumors that are in close proximity to or invading the laryngeal cartilaginous framework are typically at increased risk of developing chondronecrosis. Trauma to the mucosal surface of the larynx, especially from injudicious or random biopsies to rule out a suspected tumor, can substantially elevate the risk of chondronecrosis. Thickening and stranding of the adjacent soft tissue is commonly seen. Chondronecrosis and a recurrent tumor are both FDG avid; therefore a PET-CT scan cannot reliably differentiate the two conditions. Nonetheless, PET findings should be used to direct a biopsy, if indicated, based on the clinical context.

- The radiologist will also occasionally encounter patients who have had voice rehabilitation procedures, such as vocal fold medialization for treatment of a paralyzed vocal cord. These are expected post-treatment changes that should not be confused with abnormal foreign bodies in the larynx. The patient in Figure 18-34 has had a polytetrafluoroethylene (Gore-Tex) tape implant for right vocal fold medialization. The tape is introduced via a surgically created window

in the lamina of the thyroid cartilage, and this may mimic cartilage destruction. However, the foreign material is homogenously dense on noncontrast CT and is located submucosally in the glottic paraglottic space. If this were a rare and unusual vascular lesion such as a hemangioma or paraganglioma, it would enhance heterogeneously on a contrast-enhanced CT scan. Chunky calcification does occur with long-standing, well-differentiated papillary thyroid carcinoma, and transformation to poorly differentiated or anaplastic cancer can result in laryngeal invasion. However, the calcified component of the tumor in these situations is generally located outside the larynx within the thyroid gland itself.

- The radiographic appearance of the radiated larynx is characterized by edema and obliteration of tissue planes, which alters the appearance of the epiglottis, the aryepiglottic folds, and the paraglottic fat. Increased linear mucosal enhancement on contrast-enhanced CT is also typical. Although new onset cartilage sclerosis may represent a long-term sequela of radiation therapy, cartilage sclerosis can be caused by invasion by a tumor or reactive changes to an adjacent tumor; therefore it should prompt suspicion for recurrent disease.

- A PET scan performed before approximately 12 weeks after completion of chemoradiation therapy is susceptible to a false-positive result from a variety of reasons, including resolving mucositis or a necrotic tumor, which may have apoptotic or nonviable cancer cells. Vocal cord paralysis is seen as asymmetric FDG activity because of unopposed laryngeal muscular activity on the normal mobile side, and this should not be confused with a tumor. Later, radiation-induced bony or soft tissue necrosis can cause FDG uptake that can result in false-positive findings. When a posttreatment PET scan is evaluated, a cardinal rule is to compare it with a pretreatment study. Look for focal and asymmetric uptake that coregisters to the site of the primary tumor and/or a focal mass on anatomical imaging: diffuse uptake usually indicates postradiation inflammation and not a recurrent tumor. Increased mild-to-moderate diffuse laryngeal or oropharyngeal uptake may persist for prolonged periods after chemoradiation therapy.

- Imaging of the head and neck after treatment for cancer can be extremely challenging. Communication between the treating clinician and the radiologist is of

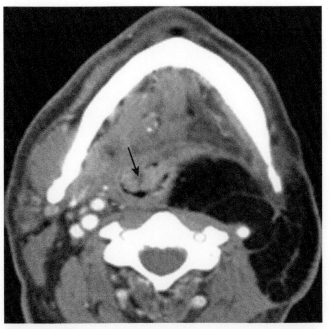

**Figure 18-65** (Courtesy of Memorial Sloan Kettering Cancer Center, New York.)

tremendous value, as is a comparison between pretreatment and posttreatment baseline imaging studies. The patient shown in Figure 18-65 had a total laryngectomy and partial pharyngectomy for locally advanced hypopharyngeal cancer. Partial defects of the pharynx are typically reconstructed with a pedicled patch, such as a pectoralis major myocutaneous flap, or a free flap, such as a radial forearm or rectus abdominis myocutaneous flap. The presence of large amounts of fat in the surgical bed in this patient point to rectus flap reconstruction. The patient had progressive difficulty swallowing, and a pharyngeal hood tube was placed, which is easily seen in the sagittal CT scan. A recurrent tumor at the superior suture line of the flap with the base of the tongue is not readily apparent *(black arrow)*.

- Image-guided biopsy (IGB) of head and neck tumors greatly aids diagnosis and subsequent treatment in the appropriate clinical setting. IGB can often be the least invasive approach to diagnosis and, in experienced hands, is a low-risk procedure that often allows a patient to avoid general anesthesia and a more complicated open surgical procedure for diagnosis. There are additional advantages in that this procedure is performed on an outpatient basis, a cytopathologist is present to ensure adequate sampling, and no residual scar is present after the procedure. Obviously, palpable lesions can easily be sampled by fine-needle aspiration by the patient's physician or a cytologist. Superficial lesions such as thyroid nodules, superficial parotid lobe lesions, and small lateral cervical lymph nodes are readily accessible with the use of real-time ultrasound guidance. Lesions that are more deeply located within the head and neck require CT or MR guidance to negotiate bone and the air–tissue interface not accessible with ultrasound guidance. CT is far less cumbersome than MRI for biopsy of these deep-seated lesions.

- The infrazygomatic intercondylar approach is an excellent option for CT-guided biopsy of lesions of the infratemporal fossa and retromaxillary region as well as for retropharyngeal lymphadenopathy at the nasopharynx level. As seen in Figure 18-66, the CT

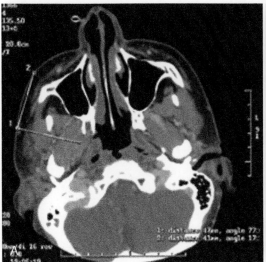
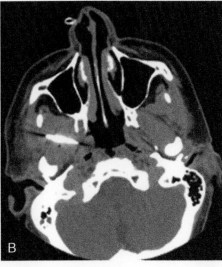

**Figure 18-66** (Courtesy of Memorial Sloan Kettering Cancer Center, New York.)

scan plan for needle localization shows the optimal site for needle entry below the zygomatic arch and in between the coronoid process and condyle of the mandible (the condylar notch) into the tumor. The outer guide needle is positioned at the edge of the lesion of interest, and a smaller needle is passed through it to sample the lesion for cytological or histological examination with a core needle, if indicated. Histopathological examination of the core biopsy in this patient revealed metastatic adenocarcinoma from a known lung primary.

## SUGGESTED READING

Ballantyne AJ. Significance of retropharyngeal nodes in cancer of the head and neck. Am J Surg 1964;108:500–4.

Hermans R, Pameijer FA, Mancuso AA, Parsons JT, Mendenhall WM. CT findings in chondroradionecrosis of the larynx. AJNR Am J Neuroradiol 1998;19(4):711–8.

McGuirt WF. Laryngeal radionecrosis versus recurrent cancer. Otolaryngol Clin North Am 1997;30(2):243–50.

Mukherji SK, Weadock WJ. Imaging of the post-treatment larynx. Eur J Radiol 2002;44(2):108–19.

Stambuk HE, Patel SG. Imaging of the parapharyngeal space. Otolaryngol Clin North Am 2008;41(1):77–101.

# 19  Pathology

## Questions

### TRUE/FALSE

1. Approximately 80% of basal cell carcinomas occur in the head and neck area. (T/F)

2. Basal cell carcinomas are never pigmented. (T/F)

3. Basal cell carcinomas can be mistaken histologically for adenoid cystic carcinoma. (T/F)

4. Basal cell carcinomas rarely metastasize. (T/F)

5. Basal cell carcinomas are associated with a good clinical outcome even when they metastasize. (T/F)

6. Melanomas are always pigmented. (T/F)

7. Histologically, melanoma tumor cells can be epithelioid or spindled. (T/F)

8. The clinical behavior of a melanoma is defined by the tumor thickness. (T/F)

9. Clark levels (microscopic extent of tumor invasion of the skin layers) are used to stage melanomas in the current American Joint Committee on Cancer (AJCC) staging system. (T/F)

10. Ulceration is not included in the staging of melanomas. (T/F)

11. The most common salivary gland neoplasm in the sinonasal region is mucoepidermoid carcinoma. (T/F)

12. Sinonasal adenocarcinoma is classified into intestinal type and nonintestinal type. (T/F)

13. The presence of in situ melanoma helps to differentiate primary mucosal melanoma in the nasal cavity from metastatic melanoma. (T/F)

14. Olfactory neuroblastoma is also called esthesioneuroblastoma. (T/F)

15. By immunohistochemical analysis, olfactory neuroblastoma is positive for S-100 (in the surrounding sustentacular cells) and negative for chromogranin and synaptophysin. (T/F)

16. Multiple endocrine neoplasia type II (MEN-II) is associated with inherited medullary carcinoma. (T/F)

17. Tumor cells in medullary carcinoma can show round, oval, plasmacytoid, and spindle cell morphology. (T/F)

18. The presence of amyloid is a characteristic feature of medullary carcinoma. (T/F)

19. Medullary carcinoma is positive for chromogranin and CEA-M immunohistochemical stains. (T/F)

20. C-cell hyperplasia is usually seen in sporadic medullary carcinoma. (T/F)

21. Papillary carcinoma is defined based on its histological nuclear features. (T/F)

22. Tall cell variant is a more aggressive histological variant than classical type papillary carcinoma. (T/F)

23. Psammoma bodies are not common in papillary carcinoma. (T/F)

24. TTF1 immunohistochemical stain can differentiate papillary carcinoma from pulmonary adenocarcinoma. (T/F)

25. The *RAS* mutation has been identified in a high proportion of papillary carcinomas. (T/F)

26. The diagnosis of keratocyst might be the first diagnosis for underlying nevoid basal cell carcinoma syndrome. (T/F)

27. Histologically, a keratocyst shows a stratified squamous epithelium. (T/F)

28. Squamous cell carcinoma has never been reported in association with a keratocyst. (T/F)

29. The recurrence rate after excision of a keratocyst is very low (<5%). (T/F)

30. The recurrence rate of a keratocyst has been correlated with the presence of odontogenic epithelium in the cyst wall. (T/F)

31. Pleomorphic adenoma is composed histologically of epithelial, mesenchymal, and stromal elements. (T/F)

32. Carcinoma ex pleomorphic adenoma is a malignant neoplasm that is associated with pleomorphic adenoma. (T/F)

33. Warthin tumor is a benign salivary gland tumor that arises in the submandibular gland. (T/F)

34. Primary squamous cell carcinoma of the parotid gland is very rare and is usually the diagnosis of exclusion in this location. (T/F)

35. Adenoid cystic carcinoma is typically a low-grade carcinoma. (T/F)

36. Adenoid cystic carcinoma is the most common malignant salivary gland neoplasm. (T/F)

37. Adenoid cystic carcinoma is composed histologically of epithelial and myoepithelial cells. (T/F)

38. Perineural spread is not common in adenoid cystic carcinoma (T/F)

39. The common histological growth patterns of adenoid cystic carcinoma are cribriform, tubular, and solid. (T/F)

40. The cribriform growth pattern of adenoid cystic carcinoma is more aggressive than the tubular and solid growth patterns. (T/F)

41. Nasopharyngeal carcinoma is classified into squamous cell carcinoma and adenocarcinoma. (T/F)

42. Nasopharyngeal carcinoma is classified into keratinizing squamous cell carcinoma, nonkeratinizing carcinoma, and basaloid squamous cell carcinoma. (T/F)

43. Nonkeratinizing squamous cell carcinoma of the nasopharynx is subclassified into undifferentiated and differentiated types. (T/F)

44. The undifferentiated type of nonkeratinizing nasopharyngeal carcinoma was previously called *lymphoepithelioma*. (T/F)

45. Approximately 85% of patients with basaloid squamous cell carcinoma of the nasopharynx have antibody to Epstein-Barr virus (EBV). (T/F)

46. Osteosarcoma can have different histological variants (e.g., chondroblastic, fibroblastic, telangiectatic, and small cell). (T/F)

47. The maxilla is the most common site of osteosarcoma. (T/F)

48. Ewing sarcoma is usually composed of large mature cells showing abundant cytoplasm. (T/F)

49. Ewing sarcoma is characterized by the t(11;22)(q24;q12) translocation, resulting in EWS-FLI fusion. (T/F)

50. *Plasmacytoma* and *myeloma* are synonymous. (T/F)

## MULTIPLE CHOICE

51. Which one of the following immunohistochemical stains is not positive in melanoma?
    A. S-100
    B. Melan A
    C. HMB45
    D. Chromogranin

52. Which of the following statements about Merkel cell carcinoma is not correct?
    A. Merkel cell carcinoma is morphologically similar to other neuroendocrine carcinomas.
    B. The differential diagnosis for Merkel cell carcinoma includes small cell carcinoma and melanoma.
    C. Merkel cell carcinoma is positive for TTF1 immunohistochemical stain.
    D. Merkel cell carcinoma is positive for CK20 immunohistochemical stain in a dotlike pattern.

53. Unfavorable prognostic indicators for ameloblastoma include all of the following except
    A. Mandibular location.
    B. Extension from the bone to the adjacent soft tissue.
    C. Nuclear pleomorphism.
    D. Tumor necrosis.
    E. Marked mitotic activities.
    F. Metastases.

54. Which of the following statements about human papillomavirus (HPV)-related squamous cell carcinoma is correct?
    A. HPV-related squamous cell carcinoma is commonly associated with nonkeratinizing basaloid morphology.
    B. p16 immunohistochemical stain can be used as a surrogate marker to identify HPV-associated oropharyngeal carcinoma.
    C. Patients are usually younger than patients with conventional squamous cell carcinoma.
    D. The tonsil is the most common location for HPV-related squamous cell carcinoma.
    E. All of the above are correct.

55. Which one of following statements is not true for thyroid cancer?
    A. Follicular carcinoma is defined histologically on the basis of capsular or vascular invasion.
    B. Follicular carcinoma lacks the nuclear features of papillary thyroid carcinoma.
    C. Hurthle cell carcinoma is composed of greater than 75% Hurthle cells.
    D. The *BRAF* mutation is the most common genetic alteration in follicular carcinoma.
    E. Colloid is usually identified in anaplastic thyroid carcinoma.

56. Which of the following histological features does not affect the prognosis in oral cavity squamous cell carcinoma?
    A. Depth of invasion
    B. Perineural invasion
    C. Lymphovascular invasion
    D. Invasive front
    E. Presence of in situ carcinoma

57. Which of the following statements regarding neurogenic tumors of the head and neck is not correct?
    A. Malignant peripheral nerve sheath tumors (MPNSTs) are positive for S-100 but not to the extent or intensity of schwannomas.

B. Paraganglioma is positive for S-100 immuno-histochemical stain in the peripheral susten-tacular cells.

C. Paraganglioma is negative for chromogranin and synaptophysin.

D. Benign and malignant paragangliomas are similar morphologically.

E. Neurofibroma is positive for S-100 immunohistochemical stain.

58. Which statement regarding soft tissue tumors of the head and neck is correct?

A. Angiosarcoma is a vascular tumor that is positive for CD31 immunohistochemical stain.

B. Sarcomatoid/spindle cell carcinoma is usually not included in the differential diagnosis of malignant soft tissue tumor.

C. Keratin markers are usually positive in soft tissue tumors.

D. Frozen section is helpful in confirming the diagnosis of low-grade liposarcoma.

E. Rhabdomyosarcoma in children is not sensitive to chemotherapy.

59. Which of the following statements is not true for mucoepidermoid carcinoma of the salivary gland?

A. Mucoepidermoid carcinoma of the salivary gland is the most common pediatric primary malignant salivary gland tumor.

B. A mucoepidermoid carcinoma of the salivary gland is histologically composed of three types of cells: epidermoid, intermediate, and mucous cells.

C. In mucoepidermoid carcinoma of the salivary gland, low-grade tumors are usually infiltrative and solid.

D. *MECT1-MAML2* fusion resulting from t(11;19) has been recently described in mucoepidermoid carcinoma.

60. From the options shown, choose the single most likely diagnosis of the tumor on the ventral tongue shown in Figure 19-1.

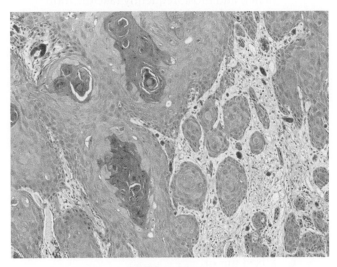

**Figure 19-1**

A. Fibrosarcoma
B. Squamous cell carcinoma
C. Adenoid cystic carcinoma
D. Melanoma
E. Pleomorphic adenoma
F. Neuroendocrine carcinoma

61. From the options shown below, choose the single most likely diagnosis of the cutaneous tumor in Figure 19-2.

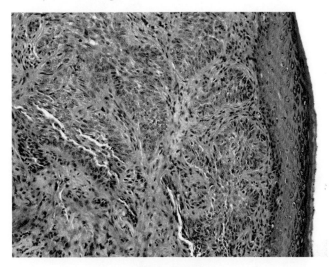

**Figure 19-2**

A. Squamous cell carcinoma
B. Basal cell carcinoma
C. Melanoma
D. Merkel cell carcinoma
E. Adenoid cystic carcinoma

62. From the options shown below, choose the single most likely diagnosis of the thyroid tumor in Figure 19-3.

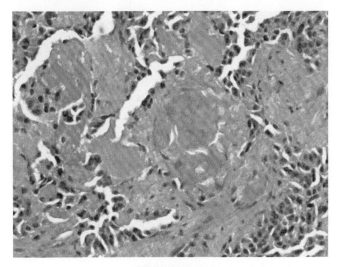

**Figure 19-3**

A. Medullary carcinoma
B. Hurthle cell carcinoma
C. Papillary thyroid carcinoma
D. Follicular carcinoma

E. Anaplastic thyroid carcinoma
F. Follicular adenoma

63. From the options below choose the single most likely diagnosis of the thyroid tumor shown in Figures 19-4 and 19-5.

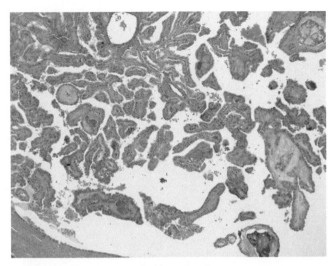

**Figure 19-4**

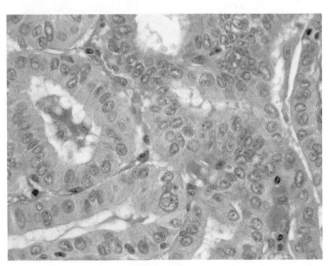

**Figure 19-5**

A. Medullary carcinoma
B. Hurthle cell carcinoma
C. Papillary thyroid carcinoma
D. Follicular carcinoma
E. Anaplastic thyroid carcinoma
F. Follicular adenoma

64. From the options below, choose the single most likely diagnosis of the parotid tumor shown in Figure 19-6.
A. Adenoid cystic carcinoma
B. Mucoepidermoid carcinoma
C. Epithelial myoepithelial carcinoma
D. Myoepithelial carcinoma
E. Acinic cell carcinoma
F. Salivary duct carcinoma

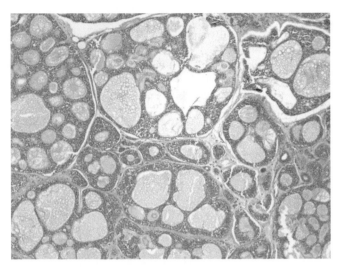

**Figure 19-6**

65. For cutaneous squamous cell carcinoma, which statement is incorrect?
A. Squamous cell carcinoma consists of nests, strands, and sheets of squamous cells that arise from the epidermis.
B. Squamous cell carcinoma can show a variable degree of keratinization.
C. Bowen disease is essentially a squamous cell carcinoma in situ that does not progress to invasive carcinoma.
D. Microscopic perineural invasion portends the same poor prognosis as invasion of major nerves.

66. Which statement is incorrect for sinonasal papillomas?
A. They are the most common benign sinonasal neoplasms.
B. They can be classified into exophytic, oncocytic, and inverted, or they can be categorized collectively as schneiderian papillomas.
C. A viral origin has been suggested for exophytic and inverted papillomas.
D. About 25% of these lesions undergo malignancy, and most frequently take the form of mucoepidermoid carcinoma.

67. Which of these statements about olfactory neuroblastoma is correct?
A. Olfactory neuroblastoma is a benign neoplasm derived from olfactory epithelium.
B. Olfactory neuroblastoma is negative for neuroendocrine markers by immunohistochemical analysis.
C. Olfactory neuroblastoma is strongly positive for cytokeratin by immunohistochemical analysis.
D. Olfactory neuroblastoma is also called *esthesioneuroblastoma*.

68. The synonym for pleomorphic adenoma is
A. Oncocytoma.
B. Ductal papilloma.
C. Mixed tumor.
D. Cystadenoma.

69. Which fusion gene has been described in adenoid cystic carcinoma?
    A. *MECT1-MAML2* fusion gene
    B. *MYB-NFIB* fusion gene
    C. *EWS-FLI* fusion gene
    D. *EWSR1-ATF1* fusion gene

70. Liposarcoma is a tumor of
    A. Vascular tissue.
    B. Fibrous tissue.
    C. Smooth muscle.
    D. Adipose tissue.

71. The term *carcinoma* is used to describe a tumor of
    A. Mesenchymal origin.
    B. Osteoid origin.
    C. Epithelial origin.
    D. Melanocytic origin.

72. The differential diagnosis of sinonasal undifferentiated carcinoma (SNUC) includes all the following except
    A. Lymphoma.
    B. Small cell carcinoma.
    C. Olfactory neuroblastoma.
    D. Well-differentiated keratinizing squamous cell carcinoma.

73. Odontogenic keratocyst is associated with
    A. Nevoid basal cell carcinoma syndrome.
    B. Neurofibromatosis.
    C. Prader-Willi syndrome.
    D. Charcot-Marie-Tooth syndrome.

74. Which of the following statements regarding lacrimal glands is true?
    A. Lacrimal gland neoplasms account for 25% of all orbital tumors.
    B. Lacrimal gland neoplasms are mostly benign.
    C. The most common benign tumor of lacrimal glands is pleomorphic adenoma.
    D. The most common malignant tumor of lacrimal glands is mucoepidermoid carcinoma.

75. Which statement about giant cell tumor of the bone is incorrect?
    A. Giant cell tumor of the bone is a malignant tumor.
    B. Giant cell tumor of the bone shows similar histological features to giant cell granuloma but with a proportionate abundance of mononuclear cells and very large giant cells.
    C. Giant cell tumor of the bone can recur and be locally destructive.
    D. Giant cell tumor of the bone metastasizes infrequently.

76. Which statement about plasmacytoma is incorrect?
    A. Plasmacytoma is a primary malignant bone tumor that is composed of plasma cells.
    B. Plasmacytoma always demonstrates kappa light chain restriction.
    C. Plasmacytoma is positive for CD138 by immunohistochemical analysis.
    D. Plasmacytoma can occur in soft tissue.

77. All of the following are variants of papillary thyroid carcinoma except
    A. Columnar cell.
    B. Tall cell.
    C. Diffuse sclerosing.
    D. Hurthle cell carcinoma.

78. Which of the following statements about papillary thyroid carcinoma is correct?
    A. *RAS* mutations are common.
    B. *RET/PTC* rearrangements are common.
    C. *BRAF* mutations are rare.
    D. None of the above are correct.

79. The histology of anaplastic thyroid carcinoma includes the following except
    A. Spindle cells.
    B. Papillary architecture.
    C. Giant pleomorphic cells.
    D. Marked increase in mitotic activity.

80. Nuclear features of papillary thyroid carcinoma include the following:
    A. Nuclear grooves.
    B. Nuclear clearing.
    C. Nuclear pseudoinclusions.
    D. All the above.

81. Medullary carcinoma is
    A. Positive for synaptophysin by immunohistochemical analysis.
    B. Positive for calcitonin by immunohistochemical analysis.
    C. Positive for monoclonal CEA by immunohistochemical analysis.
    D. All the above.

82. Which of the following statements about follicular thyroid carcinoma is correct?
    A. Follicular thyroid carcinoma shows nuclear clearing.
    B. Follicular thyroid carcinoma shows nuclear pseudoinclusions.
    C. The distinction between follicular adenoma and follicular carcinoma cannot be made on cytological or fine-needle aspiration (FNA) material in most cases.
    D. The height of follicular thyroid carcinoma cells is at least twice the width.

83. A papillary microcarcinoma measures
    A. 0.3 cm or less.
    B. 0.5 cm or less.
    C. 1 cm or less.
    D. 2 cm or less.

84. Which statement about the diffuse sclerosing variant of papillary carcinoma is incorrect?
    A. The diffuse sclerosing variant of papillary carcinoma is more common in younger patients.
    B. The diffuse sclerosing variant of papillary carcinoma shows diffuse involvement of one or two thyroid lobes by carcinoma.

C. The diffuse sclerosing variant of papillary carcinoma shows diffuse psammoma bodies and
extensive squamous metaplasia.
D. Lymph node metastases are uncommon.

85. The average weight of a normal parathyroid gland
is
A. 10 mg to 20 mg.
B. 90 mg to 100 mg.
C. 500 mg.
D. 2 g.

86. The definitive features of parathyroid carcinoma
malignancy include
A. Skeletal muscle or thyroid gland infiltration.
B. Perineural invasion.
C. Angiolymphatic invasion.
D. All the above.

87. Which statement about granular cell tumor of the
larynx is incorrect?
A. Granular cell tumor of the larynx is usually
ulcerated and soft.
B. The overlying hyperplastic squamous epithelium can be overdiagnosed as squamous cell
carcinoma.
C. Granular cell tumor of the larynx is composed
of large cells with granular cytoplasm.
D. The cells of granular cell tumor of the larynx
are positive for S-100 by immunohistochemical
analysis.

88. Which of the following statements about fibromatosis (desmoid tumor) is correct?
A. Fibromatosis is composed of moderately cellular myofibroplastic proliferation running
parallel to long vessels.
B. Fibromatosis is positive for β-catenin by immunohistochemical analysis.
C. Cytological atypia and necrosis are not common in fibromatosis.
D. All of the above are correct.

89. Angiosarcoma
A. Is a malignant vascular tumor.
B. Can have an epithelioid type.
C. Is positive for CD31 marker by immunohisto-
chemical analysis.
D. Is all of the above.

90. All of the following statements about synovial
sarcoma are correct except
A. Synovial sarcoma is a malignant vascular
tumor.
B. Histologically, synovial sarcoma can be mono-
phasic or biphasic.
C. Synovial sarcoma can occur near a nerve in the
head and neck area.
D. t(x;18) or its variants have been found in more
than 90% of synovial sarcomas.

91. Which of the following statements about Hodgkin
lymphoma is correct?
A. Hodgkin lymphoma is characterized by Reed-
Sternberg cells.

B. Hodgkin lymphoma has four histological types:
nodular sclerosis, mixed cellularity, lympho-
cytes depleted, and lymphocyte rich.
C. About 40% of Hodgkin lymphoma cases are
associated with EBV.
D. All of the above are correct.

92. Which statement about non-Hodgkin lymphoma
is incorrect?
A. Non-Hodgkin lymphoma is characterized by
Reed-Sternberg cells.
B. Diffuse large B-cell lymphoma is the most com-
mon non-Hodgkin lymphoma.
C. Diffuse large B-cell lymphoma is positive for
CD20 by immunohistochemical analysis.
D. Follicular lymphoma is the second most com-
mon non-Hodgkin lymphoma.

93. Which of the following statements about small cell
carcinoma of the head and neck is correct?
A. Small cell carcinoma of the head and neck is
similar to small cell carcinoma of the lung.
B. Small cell carcinoma of the head and neck
is negative for synaptophysin immunohistochemical stain.
C. Small cell carcinoma of the head and neck is always
negative for TTF1 immunohistochemical stain.
D. Small cell carcinoma of the head and neck is less
aggressive than small cell carcinoma of the lung.

94. Which of the following statements about mucoceles is correct?
A. Mucoceles are the least common cystic lesion of
the salivary glands.
B. Mucoceles are called *ranulae* in the base of the
tongue.
C. Microscopically, mucoceles show cysts with ill-
defined pools of mucin and inflammation.
D. All of the above are correct.

95. The most common location for polymorphous low-
grade adenocarcinoma of the salivary gland is the
A. Parotid.
B. Submandibular gland.
C. Palate.
D. Base of the tongue.

96. Which statement about acinic cell carcinoma is
incorrect?
A. The parotid is the most common location for
acinic cell carcinoma.
B. Acinic cell carcinoma shows a large range of cell
types and architectural patterns.
C. Acinic cell carcinoma cells often contain zymogen granules.
D. Acinic cell carcinoma is never high grade.

97. Salivary duct carcinoma is
A. Usually positive for estrogen receptors by im-
munohistochemical analysis.
B. Usually positive for androgen receptors by im-
munohistochemical analysis.
C. Usually positive for progesterone receptors by
immunohistochemical analysis.
D. All of the above.

98. Myoepithelial carcinoma of the salivary gland is
    A. Almost exclusively composed of myoepithelial cells.
    B. The most common malignant salivary gland tumor in the minor salivary glands.
    C. Always low grade.
    D. All of the above.

99. Which statement about oncocytoma of the salivary gland is incorrect?
    A. Oncocytoma of the salivary gland is a benign tumor.
    B. Oncocytoma of the salivary gland is composed predominately of oncocytes.
    C. The most common location for oncocytoma of the salivary gland is the submandibular gland.
    D. The differential diagnosis for oncocytoma of the salivary gland includes other salivary gland tumors with oncocytic features.

100. High-risk HPV types include
    A. HPV 16 and 11.
    B. HPV 11.
    C. HPV 18 and 16.
    D. All of the above.

## Answers

| | | |
|---|---|---|
| 1. T | 25. F | 49. T |
| 2. F | 26. T | 50. T |
| 3. T | 27. T | 51. D |
| 4. T | 28. F | 52. C |
| 5. F | 29. F | 53. A |
| 6. F | 30. T | 54. E |
| 7. T | 31. T | 55. E |
| 8. T | 32. T | 56. E |
| 9. F | 33. F | 57. C |
| 10. F | 34. T | 58. A |
| 11. F | 35. F | 59. C |
| 12. T | 36. F | 60. B |
| 13. T | 37. T | 61. B |
| 14. T | 38. F | 62. A |
| 15. F | 39. T | 63. C |
| 16. T | 40. F | 64. A |
| 17. T | 41. F | 65. C |
| 18. T | 42. T | 66. D |
| 19. T | 43. T | 67. D |
| 20. F | 44. T | 68. C |
| 21. T | 45. F | 69. B |
| 22. T | 46. T | 70. D |
| 23. F | 47. F | 71. C |
| 24. F | 48. F | 72. D |

| | | |
|---|---|---|
| 73. A | 83. C | 93. A |
| 74. C | 84. D | 94. C |
| 75. A | 85. B | 95. C |
| 76. B | 86. D | 96. D |
| 77. D | 87. A | 97. B |
| 78. B | 88. D | 98. A |
| 79. B | 89. D | 99. C |
| 80. D | 90. A | 100. C |
| 81. D | 91. D | |
| 82. C | 92. A | |

## Core Knowledge

- Basal cell carcinoma occurs in the head and neck region in approximately 80% of cases. The tumor rarely metastasizes unless it is a large tumor, but when metastases occur, basal cell carcinoma is associated with a poor clinical outcome. Histologically, basal cell carcinoma is composed of lobules of basaloid cells showing scant cytoplasm and characteristic outer palisading of the cells. The tumor can have multiple histological patterns, including an adenoid pattern, which can be mistaken for adenoid cystic carcinoma. Basal cell carcinoma can be pigmented, which makes melanoma part of the differential diagnosis.

- Melanoma may or may not be pigmented. Histologically, this tumor is usually composed of round to oval cells showing prominent nucleoli and nuclear pleomorphism. The tumor cells can be spindlelike or epithelioid. By immunohistochemical analysis, melanoma is positive for S-100, melan A, HMB45, and vimentin and is negative for keratin markers. This helps to differentiate melanoma from other malignant tumors. The clinical behavior of melanoma is typically defined by its depth of invasion, which is assessed microscopically either by direct measurement of the tumor thickness (Breslow thickness) or by Clark levels (the extent of invasion of the skin layers). Factors that are included in the current American Joint Committee on Cancer (AJCC) staging of melanoma are ulceration, nodal metastasis, distant metastasis, and Breslow thickness (except for T1 stage).

- Merkel cell carcinoma is a malignant neuroendocrine neoplasm of the skin. The tumor shows some similar morphological features to other malignant neuroendocrine tumors, and it is composed of small, round blue cells showing scant cytoplasm and dark granular chromatin. By immunohistochemical analysis, this tumor is positive for neuroendocrine markers (chromogranin and synaptophysin) and CK20 with a dotlike pattern. The differential diagnosis includes small cell carcinoma, melanoma, lymphoma, and other tumors with small, round blue cell morphology.

- Squamous cell carcinoma is the most common malignant sinonasal neoplasm, accounting for more than 80% of cases. Adenoid cystic carcinoma is the most common salivary gland–type tumor in the nasal/sinonasal region. Other tumors in the nasal/paranasal region include olfactory neuroblastoma, sinonasal undifferentiated carcinoma (SNUC), sinonasal adenocarcinoma, melanoma, lymphoma, and sarcoma. Olfactory neuroblastoma is also called esthesioneuroblastoma and is characterized by submucosal lobules of nests of tumor cells separated by fibrovascular stroma. By immunohistochemical analysis, the tumor is positive for chromogranin and synaptophysin and is usually negative for keratin. S-100 immunohistochemical stain is typically positive in the sustentacular cells surrounding the tumor lobules. Sinonasal adenocarcinoma is classified into intestinal type and nonintestinal type, which can be further divided into low-grade and high-grade subtypes.

- In 2005 nasopharyngeal carcinoma was classified by the World Health Organization (WHO) into keratinizing squamous cell carcinoma, nonkeratinizing nasopharyngeal carcinoma, which is subdivided into undifferentiated and differentiated subtypes, and basaloid squamous cell carcinoma. The nonkeratinizing nasopharyngeal carcinoma, undifferentiated subtype, often features a conspicuous lymphoid infiltrate and was previously called *lymphoepithelioma* or *lymphoepithelial carcinoma*. The undifferentiated nonkeratinizing nasopharyngeal carcinoma subtype is associated with antibodies to Epstein-Barr virus (EBV) and serum immunoglobulin A anti-EBV in 85% of cases. EBV can be detected by immunohistochemical analysis and by in situ hybridization.

- Most squamous lesions in the oral cavity have a variety of degree of histological progression from dysplasia to in situ carcinoma to invasive carcinoma. Squamous cell carcinomas range in histologic differentiation from well-differentiated to poorly or undifferentiated carcinomas. The most important histological feature of oral squamous cell carcinoma that affects treatment and, eventually, tumor prognosis is tumor depth of invasion. Other histological features that can affect prognosis include degree of differentiation, endophytic versus exophytic growth, lymphovascular invasion, perineural invasion, and invasive front.

- Approximately 80% of oropharyngeal squamous cell carcinomas are associated with high-risk human papillomavirus (HPV), most of which is HPV 16. The tonsil is the most common location of these tumors. Histologically, these tumors are usually nonkeratinizing, showing commonly basaloid morphology. Therefore, these tumors used to be classified as basaloid squamous cell carcinoma. HPV status can be tested by p16 immunohistochemical stain and by in situ hybridization. p16 immunohistochemical stain can be used as a surrogate marker to identify HPV-associated oropharyngeal carcinoma. These tumors are seen in the younger population, two to three decades earlier than usual squamous cell carcinoma of the head and neck. It is more common in males. The patients usually do not have a history of heavy alcohol consumption or smoking.

- Papillary thyroid carcinoma is the most common histological type of thyroid cancer. Papillary thyroid carcinoma is defined by its characteristic nuclear features, which include nuclear clearing, irregularity of nuclear contour, nuclear overlapping, nuclear grooves, and pseudoinclusions. Psammoma bodies, which are rounded, concentrically laminated calcifications, are commonly seen in papillary carcinoma. The classic type shows dominant complex and branching papillary architecture. Multiple histological variants can be seen including the follicular variant, tall cell variant, columnar cell variant, oncocytic variant, and others. The follicular variant is mostly encapsulated, showing a follicular growth pattern and the characteristic nuclear features of papillary carcinoma. The tall cell variant is composed predominantly of cells whose heights are two to three times their widths. The tall cell variant is more aggressive than the classic type papillary carcinoma. By immunohistochemical analysis, papillary carcinoma is typically positive for thyroglobulin, TTF1, and PAX8. The point of mutation of the *BRAF* gene has been identified in a large portion of papillary thyroid carcinomas.

- Follicular carcinoma is an invasive neoplasm of follicular cells that lacks histologically the typical nuclear features of papillary carcinoma. Follicular carcinoma is defined histologically on the basis of capsular or vascular invasion. Classically, follicular carcinoma has been divided according to its degree of capsular/vascular invasion into minimally invasive and widely invasive. Minimally invasive follicular carcinomas have limited focal capsular/vascular invasion (less than four foci), whereas widely invasive carcinomas have widespread infiltration/invasion. Mutations of *RAS* genes are found in 20% to 50% of follicular carcinomas. Hurthle cell (oncocytic) carcinoma is composed predominantly of Hurthle cells (>75% of tumor cells). The tumor cells demonstrate abundant eosinophilic cytoplasm and prominent nucleoli. Anaplastic (undifferentiated) carcinoma is a highly malignant tumor that is histologically undifferentiated, commonly exhibiting spindle and giant cell, sarcomatoid, and pleomorphic morphology. Mitotic activities are typically high in anaplastic carcinoma. Colloid is usually absent in anaplastic carcinoma. By immunohistochemical analysis, these tumors are usually positive for keratin markers and negative for thyroglobulin. TTF1 can be focally positive. PAX8 stain is positive in 50% of anaplastic thyroid carcinomas. The differential diagnosis of anaplastic thyroid carcinoma includes sarcoma, melanoma, lymphoma, and metastatic carcinoma.

- Medullary thyroid carcinoma is a malignant C-cell–derived tumor. Up to 25% of these tumors are heritable, caused by gain-of-function germline mutations of the *RET* gene. This inherited tumor has a strong association with multiple endocrine neoplasia type II (MEN-II). Histologically, the tumor is quite variable, exhibiting solid, nested, organoid, and trabecular patterns. The tumor cells are round to oval and spindled to plasmacytoid. Amyloid deposition is found in 70% to 80% of cases. The tumor stains positive for chromogranin, synaptophysin, calcitonin, TTF1, and CEA-M but negative for thyroglobulin. C-cell hyperplasia is seen in association with patients with *RET* germline mutations.

- Pleomorphic adenoma (mixed tumor) is the most common salivary gland neoplasm and is characterized histologically by a mixture of epithelial, mesenchymal, and stromal elements. Carcinoma ex pleomorphic adenoma is a malignant neoplasm that is associated with pleomorphic adenoma. Warthin tumor is a benign salivary gland tumor that arises almost exclusively in the parotid gland. This tumor usually shows cystic and papillary architecture and is composed of a bilayered epithelium: inner columnar oncocytic cells surrounded by small basal cells. Primary squamous cell carcinoma of the parotid gland is very rare, and it is essential to exclude the possibility of metastatic carcinoma. Salivary duct carcinoma is typically a high-grade carcinoma that is positive for androgen receptors by immunohistochemical analysis.

- Adenoid cystic carcinoma is a basaloid tumor consisting of epithelial and myoepithelial cells. Perineural spread is a common feature of this tumor. The tumor has three common histologic growth patterns: cribriform, tubular, and solid. The solid growth pattern is more aggressive than the cribriform and tubular patterns. Some studies have graded adenoid cystic carcinoma into low, intermediate, and high grade, and high-grade tumors have shown more than 30% solid growth pattern.

- Mucoepidermoid carcinoma is the most common primary malignant salivary gland tumor in both children and adults. The tumor is histologically composed of three types of cells: epidermoid, intermediate, and mucous cells. The tumor is usually graded into low, intermediate, and high grades. Mucoepidermoid carcinoma is usually multicystic with a solid component; sometimes the latter predominates (especially in intermediate- and high-grade tumors). *MECT1-MAML2* fusion resulting from t(11,19) has been recently described in mucoepidermoid carcinoma.

- Studies have shown the association of nevoid basal cell carcinoma syndrome (NBCCS) or *PTCH* gene in the etiology of odontogenic keratocyst. Histologically, the lesion shows a stratified squamous epithelium with a prominent palisading basal layer and surface parakeratinization. This lesion is locally aggressive and has a reported recurrence rate of 30%. The recurrence rate has been correlated with the presence of odontogenic epithelium in the cyst wall. Squamous cell carcinoma has been reported in association with keratocyst, but it is rare.

- Ameloblastoma is a slowly growing odontogenic tumor. Histologically, the tumor is composed of nests and islands of odontogenic epithelium showing peripheral palisading and a loosely arranged center. The tumor is usually solid or multicystic, but a unicystic type can be seen and is thought to be a less aggressive type. Unfavorable prognostic indicators for ameloblastoma include maxillary location, old age, extension from the bone to the adjacent soft tissue, nuclear pleomorphism, tumor necrosis, marked mitotic activities, and lymph node and distant metastases.

- Osteosarcoma is a malignant tumor of the bone and soft tissue that recapitulates the phenotype of osteoblasts and synthesizes bone. Osteosarcoma can have different histological variants (e.g., chondroblastic, fibroblastic, telangiectatic, and small cell). The mandible is the most common site of osteosarcoma. Ewing sarcoma or primitive neuroectodermal tumor (PNET) is a malignant tumor of the bone and soft tissue with small, round blue cell morphology. The tumor is usually composed of small primitive immature cells showing scant cytoplasm. It expresses CD99 immunostaining in a membranous fashion. Ewing sarcoma is characterized by t(11;22) (q24;q12) translocation, resulting in EWS-FLI fusion.

- Schwannoma is an encapsulated benign tumor of peripheral nerves. It is composed of spindle Schwann cells with alternating areas of compact elongated cells with occasional nuclear palisading (Antoni A) and less cellular, loosely textured areas (Antoni B). Schwannoma strongly expresses S-100 on immunohistochemical analysis. Malignant peripheral nerve sheath tumors (MPNSTs) are positive for S-100 but not to the extent or intensity of schwannoma.

- Paraganglioma is a usually benign neuroendocrine tumor. The tumor is composed of two types of cells—chief and sustentacular—arranged in a characteristic nested pattern. On immunohistochemical analysis, paraganglioma is positive for S-100 (in the peripheral sustentacular cells), chromogranin, and synaptophysin and negative for keratin. Benign and malignant paragangliomas are similar morphologically. A tumor is considered malignant only if regional or distant metastasis is present.

- Sarcomatoid/spindle cell carcinoma, melanoma, and lymphoma are usually included in the differential diagnosis of malignant soft tissue tumors. Soft tissue tumors are usually negative for keratin markers. Angiosarcoma is a malignant vascular tumor of the bone and soft tissue that is positive for CD31 immunohistochemical stain. Rhabdomyosarcoma is a malignant soft tissue tumor that recapitulates the features of skeletal muscle.

## SUGGESTED READING

Barnes EL, Eveson JW, Reichart P, Sidransky D, editors. World Health Organization classification of tumours. Pathology and genetics of head and neck tumours. Lyon, France: IARC Press; 2005.

El-Naggar AK, Westra WH. p16 expression as a surrogate marker for HPV-related oropharyngeal carcinoma: a guide for interpretative relevance and consistency. Head Neck 2012;34(4):459–61.

Ghossein R. Update to the College of American Pathologists reporting on thyroid carcinomas. Head Neck Pathol 2009;3(1):86–93.

Ghossein R. Problems and controversies in the histopathology of thyroid carcinomas of follicular cell origin. Arch Pathol Lab Med 2009;133(5):683–91.

Ghossein R. Encapsulated malignant follicular cell-derived thyroid tumors. Endocr Pathol 2010;21(4):212–8.

Ghossein R, Livolsi VA. Papillary thyroid carcinoma tall cell variant. Thyroid 2008;18(11):1179–81.

Griffith C, Seethala R, Chiosea SI. Mammary analogue secretory carcinoma: a new twist to the diagnostic dilemma of zymogen granule poor acinic cell carcinoma. Virchows Arch 2011;459(1):117–8.

Hunt JL. An update on molecular diagnostics of squamous and salivary gland tumors of the head and neck. Arch Pathol Lab Med 2011;135(5):602–9.

Nakayama T, Miyabe S, Okabe M, Sakuma H, Ijichi K, Hasegawa Y, et al. Clinicopathological significance of the CRTC3-MAML2 fusion transcript in mucoepidermoid carcinoma. Mod Pathol 2009;22:1575–81.

Ricarte-Filho J, Ganly I, Rivera M, Katabi N, Fu W, Shaha A, et al. Papillary thyroid carcinomas with cervical lymph node metastases can be stratified into clinically relevant prognostic categories using oncogenic BRAF, the number of nodal metastases, and extra-nodal extension. Thyroid 2012;22(6):575–84.

Seethala RR. An update on grading of salivary gland carcinomas. Head Neck Pathol 2009;3(1):69–77.

Seethala RR, Dacic S, Cieply K, Kelly LM, Nikiforova MN. A reappraisal of the MECT1/MAML2 translocation in salivary mucoepidermoid carcinomas. Am J Surg Pathol 2010;34:1106–21.

Seethala RR, Hunt JL, Baloch ZW, Livolsi VA, Leon Barnes E. Adenoid cystic carcinoma with high-grade transformation: a report of 11 cases and a review of the literature. Am J Surg Pathol 2007;31(11):1683–94.

Skálová A, Vanecek T, Sima R, Laco J, Weinreb I, Perez-Ordonez B, et al. Mammary analogue secretory carcinoma of salivary glands, containing the ETV6-NTRK3 fusion gene: a hitherto undescribed salivary gland tumor entity. Am J Surg Pathol 2010;34(5):599–608.

Westra WH. The changing face of head and neck cancer in the 21st century: the impact of HPV on the epidemiology and pathology of oral cancer. Head Neck Pathol 2009;3(1):78–81.

Westra WH. The morphologic profile of HPV-related head and neck squamous carcinoma: implications for diagnosis, prognosis, and clinical management. Value Health 2012;15(3):562–7.

# 20 Molecular Oncology

## Questions

### TRUE/FALSE

1. In patients with Fanconi anemia, head and neck squamous cell carcinoma (HNSCC) development is increased 700-fold and occurs predominantly in the oropharynx. (T/F)

2. Human papillomavirus (HPV) type 16 in SCC is more often found in intracellular episomes than integrated in the host genome. (T/F)

3. The association between HPV-positive oropharyngeal SCC development and sexual history is stronger for number of prior orogenital sexual partners than for the number of genitogenital sexual partners. (T/F)

4. Tobacco and alcohol exposure increases the likelihood of somatic *p53* mutations and loss of heterozygosity (LOH) events compared with alcohol exposure alone in patients with HNSCC. (T/F)

5. Nonsynonymous point mutations are more common than single nucleotide polymorphisms (SNPs) in HNSCC; however, the clinical relevance of SNPs has been established more firmly. (T/F)

6. Genomic microsatellite variations have successfully been exploited to shed light on the molecular tumor-progression model of HNSCC. (T/F)

7. The transcriptional progression model of HNSCC suggests that the majority of gene expression changes that characterize HNSCC occur early in its development. (T/F)

8. p53 pathway abrogation is present in virtually all HNSCCs and most commonly manifests as *p53* mutations, *human double minute-2 (HDM2)* deletions, *P14ARF* amplifications, or HPV infection. (T/F)

9. Retinoblastoma (Rb) pathway abrogation is detectable in virtually all HNSCCs and is most often due to *Rb* mutations, *p16* mutations, and *cyclin D1* amplifications or HPV integration. (T/F)

10. Phosphoinositide 3-kinase (PI3K) pathway activation in HNSCC is common and caused by amplifications of *PIK3CA*, amplification of *AKT*, or inactivation of *PTEN* by somatic mutation, homozygous deletion, or methylation. (T/F)

11. Activation of the transforming growth factor (TGF)-beta pathway results in tumor progression of HNSCC. (T/F)

12. Genetic point mutations in *epidermal growth factor receptor (EGFR)* are common in adenocarcinomas of the lung but uncommon in HNSCC. (T/F)

13. Notch1 is a transmembrane receptor, mutations of which are common in HNSCC. (T/F)

14. Mitochondrial mutations can be found in 50% of HNSCCs and contribute to the Warburg effect and apoptosis evasion. (T/F)

15. Assessment of margins for *p53* mutations is superior to classical histopathological analysis. (T/F)

16. Microarray-based analyses have convincingly established that the HNSCC primary tumor gene expression profile is a strong predictor of the presence or absence of lymph node metastases. (T/F)

17. Treatment sequelae of cetuximab include skin rashes and predict a worse response in SCC. (T/F)

18. CD44 is a stem cell marker in HNSCC. (T/F)

19. Cetuximab binds to the intracellular portion of EGFR, whereas gefitinib binds to the extracellular portion of the receptor. (T/F)

20. Resistance of HNSCC to EGFR inhibitors may be mediated through the presence of PI3K abnormalities. (T/F)

21. The following syndromes (with causative genes in parentheses) feature increased rates of thyroid neoplasia: Gardner *(APC)*, Cowden *(PTEN)*, Carney complex *(PRKAR1A)*, and Werner *(RECQL2)*. (T/F)

22. The most common recurrent alterations that have been identified in papillary thyroid carcinoma (PTC) involve *RET, BRAF,* and *NTRK1. RET* and *BRAF* alterations are typically not observed together in individual thyroid carcinomas for reasons of functional redundancy. (T/F)

23. The genomic and transcriptional profiles of radiation-induced PTC are clearly different from that of non–radiation-associated PTC when corrected for age, as evidenced by higher rates of DNA copy number abnormalities, point mutations, and transcriptional abnormalities in radiation-induced PTC. (T/F)

24. In PTC, *RET* is activated by genetic point mutations, whereas in medullary thyroid carcinomas (MTCs), *RET* is activated by fusion to an activating sequence (balanced rearrangement). (T/F)

25. *RET* activation is an early event in PTC because it can be identified in high frequency in microscopic PTC. (T/F)

26. In thyroid cancer, *RET* can be rearranged with several different fusion partners, but only a single fusion partner has been associated with *NTRK1*. (T/F)

27. In PTC, *BRAF* is typically activated by point mutations in a single codon, but activation has also been associated with balanced rearrangement. (T/F)

28. The molecular profile of encapsulated follicular variant papillary carcinomas is reminiscent of follicular adenomas/carcinomas (PPAR-gamma, RAS, PI3K involvement) rather than classic papillary carcinomas (BRAF, RET, NTRK1 involvement), which supports reclassification of these lesions as follicular thyroid tumors. (T/F)

29. PAX8 is involved in thyroid embryogenesis, its knockout in animal models results in thyroid hyperplasia, and its expression distinguishes anaplastic thyroid carcinomas from lymphomas and sarcomas. (T/F)

30. The chimeric PAX8–PPAR-gamma protein exerts a dominant negative effect on normal PPAR-gamma gene expression, which has a tumor suppressive effect when overexpressed in normal cells. (T/F)

31. *RAS* mutation in follicular thyroid carcinogenesis is an early event, commonly identifiable in follicular adenomas. (T/F)

32. *BRAF* mutation is a poor prognostic factor in thyroid cancer, and its presence can be detected preoperatively by analysis of fine-needle aspiration cytology specimens. (T/F)

33. Thyroid tumor progression is marked by increasing mitosis, necrosis, fluorodeoxyglucose positron emission tomography (FDG-PET) avidity, p53 accumulation, beta-catenin expression, *BRAF* mutation, and chromosomal complexity, and decreasing radioactive iodine (RAI) avidity, thyroglobulin detectability, and sodium–iodide symporter expression. (T/F)

34. In general, mutations in the extracellular *RET* domain are associated with more aggressive behavior than intracellular mutations in MTC. (T/F)

35. Both germline and sporadic mutations of RET are very common in MTC. (T/F)

36. Sarcomas are typically differentiated into three groups based on their genomic profile: one that features specific balanced rearrangements, one that features point mutations, and one that features

multiple, gross, imbalanced chromosomal alterations and high-level chromosomal amplifications. (T/F)

37. Well-differentiated/dedifferentiated liposarcomas are often characterized by 12q13-15 amplification, which results in overexpression of the Rb and p53 pathway members *CDK4* and *MDM2*. (T/F)

38. Angiosarcomas are often characterized by vascular-specific tyrosine kinase alterations, which provide a basis for the successful antiangiogenic therapy with bevacizumab and taxanes observed in angiosarcomas. (T/F)

39. The study of Li-Fraumeni and Rothmund-Thomson syndromes has implicated dysfunction of DNA repair genes in osteosarcoma development. (T/F)

40. Most translocation events in sarcomas affect the clinical outcome. (T/F)

41. Targeted therapy has been more successful in sarcomas featuring translocations involving transcription factor genes than sarcomas harboring translocations involving membranous receptor genes. (T/F)

42. Taxane-based chemotherapy responses are more common in rhabdomyosarcomas than in angiosarcomas. (T/F)

43. The chromosomal translocation t(11;19)(q21;p13) creates the chimeric *MEC1–MAML2* gene and is associated with high-grade mucoepidermoid carcinoma of salivary gland origin. (T/F)

44. The chromosomal translocation t(6;9) fuses the genes *NFIB* and *MYB* and is associated with 50% of adenoid cystic carcinomas of salivary gland origin. (T/F)

45. Imatinib induces significant in vitro and in vivo response rates in *c-KIT* mutated adenoid cystic carcinomas of salivary gland origin. (T/F)

46. A significant subset of Merkel cell carcinomas is associated with genetic integration of a newly identified papilloma virus. (T/F)

47. Vismodegib inhibits the Hedgehog pathway in basal cell carcinomas of the skin and results in clinical regression in familial and sporadic basal cell carcinomas. (T/F)

48. The progression-free survival rate of patients with advanced melanoma is significantly increased by dabrafenib treatment compared with reference treatment with dacarbazine. (T/F)

49. Cytotoxic T-lymphocyte antigen 4 (CTLA4) is an inhibitor of T-cell activation pathways, and inhibitors of CTLA4 increase overall and progression-free survival rates in melanoma. (T/F)

50. Secondary skin SCCs in melanoma patients treated with mitogen-activated protein kinase (MAPK) pathway inhibitors are more often seen with BRAF inhibitors than with MEK inhibitors. (T/F)

## MULTIPLE CHOICE

51. Which statements about general molecular processes involved in head and neck cancer development and progression are true?
    i. Successful establishment of sustained proliferative signaling is dependent on both mitogenic changes to malignant tumor cells and paracrine stimulation by nonmalignant cells in the tumor microenvironment.
    ii. Decreased expression of telomerase propagates replicative immortality. Telomeres are located near the centromere of human chromosomes, and their length is associated with the cellular replication span.
    iii. Tumor inflammation counteracts malignant progression.
    iv. Epithelial-to-mesenchymal transition (EMT) is commonly seen in cells near the invasive tumor border, contributes to metastasis, and produces tumor stem cells.
    v. Angiogenesis is propagated by upregulation of vascular endothelial growth factor (VEGF) and thrombospondin-1.
    vi. The molecular composition of cancer cells is typically characterized by more than 12,000 individual molecular alterations, and the majority of these genetic alterations are required for cancer development.
    A. i, ii
    B. iii, iv, v, vi
    C. i, ii, iii, iv
    D. i, iv
    E. All of the above

52. Which of the following statements are true about apoptosis in head and neck cancer?
    i. Caspases are involved in the induction of apoptosis and are often inactivated in head and neck cancers.
    ii. Tumor necrosis and autophagy are two examples of cell death mechanisms triggered by apoptosis.
    iii. Cellular senescence is a reversible, viable, nonproliferative state and precedes apoptosis.
    iv. Apoptosis is commonly triggered by increased proliferative signaling or excessive DNA damage.
    v. *HDM2* upregulation and *P14ARF* deletion are common events that facilitate apoptosis evasion in head and neck cancers.
    A. i, iv, v
    B. i, iv, iii
    C. ii, iii, iv
    D. iii, iv, v
    E. None of the above

53. Which of the statements about genomic screening of head and neck cancer are true?
    i. Balanced and unbalanced chromosomal alterations are detectable by comparative genomic hybridization.
    ii. The vast majority of genomic "mutations" detected by second generation "exome" sequencing are SNPs and nonsynonymous sequence variations.
    iii. Balanced translocations can be detected with conventional cytogenetic karyotyping, second generation "exome" sequencing, and Southern blot analysis.
    iv. LOH events may result from chromosomal gain, genomic amplification, genomic deletion, mitotic recombination, break-induced replication, or gene conversion.
    v. Spectral karyotyping is based on comparative analysis of differentially labeled test and reference DNA.
    vi. Head and neck cancers with established etiological risk factors (e.g., HNSCC and melanoma) have a greater number of genetic abnormalities than head and neck cancers without established etiological risk factors (e.g., adenoid cystic carcinomas and MTCs)
    A. iii, iv, v
    B. ii, iii, iv, vi
    C. i, iv, vi
    D. i, ii, iii
    E. i, iv, v, vi

54. Which of the following hereditary head and neck cancer syndromes are described accurately?
    i. Familial atypical multiple mole melanoma (FAMMM) syndrome: *CDKN2A* mutations, melanoma, pancreatic cancer, and HNSCC
    ii. Dyskeratosis congenita: telomere dysfunction, bone marrow failure, skin pigmentation, nail dystrophy, and thyroid cancer
    iii. Gardner syndrome: *APC* mutations, adenomatous polyps of the gastrointestinal tract, desmoid tumors, osteomas, epidermoid cysts, lipomas, dental abnormalities, and follicular variant papillary thyroid carcinomas
    iv. Multiple endocrine neoplasia type IIA (MEN-IIA): *RET* codon 634 mutations, MTC, pheochromocytoma, and mucosal (ganglio)neuromas.
    v. Fanconi anemia: *BRCA2* mutation, short stature, thumb abnormality, skin pigmentation, endocrine abnormalities, bone marrow failure, acute myeloid leukemia, HNSCC, cisplatin and radiation hypersensitivity.
    A. iii, iv, v
    B. ii, iii, iv
    C. i, iii, iv
    D. ii, iv
    E. i, v

55. Which of the statements about oncogenes and tumor suppressor genes in head and neck cancer are true?
    i. In HNSCC, inactivation of the *CDKN2A* gene often follows the classic model described by Knudson in 1971.
    ii. Promotor hypermethylation usually activates protooncogenes, whereas

hypomethylation has been shown to activate tumor suppressor genes.

iii. Genetic point mutations have been associated with activation of oncogenes and inactivation of tumor suppressor genes.

iv. The concept of oncogene addiction is applicable to the role of the chromosomal locus 3q26.3 in HNSCC, a locus with prognostic significance in HNSCC.

v. Molecular alterations that affect specific oncogenes and tumor suppressor genes functioning in a single biochemical pathway commonly occur in a mutually exclusive fashion in head and neck cancer.

A. i, iii, iv, v
B. ii, iv, v
C. i, ii, iii, iv
D. ii, iii
E. i, iii

56. Which of the following statements accurately describe the role of caretaker genes in head and neck cancer?

i. When mutated, caretaker genes typically have a direct propagative effect in head and neck carcinogenesis.

ii. HPV-induced carcinogenesis may be accelerated in the presence of p53 polymorphisms or Fanconi gene alterations.

iii. Homologous recombination is an example of single-stranded DNA repair that helps prevent tobacco-induced carcinogenesis in the upper aerodigestive tract.

iv. An increased incidence of thyroid cancer in patients with Werner syndrome suggests a role for defective DNA repair in thyroid oncogenesis.

v. Xeroderma pigmentosum is a prototypic disease implicating nucleotide excision DNA repair abnormalities in skin carcinogenesis.

A. iii, iv
B. i, ii, v
C. ii, iv, v
D. i, ii, iii
E. All of the above

57. Which of the statements about HPV are true?

i. HNSCC with deletions of the chromosomal locus 9p often contain evidence of HPV E7.

ii. In unknown primary SCC metastasis to the parotid tail region, CDKN2A overexpression is a reliable indicator of an HPV-positive oropharyngeal SCC primary tumor.

iii. The viral E6 protein is associated with the presence of p53 mutations.

iv. Serological evidence for HPV exposure is detectable in approximately 20% of individuals in the general population.

v. HPV type 16 DNA is detectable in approximately 5% of oral rinse specimens of sexually active individuals in the general population.

A. i, iii
B. i, iv, v
C. v
D. ii, iii, iv
E. iii

58. Which of the following statements about head and neck cancer development and progression are true?

i. Histological progression is paralleled by an increasing number of unbalanced chromosomal alterations in sarcomas and follicular cell–derived thyroid carcinomas.

ii. Genetic deletions of the chromosomal loci 9p21 and 3p can be detected in a minority of benign squamous hyperplasias and have a significantly higher likelihood of evolving into HNSCC (33%) than those without (6%).

iii. Accumulation of p53 and beta-catenin are late events in the progression of follicular cell–derived thyroid carcinoma.

iv. Chimeric PAX8–PPAR-gamma formation is an early event in follicular thyroid carcinoma and PTC.

v. The concept of oncogene addiction applies to amplification of the 11q13 locus in HNSCC.

A. i, iii
B. ii, iii, iv
C. i, iv
D. iii, iv, v
E. All of the above

59. Which of the following molecular alterations have independent prognostic utility in head and neck cancer?

i. p53 mutation in HNSCC
ii. RET rearrangement in PTC
iii. c-KIT mutation in adenoid cystic carcinoma
iv. t(11;19)(q21;p13) in mucoepidermoid carcinomas
v. PAX8–PPAR-gamma formation in follicular thyroid carcinoma

A. iii, iv, v
B. i
C. ii, iii
D. ii, v
E. iii, iv

60. Which of the following targeted treatment options result in a proven, statistically significant and clinically relevant survival benefit for patients with head and neck cancer?

i. Vismodegib in squamous cell skin cancer
ii. Ipilimumab in melanoma
iii. Trametinib in melanoma
iv. Vandetanib in medullary thyroid carcinoma
v. Imatinib in adenoid cystic carcinoma

A. i, ii, iii
B. v
C. iv
D. ii, iii
E. iii, iv

61. Oncogenic HPV proteins include
    A. E5 and E6.
    B. E6 and E7.
    C. E7 and E8.
    D. E8 and E9.

62. An oncogenic HPV virus is
    A. HPV type 6.
    B. HPV type 11.
    C. HPV type 35.
    D. HPV type 13.

63. A direct inhibitory effect of HPV has been corroborated for
    A. p53.
    B. Notch1.
    C. P16.
    D. FAT1.

64. The HPV-induced oropharyngeal cancer rate is increased in patients with
    A. *p53* mutations.
    B. Human immunodeficiency virus (HIV) negativity.
    C. HPV detected in sputum.
    D. A history of three or more sexual partners.

65. Which of the HNSCC susceptibility syndromes does not feature an increased risk of hematological disease?
    A. Fanconi anemia
    B. Bloom syndrome
    C. Dyskeratosis congenita
    D. FAMMM syndrome

66. In which genes are genetic polymorphisms associated with increased HPV-induced carcinogenesis?
    A. *MAML2*
    B. *RET*
    C. *p53*
    D. *NOTCH1*

67. Which molecular event occurs earliest in the progression of HNSCC?
    A. *p53* mutation
    B. Mitochondrial DNA mutations
    C. *p16* deletion
    D. Amplification of the chromosomal 3q26.3 region

68. What is the most common site of p53 mutations?
    A. Exons 3-5
    B. Exons 5-8
    C. Extracellular domain
    D. Transmembrane domain

69. Which protein is not part of the p53 apoptotic pathway?
    A. Bcl-2
    B. BAX
    C. p21
    D. RAS

70. Which of the domains below are not part of EGFR?
    A. Extracellular ligand binding domain
    B. Intracellular catalytic subunit

C. DNA binding domain
D. Transmembrane domain

71. The oncogenic Wnt signaling pathway is implicated in HNSCC by
    A. Frequent *beta-catenin* mutations.
    B. *Notch1* and *FAT1* mutations.
    C. *Notch1* and *APC* mutations.
    D. Frequent *beta-catenin, Frizzled,* and *APC* mutations.

72. Molecular detection of minimal residual HNSCC is best achieved through application of
    A. Comparative genomic hybridization and spectral karyotyping.
    B. Fluorescence in situ hybridization (FISH) and deep sequencing.
    C. Polymerase chain reaction (PCR) and methylation assays.
    D. Microarrays and tissue arrays.

73. What are the best outcome predictors of HNSCC?
    A. TNM stage and grade
    B. HPV status and chemosensitivity
    C. TNM stage and HPV status
    D. *p53* status and HPV status

74. Which factor has the biggest effect on outcome of HPV-positive oropharyngeal cancer?
    A. *p53* status
    B. *EGFR* copy number
    C. History of 15 pack-years' tobacco exposure
    D. Age

75. The negative predictive value of global gene expression analysis in the prediction of nodal metastasis in cN0 oral cavity SCC is approximately
    A. 90%.
    B. 80%.
    C. 75%.
    D. 70%.

76. The benefit of adding cetuximab to radiation therapy for HNSCC is approximately
    A. 3%.
    B. 10%.
    C. 20%.
    D. 25%.

77. Cetuximab, gefitinib, and erlotinib are examples of
    A. Monoclonal antibodies.
    B. Monoclonal antibodies against EGFR.
    C. EGFR inhibitors.
    D. EGFR activators and inhibitors.

78. Which pathway is not directly activated by signaling through EGFR?
    A. MAPK pathway
    B. PI3K pathway
    C. Rb pathway
    D. VEGF pathway

79. In completed phase III trials, HNSCC responded best to
    A. Tyrosine kinase inhibition.
    B. Tyrosine phosphatase inhibition.

C. PI3K inhibition.

D. Monoclonal antibodies.

80. The most common tumor suppressor gene mutation identified in HNSCC is
    A. *p53*.
    B. *FAT1*.
    C. *PTEN*.
    D. *Notch1*.

81. The molecular profile of radiation-induced childhood PTC is characterized by
    A. A higher rate of *RET/PTC3* rearrangements compared with sporadic PTC in adults.
    B. A higher rate of *RET/PTC1* rearrangements compared with sporadic PTC in adults.
    C. The absence of *RET/PTC* rearrangements.
    D. A higher rate of *RET/PTC* rearrangements when compared with sporadic childhood PTC.

82. RET/PTC formation is an example of
    A. Unbalanced translocation.
    B. Balanced translocation.
    C. LOH.
    D. Genetic amplification.

83. The *RET* gene is
    A. Rearranged in approximately 10% of PTC.
    B. A tumor suppressor gene.
    C. Part of the EGFR family of receptors.
    D. Affected by point mutations in Hirschsprung disease.

84. NTRK1 is
    A. Rearranged in approximately 30% of PTC.
    B. A transmembrane cell surface receptor involved in neural cell differentiation.
    C. A nuclear receptor involved in thyroid hormone metabolism.
    D. Affected by point mutations in PTC.

85. *BRAF* gene activation
    A. Is found in 10% of PTC.
    B. Is often associated with RET/PTC2-positive PTC.
    C. Has no bearing on the prognosis of PTC.
    D. Is activated by translocations in radiation-induced PTC.

86. Molecular oncogenesis of follicular thyroid carcinomas is
    A. Driven by PI3K pathway activation.
    B. Driven by MAPK pathway activation.
    C. Closely related to that of nonencapsulated follicular variant PTC.
    D. Driven by BRAF mutations.

87. *PPAR-gamma* rearrangements
    A. Usually occur in conjunction with *PAX8* rearrangements.
    B. Are not found in encapsulated follicular variant PTC.
    C. Are not found in follicular adenomas.
    D. Are typically associated with a history of irradiation.

88. The PI3K pathway
    A. Can be activated by *RAS* mutations in follicular thyroid carcinoma.
    B. Is usually inactivated in PTC.
    C. Is commonly inactivated in follicular thyroid carcinoma.
    D. Is inactivated in patients with Cowden syndrome.

89. Anaplastic thyroid carcinomas
    A. Are characterized by mutually exclusive PI3K or MAPK activation.
    B. Have a higher rate of *RET/PTC* formation than PTC.
    C. Can be differentiated from sarcomas by the presence of the *BRAF* V600E mutation.
    D. Can be differentiated from sarcomas by *PPAR-gamma* rearrangement testing.

90. Which statement is not true for thyroid cancer?
    A. PET positivity is associated with *p53* mutations.
    B. Histologically identified mitosis and necrosis are associated with *BRAF* mutations.
    C. Beta-catenin expression is associated with PET negativity.
    D. *RET/PTC* rearrangements are typical for disease with negative PET results.

91. Which of the following genes is affected by rearrangement in mucoepidermoid carcinomas?
    A. *NOTCH1*
    B. *PLAG1*
    C. *MAML2*
    D. *NTRK3*

92. Which of the following genes is commonly affected by rearrangement in pleomorphic adenomas?
    A. *PLAG1*
    B. *p53*
    C. *NTRK3*
    D. *MECT1*

93. Which of the following genes may be associated with the prognosis of salivary gland carcinomas?
    A. *c-KIT*
    B. *MECT1*
    C. *EGFR*
    D. *RET*

94. On a gross molecular level, how many distinct subgroups of sarcoma exist?
    A. 2
    B. 3
    C. 4
    D. 5

95. Balanced translocations in sarcomas
    A. Correlate well with histological subtypes.
    B. Do not correlate well with histological subtypes.
    C. Are found in 80% of sarcomas.
    D. Are found in 90% of sarcomas.

96. Translocations involving *PAX3* or *PAX7* genes are
    A. Found in many sarcomas.
    B. Pathognomonic for alveolar rhabdomyosarcoma.

C. Associated with irradiation history for sarcomas.
D. Not found in sarcomas.

97. Genetic alterations in angiogenesis genes are most typical for
    A. Angiosarcomas.
    B. Rhabdomyosarcomas.
    C. Liposarcomas.
    D. Desmoid tumors.

98. Histological progression in sarcomas is clearly associated with
    A. Increased number of balanced translocations.
    B. Increased rate of unbalanced chromosomal alterations.
    C. Increased EGFR expression.
    D. Viral integration.

99. Balanced translocation events in sarcomas can be used for
    A. Differentiating sarcomas of the central part of the neck from anaplastic thyroid carcinomas.
    B. Predicting outcome.
    C. Designation of sarcoma subtypes.
    D. Predicting the response to targeted therapy.

100. Targeted treatment has been most difficult to design for
    A. Amplified oncogenes.
    B. Mutated oncogenes.
    C. Tumor suppressor genes.
    D. Fusion genes.

## Answers

| | | |
|---|---|---|
| 1. F | 20. T | 39. T |
| 2. T | 21. T | 40. F |
| 3. T | 22. T | 41. F |
| 4. T | 23. F | 42. F |
| 5. F | 24. F | 43. T |
| 6. T | 25. T | 44. T |
| 7. T | 26. F | 45. F |
| 8. F | 27. T | 46. F |
| 9. F | 28. T | 47. T |
| 10. T | 29. T | 48. T |
| 11. F | 30. T | 49. T |
| 12. T | 31. T | 50. T |
| 13. T | 32. T | 51. D |
| 14. T | 33. T | 52. A |
| 15. T | 34. F | 53. B |
| 16. T | 35. T | 54. E |
| 17. F | 36. T | 55. A |
| 18. T | 37. T | 56. C |
| 19. F | 38. F | 57. C |

| | | |
|---|---|---|
| 58. E | 73. B | 88. A |
| 59. B | 74. C | 89. C |
| 60. D | 75. A | 90. C |
| 61. A | 76. B | 91. C |
| 62. C | 77. C | 92. A |
| 63. A | 78. C | 93. B |
| 64. C | 79. D | 94. B |
| 65. D | 80. A | 95. B |
| 66. C | 81. A | 96. B |
| 67. C | 82. B | 97. A |
| 68. B | 83. D | 98. B |
| 69. D | 84. B | 99. A |
| 70. C | 85. D | 100. C |
| 71. B | 86. A | |
| 72. C | 87. A | |

## Core Knowledge

- The molecular biological hallmarks of cancer include (1) establishment of sustained cellular proliferation, (2) inactivation of intrinsic growth suppression, (3) resistance to cell death (apoptosis), (4) establishment of replicative immortality, (5) induction of (neo) angiogenesis, (6) invasion and metastasis, (7) reprogramming energy metabolism, and (8) evasion of immunogenic destruction.

- The hallmark features can be acquired by individuals through the development of (1) biochemical alterations within malignant cells, (2) biochemical alterations of (recruited) surrounding stroma cells, and (3) the reciprocal signaling between them.

- Genetic alterations that enable hallmark features occur as activating events in cancer-promoting genes (oncogenes) and/or inactivating events in cancer-suppressing genes (tumor suppressor genes).

- Hallmark-enabling mutations are chance events among a large pool of randomly occurring, nonspecific, background, genetic alterations that develop based on the physiological balance between environmental mutagenic factors and intrinsic factors that prevent, exclude, or repair genetic damage. Hence cancer incidence is increased in the setting of increased exposure to mutagenic influences (e.g., tobacco, alcohol, sunlight, and cellular waste products) or decreased activity of protective mechanisms, the exact balance of which is typically determined by interindividual and intergeographical variability.

- (Pre)malignant cells may tip this balance even further in their favor by acquiring inactivating biochemical events in biochemical pathways that prevent, exclude, or repair genetic damage, which then provides a basis for the ultimate hallmark-enabling characteristic—genetic instability.

- The random nature of mutagenesis allows for darwinian selection of cells with genetic alterations providing a survival advantage, which are able to adapt to environmental selective pressures and outgrow their peers without the "fittest" genomic content.

- Extrapolation of screening data suggests that cancer cells contain as many as 12,000 individual aberrations, but biological and mathematical models suggest that only between 10 and 60 critical aberrations are essential in cancer pathogenesis.

- Genomic screening of cancer has evolved from large-scale chromosome-based analyses (i.e., karyotyping, comparative genomic hybridization, loss of heterozygosity [LOH] analysis, and spectral karyotyping) and secondary application of recombinant DNA and sequencing technology to identify candidate genes to high throughput sequencing and microarray-based hybridization assessments of genetic and transcriptional abnormalities, powered by the human genome project.

- Novel concepts in general molecular oncology that need better definition include the role of the surrounding tumor–stromal environment, its reciprocal interactions, the stem cell hypothesis, and epithelial-to-mesenchymal transition of cancer cells.

## HEAD AND NECK SQUAMOUS CELL CARCINOMA

- Head and neck squamous cell carcinomas (HNSCCs) develop and progress through several well-defined histopathological stages, from benign hyperplasia, through dysplasia, carcinoma in situ, and, finally, invasive cancer. The histopathological progression of HNSCC can be traced on a biochemical level by a clearly defined sequence of genetic, epigenetic, and transcriptional alterations of nuclear and mitochondrial DNA.

- Although great variability is observed in the exact sequence and profile of these alterations, the end result is almost ubiquitously shared among HNSCCs and involves biochemical dysfunction of several defined pathways, including the p53 apoptotic pathway, retinoblastoma (Rb) and transforming growth factor (TGF)-beta pathways, and the oncogenic (epidermal growth factor receptor [EGFR]-stimulated) phosphoinositide 3-kinase (PI3K), mitogen-activated protein kinase (MAPK), and Janus kinase/signal transducer and activator of transcription (JAK/STAT) pathways.

- The progression of HNSCC is driven by clearly defined extrinsic mutagenic influences (e.g., tobacco or alcohol use or human papillomavirus [HPV] infection) and/or dysfunction of intrinsic DNA protective factors that are exemplified in exaggerated form by HNSCC susceptibility syndromes such as familial atypical multiple mole melanoma (FAMMM) syndrome, Fanconi anemia, and dyskeratosis congenita but that are also present in a subtle form as normal DNA sequence variations (single nucleotide polymorphisms) among the general population.

- Little is known about the function of genetic instability genes in HNSCC, but telomerase and p53 have been associated with an increase in chromosomal alterations. Double-stranded and single-stranded DNA repair is abnormal in HNSCC cells.

- The influence of HNSCC risk factors on the development of genetic alterations is clear from studies showing that increased tobacco and alcohol exposure increase the number of detectable genetic alterations in tumor cells. Oncogenic HPV type 16 is typically present in tumor cells as nuclear episomes or in integrated form in the (pre)malignant host genome. Transcription of HPV genes exerts oncogenic effects on host cell physiology because of abrogation of p53, Rb, and other pathways. This explains the unique clinical phenotype observed in cancers harboring HPV.

- The unique presence of somatic molecular alterations in cancer cells has been shown to provide an opportunity for improved diagnostics, staging, and cancer-specific treatment of HNSCC, but further development is needed to establish these unequivocally in clinical practice. Altogether, independent prognostic significance has been attributed to HPV positivity, p53 mutation, and several other factors.

- Treatment with the EGFR inhibitor cetuximab has been heralded as the first successful targeted treatment approach for HNSCC, providing the ultimate basis for optimistic future expectations.

- Evidence for viability of targeted treatment in HNSCC has been derived from recent studies showing an improved survival rate for patients who had HNSCC treated conventionally but with the addition of cetuximab, a monoclonal antibody to EGFR.

## THYROID CANCER

- Etiological factors in thyroid cancer development include exposure to low-dose radiation, especially at a young age, and genetic syndromes associated with follicular cell–derived thyroid neoplasia, including Gardner syndrome (APC), Cowden disease (PTEN), Carney complex (PRKAR1A) and Werner syndrome (RECQL2), and nonsyndromal familial nonmedullary thyroid carcinoma. Medullary thyroid cancer is increased in multiple endocrine neoplasia syndromes (MEN-IIA and MEN-IIB), as well as in familial medullary cancer syndrome.

- The histological progression of follicular cell–derived thyroid cancer from well-differentiated papillary and follicular thyroid carcinomas to poorly differentiated thyroid carcinomas and finally to anaplastic carcinomas is paralleled by the sequential increase in number of mitosis per high-power fields (hpf), necrosis, fluorodeoxyglucose positron emission tomography (FDG-PET) avidity, p53 accumulation, beta-catenin expression, BRAF mutation, and chromosomal complexity, and decreasing radioactive iodine (RAI) avidity, thyroglobulin detectability, and sodium–iodide symporter expression.

- Characteristic genetic abnormalities in thyroid cancer include *RET/PTC* rearrangements (multiple types), *NTRK1* rearrangements (multiple types), *BRAF* mutations in (nonencapsulated follicular variant) papillary thyroid carcinomas, *PPAR-gamma* rearrangements, *RAS* mutations in follicular carcinomas and encapsulated follicular variant papillary carcinomas, *BRAF*, *beta-catenin*, *APC*, and p53 mutations in poorly differentiated and anaplastic carcinomas, and *RET*, *HRAS*, and *KRAS* mutations in medullary carcinomas.

- After adjustment for age, the genetic and transcriptional profile of radiation-induced papillary thyroid carcinomas is largely identical to that of non–radiation-induced thyroid carcinomas.

- Diagnostic and poor prognostic value in univariate analysis has been ascertained for *BRAF* mutations in papillary thyroid carcinomas, but it remains unclear whether the *BRAF* mutation is an independent predictor of outcome in these tumors. The therapeutic value of molecular alterations is unclear and largely limited to *RET*-positive medullary carcinomas that can be successfully treated with vandetanib.

- Approximately 75% of medullary thyroid carcinomas (MTCs) lack a family history or germline gene mutations and are considered sporadic MTCs. Approximately 35% to 50% of sporadic MTCs feature somatic *RET* mutations. The behavior of sporadic and hereditary MTCs is dictated by the type of *RET* mutations: increasingly aggressive behavior is associated with mutations in higher codon numbers (more intracellular locations of mutations).

## SALIVARY GLAND CANCERS, SKIN CANCERS, AND SARCOMAS

- Balanced translocations have been found in salivary gland carcinomas; for example, the t(11;19)(q21;p13) *MEC1-MAML2* translocation is found in mucoepidermoid carcinomas, and t(6;9) fuses the *NFIB* gene to the *MYB* gene in adenoid cystic carcinomas. These translocations are potential treatment targets, but no agents have been developed yet.

- On a molecular level, sarcomas can largely be differentiated into three molecular groups: a near diploid karyotype with specific translocations (20% to 30%) or activating mutations, an intermediate complexity karyotype with specific amplifications, and, finally, a group with unstable karyotypes and multiple DNA copy number changes (66%). Translocations in sarcomas are not clearly associated with subtype, prognosis, or response to the targeted treatment. The therapeutic benefit associated with translocation-positive sarcomas is limited to the small proportion with translocations affecting *EGFRs*; no benefit has been found in the majority with translocations affecting nuclear transcription factors. Targeted treatment with angiogenesis inhibitors such as bevacizumab and taxanes is of clinical benefit in patients with angiosarcoma, who often display vascular endothelial growth factor upregulation, *KDR* gene (encodes vascular *EGFR-2*) mutations, and abnormalities in other vascular-specific tyrosine kinase enzymes.

- In recent years, molecular analysis of skin cancers has led to the development of several targeted treatment agents, including the Hedgehog pathway inhibitor, vismodegib, for basal cell carcinomas and the MAPK pathway inhibitors vemurafenib, dabrafenib, and trametinib.

## SUGGESTED READING

Adelstein DJ, Koyfman SA, El-Naggar AK, Hanna EY. Biology and management of salivary gland cancers. Semin Radiat Oncol 2012;22(3):245–53.

Ball DW. Medullary thyroid cancer: therapeutic targets and molecular markers. Curr Opin Oncol 2007;19(1):18–23.

Ha PK, Chang SS, Glazer CA, Califano JA, Sidransky D. Molecular techniques and genetic alterations in head and neck cancer. Oral Oncol 2009;45(4–5):335–9.

Hanahan D, Weinberg RA. Hallmarks of cancer: the next generation. Cell 2011;144(5):646–74.

Hanahan D, Weinberg RA. The hallmarks of cancer. Cell 2000;100(1): 57–70.

Stratton MR. Exploring the genomes of cancer cells: progress and promise. Science 2011;331(6024):1553–8.

Taylor BS, Barretina J, Maki RG, Antonescu CR, Singer S, Ladanyi M. Advances in sarcoma genomics and new therapeutic targets. Nat Rev Cancer 2011;11(8):541–57.

Tsao H, Chin L, Garraway LA, Fisher DE. Melanoma: from mutations to medicine. Genes Dev 2012;26(11):1131–55.

Vogelstein B, Kinzler KW. Cancer genes and the pathways they control. Nat Med 2004;10(8):789–99.

Wreesmann VB, Singh B. Clinical impact of molecular analysis on thyroid cancer management. Surg Oncol Clin N Am 2008;17(1):1–35. vii.

# 21 Surgical Anatomy

## Questions

### TRUE/FALSE

1. The facial nerve offers no innervation to the parotid gland. (T/F)

2. The Stensen duct passes deep to the masseter and superficial to the buccinator. (T/F)

3. The Stensen duct emerges opposite the third maxillary molar. (T/F)

4. The preganglionic fibers involved in the parotid gland parasympathetic supply travel from the superior salivatory nucleus through the glossopharyngeal nerve, the tympanic plexus, and the greater petrosal nerve, and the postganglionic fibers travel through the otic ganglion and the auriculotemporal nerve to the parotid. (T/F)

5. The preganglionic fibers involved in the parotid gland sympathetic supply begin in the interomediolateral horn nucleus between T1 and T3 and enter the sympathetic chain; postganglionic fibers begin at the superior cervical ganglion and follow the external carotid to the parotid. (T/F)

6. The geniculate ganglion branches are the greater superficial petrosal nerve, the lesser petrosal nerve, and the external petrosal nerve. (T/F)

7. In the pterygoid canal, the greater petrosal nerve joins the deep petrosal nerve to become the nerve of the pterygoid canal. (T/F)

8. The nerve of the pterygoid canal synapses in the pterygopalatine ganglion, and postsynaptic fibers via $V_2$ (the maxillary nerve) supply the lacrimal gland and mucous glands of the nasal and oral cavities. (T/F)

9. The external petrosal nerve is a constant neural branch. (T/F)

10. The lesser petrosal nerve carries postganglionic parasympathetic secretory fibers to the parotid gland via the otic ganglion. (T/F)

11. Removal of bone along the lateral surface of the digastric ridge is a useful technique for identification of the facial canal at the stylomastoid foramen. (T/F)

12. The cochleariform process is the insertion point for the stapedius tendon. (T/F)

13. The pyramidal ridge gives rise to the tensor tympani. (T/F)

14. The facial recess and sinus tympani are divided by the pyramidal ridge. (T/F)

15. Key landmarks to the posterior tympanic segment are the stapes and round window. (T/F)

16. $V_3$ exits at the foramen ovale and innervates the lateral pterygoid muscle before branching into the anterior and posterior divisions. (T/F)

17. Lateral medullary syndrome exhibits ipsilateral loss of pain/temperature sensation from one side of the face and the contralateral side of the body. (T/F)

18. The ophthalmic nerve is a sensory branch of $V_1$. (T/F)

19. The maxillary nerve passes through the foramen rotundum and carries only sensory fibers from the teeth, palate, paranasal sinus, and part of the meninges. (T/F)

20. The gasserian ganglion is a sensory ganglion. (T/F)

21. The distal third of the internal maxillary artery terminates as the sphenopalatine artery. (T/F)

22. The foramen rotundum lies in the posterior wall, connecting the pterygopalatine fossa (PPF) to the middle cranial fossa. (T/F)

23. The PPF connects inferiorly with the superior orbital fissure. (T/F)

24. The PPF extends into the infratemporal fossa through the pterygopalatine fissure. (T/F)

25. The greater petrosal nerve (preganglionic sympathetics) joins the deep petrosal nerve (postganglionic parasympathetics) to form the nerve of the pterygoid canal. (T/F)

26. The thyroid gland begins embryological development within the fetal oropharynx at 3 weeks. (T/F)

27. The thyroidea ima is a branch of the thyrocervical trunk. (T/F)

28. The Cernea classification describes the course of the external branch of the superior laryngeal nerve in relation to the cricothyroid muscle. (T/F)

29. The right recurrent laryngeal nerve is the nerve of the fourth pharyngeal arch. (T/F)

30. The right recurrent laryngeal nerve loops around the right innominate artery. (T/F)

31. The infratemporal fossa is bounded posteriorly by the spine of the sphenoid and the articular tubercle of the temporal bone. (T/F)

32. The medial pterygoid plate lies in the medial aspect. (T/F)

33. The infratemporal fossa is bounded superiorly by the greater wing of the sphenoid and the undersurface of the squamous portion of the temporal bone. (T/F)

34. The lateral pterygoid muscle originates on the infratemporal surface of the greater wing of the sphenoid bone and the medial aspect of the lateral pterygoid plate. (T/F)

35. The mandibular nerve innervates the lateral but not the medial pterygoid muscle. (T/F)

36. The inferior parathyroid gland originates from the third pharyngeal pouch. (T/F)

37. The parathyroid glands are both exclusively supplied by the inferior thyroid artery of the thyrocervical trunk. (T/F)

38. The oxyphilic cells are the dominant histopathological cells and produce parathyroid hormone (PTH). (T/F)

39. Each parathyroid gland weighs approximately 2 g. (T/F)

40. Treatments of hypoparathyroidism include calcium, PTH, and vitamin D supplements.

41. PTH has a half life of approximately 15 minutes. (T/F)

42. Vitamin D activation by 1-alpha-hydroxylase occurs in the intestine under the direct action of PTH. (T/F)

43. Osteoclastic action is directly stimulated in bone by PTH, thereby increasing calcium levels in the bloodstream. (T/F)

44. In the kidney, PTH enhances resorption of calcium and magnesium within the proximal tubules and thick descending limb. (T/F)

45. In the intestine, the activated form of vitamin D increases calcium absorption via the calcium-binding protein calbindin. (T/F)

46. The Reinke space is a "potential" anatomical space. (T/F)

47. The squamous epithelium and superficial lamina propria serve as the vocal mucosal vibratory component in phonation. (T/F)

48. The posterior cricoarytenoid muscle abducts the vocal cords by adducting the rima glottidis. (T/F)

49. The vocal ligament is composed of the superficial and intermediate layers of the lamina propria. (T/F)

50. The "body" of the vocal cord is composed of the thyroarytenoid and vocalis muscles. (T/F)

## MULTIPLE CHOICE

51. Assign the regions (a) through (j) to one of the following American Joint Committee on Cancer (AJCC)-classified anatomical sites.
    i. Supraglottis
    ii. Glottis
    iii. Subglottis
    iv. Oropharynx
    v. Hypopharynx
    vi. Nasopharynx
    vii. Oral cavity
    (a) The superior surface of the soft palate
    (b) Vallecula
    (c) Aryepiglottic folds
    (d) Fossa of Rosenmüller
    (e) Postcricoid
    (f) Glossotonsillar sulci
    (g) Retromolar trigone
    (h) Upper margin of the cricoid
    (i) Posterior hard palate
    (j) Lingual aspect of the epiglottis

52. Select the structure associated with the tongue or floor of the mouth that is the single best match for options (a) through (j).
    i. Mylohyoid muscle
    ii. Anterior belly of the digastric
    iii. Lingual nerve
    iv. Genioglossus
    v. Hypoglossal nerve
    vi. Submandibular gland
    vii. Mandibular canal
    viii. Intrinsic tongue musculature
    ix. Thyroglossal duct cyst
    x. Afferent fibers of the glossopharyngeal nerve
    xi. Sublingual gland
    (a) Gag reflex
    (b) Protrudes the tongue
    (c) Somatic information from the mucous membranes of the anterior two thirds of the tongue
    (d) First pharyngeal arch
    (e) Ducts of Rivinus
    (f) Papillary thyroid cancer
    (g) Separates the deep and superficial lobes of the submandibular gland
    (h) Passes deep to the belly of the digastric
    (i) The superficial component comprising the majority of the gland
    (j) Inferior alveolar artery

53. Match the tooth number to the name of that tooth.
    - i. Tooth number 18
    - ii. Tooth number 28
    - iii. Tooth number 6
    - iv. Tooth number 1
    - v. Tooth number 24
    - (a) Canine
    - (b) Incisor
    - (c) Bicuspid
    - (d) Wisdom
    - (e) Molar

54. Assign true (T) or false (F) to the following statements:
    - (a) The larynx ascends as a child grows.
    - (b) The laryngeal cartilaginous skeleton consists of three paired and three single cartilages.
    - (c) The vocal process provides attachment to the posterior end of the true vocal cords.
    - (d) The corniculate and cuneiform cartilages are nonfunctional in humans.
    - (e) The quadrangular cartilage is an extrinsic ligament from the epiglottic cartilage to the corniculate and arytenoid cartilages.
    - (f) The superior border of the conus elasticus is free bilaterally and thickens to form the vocal ligament.
    - (g) The aryepiglottic folds are formed by the inferior free edges of the quadrangular ligament.
    - (h) Cricothyroid muscle contraction tilts the larynx forward, causing increased tension and elongation of the vocal cords.
    - (i) The external branch of the superior laryngeal nerve innervates the cricothyroid muscle and offers a branch to the inferior constrictor muscle.
    - (j) The Semon law states that injury to the recurrent laryngeal nerve has a greater effect on the adductor muscles than on other muscles of the larynx.

55. Assign true (T) or false (F) to the following statements:
    - (a) The second lamella forms the ethmoid bulla.
    - (b) The third lamella separates the anterior from the posterior ethmoidal cells.
    - (c) The Keros classification measures the depth of the olfactory fossa.
    - (d) The anterior ethmoidal artery is usually located superior to the ethmoidal fovea and is rarely a source of significant bleeding.
    - (e) An isolated cell in the frontal sinus is a Kuhn type 1.
    - (f) Bleeding during a sphenoidotomy is commonly due to trauma to the posterior nasal artery.
    - (g) The sphenoid ostium is located posterolaterally to the superior turbinate in 85% of the population and should be safely opened inferolaterally.
    - (h) A Haller cell exists between the maxillary sinus and the floor of the orbit.
    - (i) The anterior and middle ethmoidal cells are innervated by the maxillary division of the trigeminal nerve.
    - (j) The intersphenoidal septum may insert into the external carotid artery.

56. Match each branchial arch to its parts.
    - i. First branchial arch
    - ii. Second branchial arch
    - iii. Third branchial arch
    - iv. Fourth branchial arch
    - (a) Internal carotid artery (ICA)
    - (b) Posterior belly of the digastric muscle
    - (c) Mandibular arch
    - (d) Stapes
    - (e) Parotid, submandibular, and sublingual glands

*For Questions 57 through 70, a clinical examination including panendoscopy reveals the following tumor characteristics. Provide the correct TNM staging (per AJCC/UICC).*

57. A 2.5-cm tumor on the soft palate involving the left tonsil with two cervical nodes approximately 3 cm in size on the left at levels II and III revealed by palpation
    - A. T4N2B
    - B. T4N2C
    - C. T2N2C
    - D. T2N2B

58. A 3.0-cm tumor on the floor of the mouth with evidence of mandibular erosion and cervical lymph nodes in bilateral levels I and II
    - A. T4aN2B
    - B. T2N2C
    - C. T4aN2C
    - D. T4aN3

59. A 1.5-cm tumor on the superior and inferior aspects of the right vocal cord without palpable cervical lymph node disease
    - A. T1aN0
    - B. T4N0
    - C. T2N0
    - D. T1bN0

60. A 3.5-cm tumor in the postcricoid region extending to the left pyriform fossa with one 4-cm cervical node on the left at level III
    - A. T2bN2a supraglottic tumor
    - B. T2N2a hypopharyngeal tumor
    - C. T3N2a supraglottic tumor
    - D. T2aN2b hypopharyngeal tumor

61. A right-sided 2.5-cm anterolateral tongue tumor with extension onto the lower alveolar margin and multiple cervical nodes along the right jugular chain
    - A. T4aN2B
    - B. T3N2C
    - C. T2N2C
    - D. T2N2B

62. A 2.0-cm central nasopharyngeal mass extending to the right lateral oropharyngeal wall with two cervical lymph nodes (3 cm and 2 cm) that can be palpated on the right at levels III and IV
    A. T1N1
    B. T2N2B
    C. T1N2B
    D. T3N2B

63. A 1.5-cm squamous cell carcinoma on the lingual surface of the epiglottis with bilateral nodal disease less than 6 cm
    A. T1N2C oropharyngeal
    B. T1N2C supraglottic
    C. T1N2B oropharyngeal
    D. T1N2B supraglottic

64. A 3.5-cm nasopharyngeal tumor with extension into the left nasal cavity and a 4.5-cm mass in the left supraclavicular region
    A. T1N1
    B. T1N3
    C. T2N3
    D. T2N1

65. A 3.0-cm maxillary sinus tumor with extension into the posterior maxillary sinus wall and the pterygoid fossa
    A. T3N0
    B. T4aN0
    C. T4bN0
    D. T2N0

66. A 2.5-cm ethmoidal squamous cell carcinoma with extension and erosion of the medial wall and floor of the orbit
    A. T2N0
    B. T4aN0
    C. T3N0
    D. T2bN0

67. A 3-cm glottic tumor, involving both cords, with radiological evidence of paraglottic space invasion, normal vocal fold movement on fiberoptic endoscopy, and two cervical lymph nodes on the right at levels II and III
    A. T3N2B
    B. T1bN2B
    C. T4aN2B
    D. T3N1

68. A 2.5-cm papillary thyroid carcinoma with extrathyroidal extension and four positive nodes in level VI in a 55-year-old woman
    A. T3N1A
    B. T2N2B
    C. T2N1
    D. T3N2B

69. A 2.5-cm medullary thyroid carcinoma with extrathyroidal extension and four positive nodes in level VI in a 55-year-old woman
    A. T3N1A
    B. T2N2B
    C. T2N1
    D. T3N2B

70. A 3.0-cm anaplastic thyroid carcinoma with no extrathyroidal extension and multiple bilateral cervical lymph node disease less than 6 cm is likely
    A. T2N2C.
    B. T4bN2C.
    C. T4aN1B.
    D. T4aN2C.

71. The Chandler classification for the patient shown in Figure 21-1 is likely
    A. Chandler I.
    B. Chandler II.
    C. Chandler III.
    D. Chandler IV.

72. *Preseptal cellulitis* anatomically refers to a cellulitic insult
    A. Anterior to the orbital septum.
    B. Posterior to the orbital septum.
    C. Both anterior and posterior to the orbital septum.
    D. Resulting in cavernous sinus thrombosis.

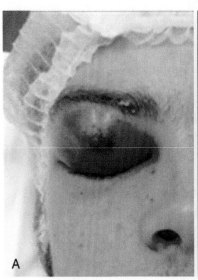
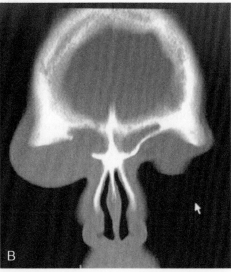

**Figure 21-1**

73. The orbital septum is best described as
    A. A perforated membranous sheet extending from the orbital rim to the eyelid, incorporating superiorly the levator palpebrae superioris and inferiorly the tarsal plate in the lower eyelid.
    B. A membranous sheet extending from the orbital rim to the eyelid anastomosing with the superior and inferior tarsal plates.
    C. A continuous fibrous sheet extending from the orbital rim to the lower tarsal plate.
    D. A perforated membranous sheet extending posterior to the levator palpebrae superioris and lower tarsal plate.

74. The cavernous sinus lateral wall contains
    A. Cranial nerves (CNs) III, IV, $V_2$, $V_3$, and VI.
    B. CNs IV, $V_1$, $V_2$, and VI.
    C. CNs III, IV, $V_1$, and $V_2$.
    D. CNs III, IV, $V_1$, $V_2$, and VI.

75. The following structures pass through the cavernous sinus:
    A. Medially the ICA with its sympathetic plexus and laterally CN VI.
    B. Medially the ICA and laterally CN VI.
    C. Laterally the ICA with its sympathetic plexus and medially CN VI.
    D. Medially the sympathetic plexus and laterally CN VI.

76. Thrombosis of the cavernous sinus readily occurs due to infection of the
    A. Maxillary sinus.
    B. Ethmoid sinus.
    C. Agger nasi cell.
    D. Sphenoid sinus.

77. Gradenigo syndrome is
    A. Otorrhea, CN VI paralysis, and retroorbital pain due to involvement of CN $V_1$.
    B. Otorrhea, CN IV palsy, and retroorbital pain due to involvement of CN $V_1$.
    C. Otorrhea, CN VII paralysis, and retroorbital pain due to involvement of CN $V_1$.
    D. Otorrhea, CN X palsy, and retroorbital pain due to involvement of CN V.

78. Gradenigo syndrome is also known as
    A. Temporal bone osteomyelitis.
    B. Sphenoiditis.
    C. Petrous apicitis.
    D. Pterygoid osteomyelitis.
    E. Sellar osteomyelitis.

79. Regarding the superficial muscular aponeurotic system (SMAS), which of the following statements is incorrect?
    A. In the parotid region, SMAS is superficial to the branches of the facial nerve.
    B. In the mandibular area, loose fibrous connections exist between the SMAS and the platysma muscle.
    C. The main facial artery and vein are located deep to the SMAS.
    D. In the pretragal region, it is completely separate from the parotid fascia.

80. Sensation in the tongue is
    A. Largely mediated by CN $V_1$ and taste by the chorda tympani (VII).
    B. Largely mediated by CNs $V_3$ and IX and taste by the chorda tympani (VII).
    C. Mediated by CNs $V_2$ and IX and taste by the lingual nerve (VII).
    D. Mediated by the chorda tympani and taste by the lingual nerve (VII).

81. A paralyzed tongue protrudes to the ipsilateral side of nerve injury because of unopposed
    A. Intrinsic tongue muscle action on the nonparalyzed side.
    B. Mylohyoid muscle contraction on the nonparalyzed side.
    C. Intrinsic and extrinsic muscle action on the paralyzed side.
    D. Intrinsic and extrinsic muscle action on the nonparalyzed side.

82. Taste loss after a tonsillectomy is likely related to a damaged
    A. Lingual nerve.
    B. Vagus nerve.
    C. Glossopharyngeal nerve.
    D. Chorda tympani.

83. The glossopharyngeal nerve is commonly damaged
    A. Near the superior pole of the tonsil.
    B. Near the inferior pole of the tonsil.
    C. Near the middle of the tonsil.
    D. Deep to the tonsil.

84. Which of the following statements is incorrect regarding the hypoglossal nerve?
    A. The nerve emerges between the ICA and the internal jugular vein.
    B. The nerve travels superficial to the anterior belly of the digastric muscle.
    C. The nerve travels deep to the stylohyoid and posterior belly of the digastric muscle.
    D. The nerve offers innervation to the intrinsic and extrinsic muscles of the tongue.

85. The sublingual gland
    A. Lies between the mucosa of the floor of the mouth and above the mylohyoid muscle.
    B. Is drained by the Wharton duct.
    C. Contains the duct of Rivinus, which is formed when anterior sublingual ducts fuse into a single duct.
    D. Abuts the hyoid bone.

86. Which of the following statements is incorrect?
    A. There are 20 deciduous teeth.
    B. There are 32 permanent teeth.
    C. Dental disease may cause maxillary sinusitis.
    D. The maxilla is almost completely innervated by the mandibular nerve.

87. Regarding the middle ear, which of the following statements is incorrect?
    A. The stapedius muscle is innervated by CN VII.
    B. The tensor tympani is innervated by CN V.

C. The tegmen tympani separates the tympanic cavity from the middle cranial cavity.

D. The tegmen tympani may be dehiscent in up to 15% of people.

88. Which of the following statements about the eustachian tube is correct?
   A. The eustachian tube is 52 mm in length in adults.
   B. The bony portion is in the posterolateral third.
   C. The fibrocartilaginous portion is in the posterolateral third.
   D. The fossa of Rosenmüller is situated anterior to the torus tubaris.

89. Eustachian tube dysfunction may cause the following, except
   A. Autophony.
   B. Serous otitis media.
   C. Nasal polyposis.
   D. Palatal myoclonus.

90. The eustachian tube opens during swallowing or yawning because of the following muscles, except the
   A. Palatopharyngeus.
   B. Tensor veli palatini.
   C. Salpingopharyngeus.
   D. Levator veli palatini.

91. True Ludwig angina is an infection of the
   A. Buccal space.
   B. Submandibular space.
   C. Parotid space.
   D. Digastric space.

92. Ludwig angina is commonly caused by
   A. Alpha-hemolytic streptococci.
   B. *Streptococcus agalactiae*.
   C. Rhinovirus.
   D. *Haemophilus influenzae* type B.

93. Ludwig angina is commonly seen in
   A. Individuals with tongue piercings.
   B. Immunocompromised patients.
   C. Premature babies.
   D. Smokers.

94. A 52-year-old patient with right-sided Bell palsy cannot close his right eye, which means that the patient's House-Brackmann score is
   A. 2.
   B. 3.
   C. 4.
   D. 5.

95. Common causes of seventh nerve palsy include the following, except
   A. Herpes zoster oticus.
   B. Neurosarcoidosis.
   C. Acoustic neuroma.
   D. Amyloidosis.

96. Which of the following pairings is incorrect?
   A. CN III and Edinger-Westphal nucleus
   B. CN VII and inferior salivatory nucleus
   C. CN X and dorsal motor nucleus
   D. CM IX and inferior salivatory nucleus

97. Which of the following pairings is incorrect?
   A. CN VII and greater superficial petrosal nerve
   B. CN IX and greater superficial petrosal nerve
   C. CN IX and tympanic plexus
   D. CN VII and chorda tympani

98. The brachial plexus extends from
   A. C5 to T1.
   B. C6 to T2.
   C. C4 to T1.
   D. C4 to T2.

99. The brachial plexus contains
   A. Three trunks, six divisions, and numerous branches.
   B. Six trunks, three cords, and numerous branches.
   C. Three trunks, three divisions, and numerous branches.
   D. Three trunks, three cords, and three divisions.

100. Regarding the brachial plexus, which of the following pairings is incorrect?
   A. Posterior cord and radial nerve
   B. Medial cord and ulnar nerve
   C. Posterior cord and median nerve
   D. Lateral cord and musculocutaneous nerve

## Answers

| | | |
|---|---|---|
| 1. F | 25. F | 49. F |
| 2. F | 26. T | 50. T |
| 3. F | 27. F | 51. (a) vi (b) iv |
| 4. F | 28. F | (c) i (d) vi |
| | | (e) v (f) iv |
| 5. T | 29. F | (g) vii (h) iii |
| 6. T | 30. F | (i) vii (j) i |
| 7. T | 31. T | 52. (a) x (b) iv |
| 8. T | 32. F | (c) iii (d) ii |
| 9. F | 33. T | (e) xi (f) ix |
| | | (g) i (h) v |
| 10. F | 34. F | (i) vi (j) vii |
| 11. T | 35. F | 53. (a) iii (b) v |
| 12. F | 36. T | (c) ii (d) iv |
| 13. F | 37. T | (e) i |
| 14. T | 38. F | 54. (a) F (b) T |
| | | (c) T (d) T |
| 15. F | 39. F | (e) F (f) T |
| 16. T | 40. F | (g) F (h) T |
| 17. T | 41. F | (i) T (j) F |
| 18. F | 42. F | 55. (a) T (b) T |
| | | (c) T (d) T |
| 19. T | 43. F | (e) F (f) T |
| 20. T | 44. F | (g) F (h) T |
| 21. T | 45. T | (i) F (j) F |
| 22. T | 46. T | 56. (a) iii (b) ii |
| 23. F | 47. T | (c) i (d) ii |
| | | (e) i |
| 24. T | 48. F | 57. D |
| | | 58. C |

| | | |
|---|---|---|
| 59. A | 73. A | 87. D |
| 60. B | 74. C | 88. B |
| 61. D | 75. A | 89. C |
| 62. A | 76. D | 90. A |
| 63. B | 77. A | 91. B |
| 64. B | 78. B | 92. A |
| 65. A | 79. D | 93. B |
| 66. C | 80. B | 94. C |
| 67. A | 81. D | 95. D |
| 68. A | 82. C | 96. B |
| 69. A | 83. B | 97. B |
| 70. C | 84. B | 98. A |
| 71. D | 85. A | 99. A |
| 72. A | 86. D | 100. C |

## Core Knowledge

- Oral cavity subsites include the hard palate, the floor of the mouth, alveolar margin, anterolateral tongue, and buccal mucosa.

- The pharynx is divided into three parts.
  - The nasopharynx begins anteriorly at the posterior choana and extends to the free border of the soft palate. It includes the vault, the lateral wall (including the fossa of Rosenmüller and the mucosa covering the torus tubaris), and the posterior wall.
  - The oropharynx extends from the superior border of the soft palate to the vallecula (hyoid). The structures in the oropharynx include the base of the tongue, the inferior (anterior) surface of the soft palate, uvula, anterior and posterior tonsillar pillars, pharyngeal tonsils, posterior wall, and lateral wall.
  - The hypopharynx extends from the vallecula (superior border of the hyoid) to the lower border of the cricoid. The structures in the hypopharynx include the pyriform sinus, lateral wall, posterior wall, and postcricoid wall (which is the anterior wall of the hypopharynx).

- The larynx is divided into three parts.
  - The supraglottic larynx includes the epiglottis (both the lingual and the laryngeal aspects), the suprahyoid epiglottis, the infrahyoid epiglottis, the laryngeal aspect of the aryepiglottic fold, arytenoids, and false cords. The inferior boundary of the supraglottis is the horizontal plane through the lateral margin of the ventricle at its junction with the superior surface of the vocal cord.
  - The glottic larynx includes the superior and inferior aspects of the true cords and the anterior and posterior commissures. It occupies a horizontal plane 1 cm thick.
  - The subglottic larynx extends from the lower boundary of the glottis to the lower margin of the cricoid cartilage.

- The parts of the esophagus are as follows: the cervical esophagus starts 15 to 20 cm from the incisors, the upper thoracic esophagus starts 20 to 25 cm from the incisors, the middle thoracic esophagus starts 25 to 30 cm from the incisors, and the lower thoracic esophagus and esophagogastric junction start 30 to 40 cm from the incisors.

- The cervical fascia consists of several layers. The superficial fascia is a continuous layer of fatty subcutaneous tissue. In the face, this invests the muscles of expression. In the neck, it invests the platysma muscle. The deep cervical fascia is broken up into the superficial layer of the deep cervical fascia (SLDF), the middle layer of the deep cervical fascia (MLDF), which has muscular and visceral subdivisions, and the deep layer of the deep cervical fascia (DLDF), which is also subdivided into the prevertebral and alar divisions. The SLDF arises from the spinous process of the vertebral column and encases the neck. It envelopes the trapezius and sternocleidomastoid muscles. A single sheet of fascia covers the posterior belly of the omohyoid, fixing it to the clavicle, and a thin sheet passes in front of the strap muscles. Above the hyoid, it covers the mylohyoid and the anterior belly of the digastric and splits into two layers, investing the mandible. It envelops the parotid gland and submandibular gland before extending up to cover the masseter and ultimately inserts into the zygomatic arch. The MLDF forms a continuous sheet deep to the SLDF and has muscular and visceral divisions. The muscular division invests the sternohyoid, sternothyroid, thyrohyoid, and omohyoid muscles. This layer extends from the hyoid and thyroid cartilages to the sternum, clavicle, and scapula. The visceral layer invests the thyroid gland, trachea, pharynx, and esophagus. Included within the MLDF is the buccopharyngeal fascia, which lies posterior to the pharynx and covers the constrictor muscles, extending from the outer buccinator muscle fascia downward and continuing as the fibrous pericardium and covering to the thoracic esophagus and trachea. The DLDF is a complete fascial ring around the neck. This covers the posterior compartment of the neck deep to the more superficial visceral compartment. It lies deep to the great vessels of the neck but superficial to the phrenic nerve. The prevertebral division is anterior to the vertebral bodies, enclosing the vertebral musculature and inserting into the transverse processes. It extends from the skull base to the coccyx. The alar division extends across the midline, from transverse process to transverse process. This extends from the skull base to T2, where it fuses with the MLDF. In the neck from the midline, it extends in an anterolateral direction to form the medial, posterior, and lateral border of the carotid sheath (the anterolateral aspect consists of the SLDF and, to a lesser degree, the MLDF).

- The parapharyngeal space (PPS) was previously divided into the prestyloid and poststyloid spaces. This terminology is now incorrect. The prestyloid space is the true PPS. The PPS is an inverted cone-shaped space that extends from the skull base to the level of the hyoid bone on either side of the pharynx. The carotid space (CS) is the designation given to the previously named poststyloid space and is separated from the prestyloid space by the tensor-vascular-styloid fascia overlying the tensor veli palatini muscle.

- The CS is contained by the carotid sheath and is formed from all three layers of the deep cervical fascia spanning the entire neck, extending from the skull base to the aortic arch. The CS communicates with the carotid canal and jugular foramen superiorly at the skull base and contains the carotid artery, internal jugular vein, cranial nerves IX, X, XI, and XII, and the sympathetic chain.

- The masticator space is enclosed by the split layers of the SLDF and extends from the skull base to the inferior border of the mandible. It contains the ascending mandibular ramus, the posterior body of the mandible, and the muscles of mastication (i.e., masseter, medial and lateral pterygoids, and temporalis), the motor and sensory branches of the mandibular branch of the trigeminal nerve ($V_3$), and the inferior alveolar artery and vein.

- The pterygopalatine fossa (PPF) is bounded by the pterygopalatine fissure laterally and the perpendicular plate of the palatine bone and orbital sphenoidal process medially. Anteriorly is the infratemporal face of the maxilla and posteriorly the root of the pterygoid process and the greater wing of the sphenoid. The distal or terminal third of the internal maxillary artery (IMAX) crosses the PPF, terminating as the sphenopalatine artery. The PPF connects with seven anatomical zones: anteriorly, the inferior orbital fissure; inferiorly, the palatine foramen; posteriorly, the foramen rotundum, vidian canal, and palatovaginal canal; laterally, the pterygomaxillary fissure; and medially, through the sphenopalatine foramen.

- The boundaries of the infratemporal fossa are the ramus of the mandible laterally, the lateral pterygoid plate medially, the infratemporal surface of the maxilla anteriorly, the superior wing of the sphenoid and undersurface of the squamous portion of the temporal bone superiorly, and the spine of the sphenoid and the articular tubercle of the temporal bone posteriorly. The inferior aspect is the medial pterygoid muscle. The contents include the chorda tympani, otic ganglion, the mandibular nerve, which supplies all muscles of mastication (and the mylohyoid, digastric anterior belly, and tensors veli palatini and tympani), the IMAX, which runs on the lower border of the lateral pterygoid muscle only to cross through its two heads of origin, the pterygoid venous plexus, the medial and lateral pterygoid muscles, and the lower aspect of the temporalis muscle.

- The parotid is innervated by both parasympathetic and sympathetic fibers.
  - For the parasympathetic supply, preganglionic fibers travel from the inferior salivatory nucleus through the glossopharyngeal nerve, tympanic plexus, and lesser petrosal nerve, and postganglionic fibers travel through the otic ganglion and auriculotemporal nerve to the parotid.

- For the sympathetic supply, preganglionic fibers begin in the interomediolateral horn nucleus between T1 and T3 and enter the sympathetic chain; postganglionic fibers begin at the superior cervical ganglion and follow the external carotid to the parotid.

- The geniculate ganglion has three branches: the greater superficial petrosal nerve, the lesser petrosal nerve, and the external petrosal nerve. In the pterygoid canal, the greater petrosal nerve (preganglionic parasympathetics) joins the deep petrosal nerve (postganglionic sympathetics) to become the nerve of the pterygoid canal. The nerve of the pterygoid canal synapses in the pterygopalatine ganglion, and postsynaptic fibers via the $V_2$ maxillary nerve supply the lacrimal and mucous glands of the nasal and oral cavities. The external petrosal nerve is an inconstant neural branch. The lesser petrosal nerve carries preganglionic secretory fibers, joins the otic ganglion, and then proceeds to the parotid gland as postganglionic fibers that travel with the (mixed) auriculotemporal nerve. This is a branch of $V_3$ that carries sympathetic nerves to the vasculature and sweat glands of the scalp and parasympathetic fibers to the parotid. Frey syndrome occurs when aberrant regeneration of parasympathetic nerves to local vessels and sweat glands after superficial parotidectomy results in a "sympathetic response" of facial sweating and erythema instead of the normal gustatory response; hence it is called *gustatory sweating*.

- The facial nerve within the epitympanum passes medial to the necks of the malleus and incus. The posterior portion of the tympanic segment has a constant anatomical association with the inferior margin of the lateral semicircular canal. The most common sites of facial nerve injury are at the second genu and mastoid segment. Removal of bone along the lateral surface of the digastric ridge is a useful technique for identification of the facial canal at the stylomastoid foramen. The cochleariform process is the attachment point for the tensor tympani muscle ($V_3$), which inserts into the manubrium of the malleus and pulling it medial, thereby reducing the vibration and amplitude of sound. The pyramidal ridge (a cone-shaped bony prominence in the posterior wall of the tympanic cavity) gives rise to the stapedius tendon (VII). The facial recess and sinus tympani are divided by the pyramidal ridge. The sinus tympani is of variable depth, extending posterior to the facial nerve. Key landmarks to the posterior tympanic segment are the stapes and oval window. The facial nerve exits the stylomastoid foramen and gives rise to the posterior auricular nerve, entering the parotid fossa and passing between the stylohyoid and the posterior belly of the digastric. The superior aspect of the posterior belly of the digastric is the key surgical landmark in the identification of the pes anserinus. The trajectory of the posterior belly indicates the anatomical level of dissection for the pes.

- The trigeminal nerve consists of three major branches: $V_1$, $V_2$, and $V_3$. The gasserian ganglion is a sensory ganglion within the Meckel cave or cavity of the dura at the apex of the petrous temporal bone. $V_1$ is the ophthalmic branch and passes through the superior orbital fissure and is exclusively sensory. $V_2$ is the maxillary branch and passes through the foramen rotundum and is also exclusively sensory. $V_3$, the mandibular nerve, is a mixed nerve and passes through the foramen ovale. The motor component joins the mandibular nerve outside the cranium. Within the infratemporal fossa, it gives off the meningeal nervus spinosus and the nerve to the medial pterygoid muscle. $V_3$ then branches into four anterior and four posterior branches.

- Muscles of note in the neck include the anterior and posterior digastric, the sternocleidomastoid (SCM), and the omohyoid muscles.
  - The anterior digastric originates from the first pharyngeal arch and innervation is from the mandibular nerve. The anterior digastric arises from the digastric fossa on the lower border of the mandible.
  - The posterior digastric arises from the mastoid process and the digastric groove (between the styloid process and the mastoid process), originates from the second pharyngeal arch, and innervation is from the facial nerve. Contraction of the digastric elevates the hyoid.
  - The SCM arises from the sternal manubrium and the clavicle to insert into the mastoid. Innervation is via cranial nerve XI. The blood supply to the SCM muscle can be divided into three parts: upper, middle, and lower. The upper third of the SCM muscle is supplied by branches of the occipital artery. The middle third is supplied by the superior thyroid artery, the external carotid, or branches of both, and the lower third is supplied by the suprascapular artery (thyrocervical trunk).
  - The omohyoid muscle extends from the scapula to the hyoid. It is innervated by ansa cervicalis (cervical plexus) and is an important landmark in neck surgery.

- A pharyngeal pouch or Zenker diverticulum is a pharyngeal mucosal herniation at the Killian dehiscence, which occurs between the propulsive oblique fibers of the thyropharyngeus and the horizontal fibers of the cricopharyngeus, which have a sphincteric action.

- The thyroid gland begins embryological development between the first and second pouches at 18 to 24 days, between the tuberculum impar and the copula at the foramen cecum, which is the opening of the thyroglossal duct into the tongue. This duct is obliterated by week 7 to 10 after the descent of the thyroid. The pyramidal lobe represents persistence of the inferior aspect of the thyroglossal duct. The ultimobranchial body originates from the ventral portion of the fourth pharyngeal pouch. Neural crest cells infiltrate the ultimobranchial body. This then fuses with the thyroid, and its parafollicular C cells disperse within it and hence are of neural crest origin.

- The parathyroid glands include the superior and inferior glands. The superior parathyroid gland originates from the fourth pouch, and the inferior parathyroid originates from the third pouch. The blood supply for both glands is from the inferior thyroid artery, a branch of the thyrocervical trunk. The parathyroids weigh between 25 and 40 mg and produce parathyroid hormone (PTH), which is a polypeptide containing 84 amino acids. PTH acts in the bones, kidneys, and intestine. In bone, it acts by indirectly stimulating osteoclasts, thereby increasing calcium resorption, and by directly stimulating osteoblastic activity. PTH results in osteoblasts binding to a protein called *receptor activator of nuclear factor kappa-B ligand* (RANKL). This reduces their expression of a protein called *osteoprotegerin*, which inhibits osteoclasts. RANKL then binds with its receptor RANK, resulting in increased osteoclastic formation. In the intestine, PTH results in 1-alpha-hydroxylase activating vitamin D to 1,25-dihydroxycholecalciferol. This acts with the protein calbindin to increase calcium absorption. In the kidneys, PTH increases resorption of calcium and magnesium in the proximal tubules and thick ascending limb and reduces the resorption of phosphate. The treatment of hypoparathyroidism is limited by the fact that there is no artificial replacement form of the hormone.

- The vocal cords are composed of five layers: the epithelial layer, the superficial, intermediate, and deep layers of the lamina propria, and the muscular layer. The Reinke space is only a potential space, but it becomes pathological, and hence a space, when fluid accumulates within the superficial lamina propria. This is commonly attributed to smoking. Speech is impaired because the vibratory components of the cords are the epithelial and superficial lamina propria layers. The vocal ligament is composed of the intermediate and deep layers of the vocal fold, and the "body" is the thyroarytenoid and vocalis muscles. The superior laryngeal nerve has an external branch that supplies the cricothyroid muscle and an internal branch that pierces the thyrohyoid membrane, offering sensory innervation above the glottis. The vocal cords receive dual sensory innervation between the recurrent laryngeal nerve and the internal branch of the superior laryngeal nerve. The recurrent laryngeal nerve is named as such because it loops around the arch of the aorta on the left and around the right subclavian artery on the right. It supplies sensation at and below the cords and also has a motor function, supplying all laryngeal muscles except for the cricothyroid.

- The laryngeal superstructure is composed of the cartilaginous structure, which is made up of three paired cartilages (arytenoid, cuneiform, and corniculate), and three single structures (the cricoid, thyroid, and epiglottis). The intrinsic membranes of the larynx include the conus elasticus (cricovocal membrane), which extends laterally deep to the cricothyroid ligament attaching inferiorly to the cricoid cartilage and extending to the inner surface of the thyroid cartilage and posteriorly to the arytenoid cartilage. The superior free edge bilaterally forms the vocal ligament. The quadrangular membrane extends from the side of the epiglottic cartilage to the corniculate and arytenoid cartilages. This forms the aryepiglottic fold of the larynx and false (vestibular) folds. There are two spaces of importance within the larynx: the preepiglottic and paraglottic spaces. The preepiglottic space is bounded by the thyrohyoid membrane anteriorly, the thyroepiglottic ligament and valleculae superiorly, and the anterior surface of the epiglottis and petiole posteriorly. The paraglottic space is bounded anterolaterally by the conus elasticus, the quadrangular membrane, and the thyroid cartilage. Posteriorly lies a reflection of the pyriform sinus mucosa. The paraglottic space extends anterosuperiorly into the preepiglottic space and is a route for extralaryngeal progression of glottic cancer.

- The arterial supply to the nose is from the anterior and posterior ethmoid arteries, which are branches of the ophthalmic artery. The sphenopalatine artery (terminal branch of the IMAX) branches into the posterior septal artery and the posterior lateral nasal artery. The greater palatine arteries originate from the IMAX, and the sublabial artery is a branch of the facial artery.

- The maxillary sinus grows according to a biphasic pattern, between 0 and 3 years of age and between 6 and 12 years of age. The roof of the maxillary sinus is the floor of the orbit, and there is a pyramidal orientation to the sinus. The posteromedial wall aspect of the sinus is the PPF, and the infratemporal fossa lies behind the posterolateral wall. The maxillary sinus is supplied by branches of the IMAX, including the infraorbital, alveolar, greater palatine, and sphenopalatine arteries. Innervation is through branches of $V_2$ (infraorbital nerve) and the greater palatine nerves.

- The ethmoid sinuses are present at birth and grow and pneumatize up to the age of 12 years. The agger nasi is the first anterior ethmoidal cell to undergo pneumatization. The ethmoid sinuses are supplied by the anterior and posterior ethmoidal arteries (ophthalmic artery) and the sphenopalatine artery (terminal branches of the IMAX). The Keros classification divides the ethmoid roof into three configurations: shallow type I (1 to 3 mm), medium type II (4 to 7 mm), and deep type III (8 to 16 mm). A Haller cell, or infraorbital cell, is an anterior ethmoidal cell that pneumatizes into the maxillary sinus ostium below the inferior orbital wall. The ethmoid bulla lies posterior to the uncinate process, superior to the infundibulum, and anterior to the basal lamella. The two-dimensional space between the bulla and the uncinate is the hiatus semilunaris. Anterior ethmoidal cells drain into the middle meatus via the ethmoid infundibulum. Posterior ethmoidal cells drain into the superior meatus. The osteomeatal complex is lamina papyracea laterally, the middle turbinate medially, the frontal recess superiorly, and the maxillary sinus ostium inferiorly.

- The middle turbinate has an anterior and posterior buttress and a horizontal and a vertical lamella. The anterior buttress is a point of attachment of the turbinate to the lateral nasal wall in the agger nasi region. The posterior buttress is a point of attachment to the lateral nasal wall near the posterior end of the middle turbinate. The vertical lamella attaches to the lateral cribriform plate lamella and marks the boundary between the cribriform plate and the ethmoid roof. The horizontal lamella (also called the *ground lamella*) attaches to the lateral nasal wall and marks the division between the anterior and posterior ethmoid air cells. The uncinate process originates from ethmoid bone and has three potential attachments. It usually attaches to the medial orbital wall superiorly but may attach to the skull base or the middle turbinate.

- The frontal sinus is formed by the upward movement of anterior ethmoid cells after the age of 2 years. The growth of the sinus is largely between ages 6 years to the teenage years. The frontal sinus is supplied by the supraorbital and supratrochlear arteries of the ophthalmic artery (the first branch of the supraclinoid internal carotid artery). It is innervated by the supraorbital and supratrochlear nerves of $V_1$. The frontal recess is bounded anteriorly by the posterior wall of the agger nasi cell, superiorly by the frontal sinus, medially by the lateral cribriform plate lamella, laterally by the lamina papyracea, and posteriorly by the anterior wall of the ethmoidal bulla.

- The sphenoid sinus has three potential orientations: sellar (67%), presellar, and conchal. This sinus does not reach full size until the teenage years. The ostium is located on the anterosuperior surface of the sphenoid face, usually medial to the superior turbinate. The sphenopalatine artery supplies the sinus, except for the planum sphenoidale, which is supplied by the posterior ethmoidal artery. Innervation of the sphenoid sinus comes from branches of $V_1$ and $V_2$.

## SUGGESTED READING

Janfaza P. Surgical anatomy of the head and neck. Philadelphia: Lippincott Williams & Wilkins; 2001.

Mohebati A, Shaha AR. Anatomy of thyroid and parathyroid glands and neurovascular relations. Clin Anat 2012;25(1):19–31.

Netter F. Atlas of human anatomy. 5th ed. Philadelphia: Saunders; 2010.

O'Neill JP, Fenton JE. The recurrent laryngeal nerve in thyroid surgery. Surgeon 2008;6(6):373–7.

Patel SG, Meyers P, Huvos AG, Wolden S, Singh B, Shaha AR, et al. Improved outcomes in patients with osteogenic sarcoma of the head and neck. Cancer 2002;95(7):1495–503.

Pinheiro-Neto CD. Anatomical correlates of endonasal surgery for sinonasal malignancies. Clin Anat 2012;25(1):129–34.

Pravin KP, Shyamsunder NB. Head and neck embryology, <http://emedicine.medscape.com/article/1289057-overview>; [accessed 14.30.01].

Rhoton Jr AL. The anterior and middle cranial base. Neurosurgery 2002;51(4 Suppl.):S273–302.

Shah J, Patel SG, Singh B. Jatin Shah's head and neck surgery and oncology. 4th ed. Philadelphia: Mosby; 2012.

Stambuk H, Patel S. Imaging of the parapharyngeal space. Otolaryngol Clin North Am 2008;41(1):77–101.

# 22 Nutrition

## Questions

### TRUE/FALSE

1. Available evidence is insufficient for drawing definitive conclusions about the effectiveness of prophylactic feeding tubes in the patient population with head and neck cancer or for supporting an evidence-based practice guideline. (T/F)

2. The stages of oropharyngeal swallowing are under involuntary control. (T/F)

3. Acute mucositis is a major dose-limiting side effect of chemoradiation therapy. (T/F)

4. Nothing-by-mouth (*nil per os*; NPO) intervals as short as 2 weeks have been shown to predict poor long-term swallowing outcomes. (T/F)

5. Based on population data from the Surveillance, Epidemiology, and End Results (SEER) database, swallowing outcomes (i.e., rates of dysphagia, stricture, and pneumonia) are worse for patients with head and neck cancer treated with surgery and irradiation than for patients treated with other modalities. (T/F)

6. Reported aspiration rates of 24% to 31% after chemoradiation therapy likely underestimate the true incidence of aspiration. (T/F)

7. Postural changes improve swallowing for patients with unilateral pharyngeal weakness. The head turn rotates the head to the strong side, whereas the head tilt angles the head to the weak side. (T/F)

8. The minimum time period for when percutaneous endoscopic gastrostomy (PEG) tube feedings are preferred over nasogastric (NG) tube feedings is 2 months. (T/F)

9. More than 40% of patients successfully treated for head and neck cancer have fair to poor dental status at a 5-year follow-up. (T/F)

10. Patients being fed via a PEG tube tend to have less weight loss and, more commonly, a beneficial weight gain compared with patients fed via an NG tube at 6 months after treatment. (T/F)

11. Megestrol acetate is a progestational agent that has been shown to reduce weight loss and improve appetite in patients with head and neck cancer who are not receiving enteral tube feeding. (T/F)

12. Approximately 90% of patients who undergo prophylactic PEG tube placement while undergoing chemoradiation treatment for head and neck cancer return to a virtually normal oral diet and are weaned from enteral feeding by 2 months after treatment. (T/F)

13. Prophylactic PEG tube placement is superior to NG tube placement or oral feedings in terms of nutrition and weight outcomes and results in fewer treatment interruptions in patients with head and neck cancer. (T/F)

14. Regular consultation with a dietitian has been shown to improve outcomes and quality of life in patients undergoing chemoradiation treatment for head and neck cancer. (T/F)

15. Amifostine concentrates in salivary glands, scavenges radiation-induced free radicals, and has been shown to reduce acute and chronic xerostomia without compromising the efficacy of chemoradiation treatment. (T/F)

16. Grade 5 oral mucositis as defined by the World Health Organization (WHO) and National Cancer Institute (NCI) is tissue necrosis with significant spontaneous bleeding and life-threatening consequences (Figure 22-1). (T/F)

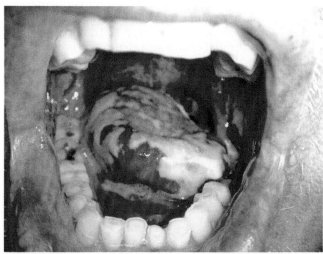

**Figure 22-1** (From Shah JP, Patel SG, Singh B. Jatin Shah's head and neck: surgery and oncology, 4th ed. Philadelphia: Mosby; 2012, [Figure 20-19].)

17. The incidence of grade 3 to 4 oral mucositis is higher in patients treated with accelerated fraction radiation therapy than in those treated with conventionally fractionated radiation therapy. (T/F)

18. Patients with head and neck cancer with 10% weight loss in the 6 months prior to surgery are at a significantly higher risk of major complications. (T/F)

19. An immune-enhancing enteral diet with arginine significantly decreases the rate of postsurgical wound infections, the incidence of fistula development, and the length of hospital stay. (T/F)

20. The prevalence of malnutrition in patients with newly diagnosed head and neck cancer is as high as 75%, and more than 80% are expected to experience further weight loss during treatment. (T/F)

21. Albumin levels are a reliable and sensitive marker for nutritional status. (T/F)

22. Severe malnutrition is associated with weight loss of more than 5% in 1 month or more than 10% in 6 months. (T/F)

23. Appropriate daily fluid intake for postoperative patients is 30 to 40 mL/kg/day. (T/F)

24. Delayed oral feeding (greater than 7 days postoperatively) after primary total laryngectomy reduces the incidence of fistula formation. (T/F)

25. Cetuximab given with radiation therapy has been shown to produce significantly lower rates of weight loss, oral mucositis, and the need for tube feeding compared with conventional chemoradiation therapy using cisplatin. (T/F)

26. Intensity-modulated radiation therapy (IMRT) has been shown to produce significantly lower rates of acute side effects, including weight loss, oral mucositis, and the need for tube feeding compared with three-dimensional conformal radiation therapy. (T/F)

27. Weekly nutritionist counseling, intervention, and posttreatment follow-up lead to improved patient-centered outcomes. (T/F)

28. Esophageal strictures occur in 33% to 50% of patients with head and neck cancer undergoing definitive chemoradiation therapy. (T/F)

29. Severe weight loss (more than 10% of body weight in 6 months) during chemoradiation treatment has been observed in more than half of patients with head and neck cancer in the absence of adequate nutritional support. (T/F)

30. Ulcerative mucositis typically develops earlier after chemotherapy infusion (by days 5 to 10) than with radiation treatment (days 21 to 28) but resolves sooner. (T/F)

31. The push PEG technique appears to have a significantly lower risk of complications when compared with the pull PEG technique. (T/F)

32. The possibility of tumor implantation at the gastrostomy site is controversial and has not been conclusively demonstrated to seed from the primary head and neck tumor. (T/F)

33. With appropriate pretreatment counseling, the use of enteral feeding, and intensive intervention during treatment, patients can expect to maintain their body weight. (T/F)

34. In the terminal phase of palliative patients, anorexia (lack of appetite) is often the first in a series of expected issues. (T/F)

35. Chemotherapy-induced mucositis that is clinically significant results in unanticipated dose reduction in approximately 25% of cycles. (T/F)

36. For mild to moderate oral mucositis, normal saline rinses are no less effective than combination "magic mouthwash" rinses for pain management. (T/F)

37. The Mendelsohn swallow maneuver is performed by consciously elevating the larynx and swallowing while holding this position, thereby stretching the cricopharyngeal muscle open. (T/F)

38. Metoclopramide is a serotonin agonist that accelerates gastric emptying, thereby treating nausea. (T/F)

39. Dilation of esophageal strictures secondary to chemoradiation therapy with Maloney dilators up to 42F is sufficient for resolving dysphagia. (T/F)

40. The majority of esophageal strictures will resolve with multiple dilation procedures. (T/F)

41. Body mass index (BMI) less than 18.5 $kg/m^2$ is highly suggestive of clinically significant malnutrition in patients with head and neck cancer and is a strong indicator for prophylactic PEG tube placement. (T/F)

42. Refeeding syndrome consists of metabolic disturbances that occur with reintroduction of nutrition via highly concentrated feedings such as total parenteral nutrition (TPN), as opposed to peripheral parenteral nutrition (PPN), PEG, or NG tube feedings. (T/F)

43. Refeeding syndrome can be prevented by limiting enteral feedings to 15 to 20 kcal/kg/day for the first several days before advancing to standard levels. (T/F)

44. Fluid triglyceride levels of 75 mg/dL from the neck drain effectively rule out a chyle leak. (T/F)

45. A middle chain triglyceride diet is sufficient nutrition for patients being treated for a chyle leak. (T/F)

46. Preoperative or postoperative use of immunonutrition (e.g., arginine or glutamine-enhanced formulations) has not been conclusively shown to improve survival outcomes. (T/F)

47. Malnutrition affects the tumor response to chemoradiation therapy and is a correspondingly significant negative predictor of prognosis and outcome. (T/F)

48. Patients with head and neck squamous cell carcinoma (HNSCC) who initially refuse a PEG tube but later require one during treatment have no difference in outcomes compared with patients undergoing prophylactic PEG tube placement before the start of treatment. (T/F)

49. Cancer cachexia is characterized by a decreased metabolic rate and resting energy expenditure. (T/F)

50. Patients with PEG tube feeding who continue to lose weight, have diarrhea with feeding, or have early satiety have indications for TPN. (T/F)

## MULTIPLE CHOICE

51. PEG tube dependency can occur as a result of
    A. The length of time or effort to consume food.
    B. Patient difficulty in enjoying or tasting food in a social setting.
    C. Psychological perceptions of fragility and pain from treatment side effects.
    D. Development of a stricture that is not correctable.
    E. All of the above.

52. Tube feeding has been reported to lead to all of the following, except
    A. Maintenance of weight or less weight lost.
    B. Fewer chemotherapy or radiation treatment breaks.
    C. A higher hospital admission rate.
    D. A lower infection rate.
    E. Better survival outcomes.

53. The modified barium swallow (MBS) is the gold standard modality for evaluating the swallowing mechanism. What is the MBS able to detect that the fiberoptic endoscopic evaluation of swallowing (FEES) tool cannot?
    A. Extent of aspiration
    B. Laryngeal penetration
    C. Presence of residual bolus
    D. Presence of aspiration
    E. Mobility of the vocal cords

54. Advantages of FEES over an MBS or barium esophagram include
    A. Assessment of oral stage and movement of the base of the tongue.
    B. Examination of structural movement at the height of swallowing.
    C. Visualization of surface anatomy and mucosal abnormalities.
    D. Detection of a postsurgical fistula.
    E. Detection of an esophageal stricture.

55. Early swallowing exercise regimens remain the best method for preventing long-term dysphagia and poor swallowing outcomes. What is not a primary goal of such regimens?
    A. Strengthen oropharyngeal and pharyngeal musculature
    B. Improve precision of oropharyngeal movements
    C. Maintain pharyngeal and cricopharyngeal muscle range of motion

D. Prevent the need for enteral feeding
E. Decrease the risk of esophageal strictures

56. Dysphagia after chemoradiation therapy typically results from
    A. Dysregulated wound healing mechanisms leading to fibrosis and compression of swallowing muscles.
    B. Neuropathy from chemotoxicity or late effects from radiation.
    C. Devascularization from radiation injury.
    D. Formation of esophageal strictures.
    E. All of the above.

57. The super-supraglottic swallow is performed by
    A. Holding one's breath, then swallowing, coughing, and swallowing again before inhaling.
    B. Holding one's breath while bearing down, swallowing, coughing, and swallowing again before inhaling.
    C. Consciously keeping the larynx elevated while swallowing.
    D. Consciously squeezing one's swallowing muscles while swallowing.
    E. Consciously closing the false cords to prevent aspiration during swallowing.

58. The chin tuck maneuver brings the patient's chin to his or her chest. This action helps prevent aspiration during swallowing by
    A. Pushing the base of the tongue to the pharyngeal wall and moving the epiglottis posteriorly.
    B. Tilting the arytenoids forward.
    C. Stretching open the cricopharyngeus muscle.
    D. Keeping the vocal cords closed.
    E. Stretching the base of the tongue to improve the pharyngeal phase of swallowing.

59. Disadvantages of TPN include all of the following, except
    A. Difficulty attaining nutritional requirements because of fluid overload.
    B. Major infection or sepsis.
    C. Small bowel obstruction or paralytic ileus.
    D. Cholelithiasis, liver dysfunction, and gastrointestinal tract atrophy.
    E. Central venous access if required.

60. Palifermin is a human recombinant keratinocyte growth factor that stimulates growth of oral surface mucosa and has been studied for the prevention and treatment of oral mucositis during chemoradiation treatment. Which of the following statements is true for patients with HNSCC receiving definitive chemoradiation?
    A. Palifermin significantly reduces the incidence of severe oral mucositis.
    B. Palifermin significantly reduces patient-reported symptoms of mucositis.
    C. Palifermin significantly reduces the incidence of treatment interruptions.
    D. Palifermin significantly increases the time to development of severe mucositis.
    E. All of the above are true.

61. Appropriate screening criteria in favor of prophylactic PEG tube placement include
    A. Heavy alcohol intake.
    B. Preexisting dysphagia or aspiration.
    C. Noncompliant persona.
    D. Presence of odynophagia.
    E. Both A and B.

62. Although prealbumin is used as a marker for nutritional status, values are significantly affected by
    A. Hydration status.
    B. Renal function.
    C. Mild to moderate liver disease.
    D. Acute alcohol intoxication.
    E. Hyperthyroidism.

63. Which of the following is not a limitation of body weight as a measure of nutritional status?
    A. A patient can be malnourished without demonstrating weight loss.
    B. Water accumulation via third-spacing may mask true body weight.
    C. Serial weight measurements are usually inconsistent and cannot reliably identify trends.
    D. Weight loss does not distinguish between the type of loss (e.g., fat or lean muscle mass).

64. What is the recommended daily energy intake and protein intake for HNSCC patients undergoing surgery or chemoradiation therapy?
    A. 30 kcal/kg/day and 1.2 g protein/kg/day
    B. 1.2 kcal/kg/day and 30 g protein/kg/day
    C. 10 kcal/kg/day and 1.2 g protein/kg/day
    D. 30 kcal/kg/day and 10 g protein/kg/day

65. What is the most commonly recommended type of enteral feeding for postoperative patients?
    A. Monomeric feeding (predigested carbohydrate, protein, and small amounts of fat)
    B. Polymeric feeding (intact protein, triglycerides, vitamins, minerals, essential trace elements, and $H_2O$)
    C. Immune-enhancing formulas (immunostimulants such as arginine, in addition to protein, carbohydrates, and triglycerides)
    D. Hydration solutions (water, minerals, and carbohydrates)

66. What percentage of HNSCC patients receiving long-term enteral feeding eventually resume oral intake and can discontinue home enteral nutrition?
    A. Up to 10%
    B. Up to 25%
    C. Up to 50%
    D. Up to 75%

67. What percentage of patients with HNSCC undergoing chemoradiation therapy requires permanent enteral nutrition?
    A. 2%
    B. 10%
    C. 25%
    D. 50%

68. Although controversial, which factors have been associated with the eventual use of tube feeding during treatment?
    A. Advanced stage tumor
    B. Multimodality chemoradiation treatment
    C. Hypopharyngeal tumor site
    D. All of the above

69. How does cancer cachexia differ from starvation?
    A. Metabolism shifts to a slow catabolic mode to minimize energy expenditure.
    B. There is roughly equal loss of muscle and fat.
    C. Refeeding enterically or by TPN replenishes some body mass and increases survival outcomes.
    D. There is decreased protein breakdown.

70. Which agents are not used as appetite stimulants in patients with cancer?
    A. Megestrol acetate
    B. Dexamethasone
    C. Lorazepam
    D. Dronabinol

71. Which is not a complication of NG tube feeding?
    A. Laryngeal ulceration
    B. Esophageal reflux and stricture
    C. Alar necrosis
    D. Vocal cord palsy

72. In the absence of clear indicators for use of prophylactic PEG tubes, what are common influential factors in determining use?
    A. Pretreatment of swallowing function
    B. Pretreatment weight loss
    C. Patient choice
    D. All of the above

73. The systemic agent with the lowest risk of producing oral mucositis is
    A. Docetaxel
    B. Cisplatin
    C. 5-Fluorouracil
    D. Methotrexate

74. Which of the following topical agents for oral mucositis has relatively strong supporting data?
    A. Chlorhexidine
    B. Antibiotic rinses
    C. Ice chip therapy (cryotherapy)
    D. Disinfectant lozenges

75. The per os intake of tolerable foods for patients receiving NG tube feeding is
    A. Discouraged when it causes symptomatic aspiration.
    B. Discouraged because it may cause NG tube dislodgement.
    C. Encouraged when possible because it prevents swallowing muscle atrophy and future dysphagia.
    D. Both A and C.

76. Which is not an appropriate indication for jejunostomy instead of gastrostomy tube placement?
    A. Gastric ileus
    B. Significant or symptomatic aspiration

C. History of peptic ulcer disease
D. Significant gastroesophageal reflux

77. How does PPN differ from TPN?
   A. Higher glucose concentration
   B. Lower osmolarity
   C. Requires a peripherally inserted central catheter (PICC)
   D. Causes hepatic steatosis given the high volumes and density of nutrition given

78. Successful resolution of esophageal strictures occurs for the majority of patients with HNSCC when the esophagus can be dilated to
   A. 24F.
   B. 28F.
   C. 32F.
   D. 42F.

79. Which of the following has been shown to be associated with malnutrition in patients with HNSCC?
   A. Increased mortality rate
   B. Depression
   C. Reduced response to chemotherapy and/or radiation therapy
   D. All of the above

80. Midarm muscle circumference (MAMC) is an indicator for
   A. Fat stores.
   B. Lean muscle mass.
   C. Weight adjusted for age.
   D. BMI.

81. Significant aspects of refeeding syndrome include all of the following, except
   A. Hyperphosphatemia.
   B. Thiamine deficiency.
   C. Hypokalemia.
   D. Cardiac arrhythmia.

82. Which of the following laboratory values from a neck drain are not diagnostic for a chyle leak?
   A. Presence of chylomicrons
   B. Drain triglyceride levels greater than 110 mg/dL
   C. Drain triglyceride/drain cholesterol levels less than 1
   D. Drain triglyceride/serum triglyceride levels greater than 1

83. Alternative dietary strategies for managing a chyle leak if middle-chain triglycerides are unavailable include
   A. A fat-free diet (less than 0.5 g of fat per serving).
   B. NG tube feeding.
   C. PEG tube feeding.
   D. Feeding with small-chain triglycerides.

84. Which patient-related issues are commonly underestimated by treating physicians?
   A. Patient motivation
   B. Social support
   C. Patient compliance
   D. Effects of oral mucositis

85. According to the American Dietetic Association, how does a pureed dysphagia diet differ from a mechanically altered dysphagia diet?
   A. The pureed diet consists of homogenous, cohesive, pudding-like food that does not require chewing.
   B. The pureed diet consists of cohesive, moist, semisolid food that requires some chewing.
   C. The mechanically altered diet consists of soft-solid food that does not require chewing.
   D. The mechanically altered diet consists of homogenous, cohesive, pudding-like food that does not require chewing.

86. How does swallowing larger boluses primarily address dysphagia as a behavioral strategy?
   A. It facilitates better clearing of residual material before the next bolus is attempted.
   B. It is easier to sense for patients who have impaired sensation and delayed triggering of the swallowing mechanism.
   C. It increases laryngeal elevation to better open the cricopharyngeal muscle.
   D. It increases posterior movement of the base of the tongue.

87. What is an advantage of a jejunostomy tube over a gastrostomy tube?
   A. Decreased aspiration
   B. Possibility of larger bolus feedings
   C. Lower complication rate
   D. Greater patient comfort and maintenance

88. Qualitative changes in saliva composition during radiation treatment include a
   A. More basic pH.
   B. Decrease in immunoprotein concentration.
   C. Decrease in salivary flow rate and increased viscosity.
   D. Decrease in *Streptococcus*, *Lactobacillus*, and *Candida* species.

89. Radiation increases the rate of dental caries for all of the following reasons, except
   A. Decreased salivary flow rate.
   B. Increased cariogenicity of altered oral flora.
   C. Altered salivary composition, including decreased buffer capacity and more acidic character.
   D. Decreased chewing caused by temporary mucositis and dysphagia.

90. Trismus due to radiation therapy is most commonly caused by
   A. High radiation doses to the temporomandibular joint.
   B. Fibrosis and scarring of the masseter muscles.
   C. Inclusion of the pterygoid muscles in the treatment portals.
   D. None of the above.

91. The risk of osteoradionecrosis has been shown to be increased by all of the following factors, except
   A. Dental implants.
   B. Preradiation dental extraction followed by inadequate healing time.

C. Postradiation dental extraction.
D. Prosthetic appliances in edentulous patients.

92. A liquid or soft diet, although easier for patients with HNSCC to eat, is less desirable because
    A. Such diets exacerbate the risk of oral cavity infections compared with solid foods.
    B. Such diets contain less energy and protein density and require additional dietary supplements.
    C. Patients on such diets are more likely to require enteral feeding.
    D. Patients on such diets are more likely than those on solid diets to have permanent dysphagia after treatment.

93. From a patient quality-of-life perspective, what is the most burdensome oral cavity symptom listed below?
    A. Restricted mouth opening
    B. Lack of saliva
    C. Restricted tongue mobility
    D. Reduced oral cavity sensation

94. Although various techniques exist to address trismus, which of the following has been shown to be effective for long-term treatment?
    A. Unassisted exercise
    B. Manual exercises with stacked tongue blades
    C. Therabite system
    D. Coronoidectomy

95. Lean muscle mass loss in patients with cancer, in contrast to fat loss alone, is associated with all of the following, except
    A. Impaired immune functioning.
    B. Reduced physical activity and quality of life.
    C. Decreased energy expenditure needs.
    D. A prolonged hospital stay.

96. Which head and neck tumor site has the highest incidence of critical weight loss?
    A. Hypopharynx
    B. Oral cavity
    C. Larynx
    D. Oropharynx

97. Taste disturbance, including a metallic aftertaste that leads to food aversion, generally returns in some form after radiation treatment within
    A. 3 months.
    B. 6 months.
    C. 12 months.
    D. 5 years.

98. After cancer treatment, the gain in weight is most predominantly from
    A. Fat.
    B. Lean muscle mass.
    C. An equal amount of fat and lean muscle mass.
    D. Fluid.

99. Difficulty swallowing liquids is most commonly due to
    A. Neurological impairment leading to poor muscular control before swallowing.
    B. Reduced cricopharyngeal opening at the esophageal stage of swallowing.

C. A delayed involuntary swallow reflex.
D. Anatomical and physiological impairment during swallowing.

100. Difficulty swallowing solids is most commonly caused by
    A. Neurological impairment leading to poor muscular control before swallowing.
    B. Reduced cricopharyngeal opening at the esophageal stage of swallowing.
    C. A delayed involuntary swallow reflex.
    D. Anatomical and physiological impairment during swallowing.

## Answers

| | | |
|---|---|---|
| 1. T | 32. F | 63. C |
| 2. F | 33. F | 64. A |
| 3. T | 34. T | 65. B |
| 4. T | 35. T | 66. B |
| 5. F | 36. T | 67. B |
| 6. T | 37. T | 68. D |
| 7. F | 38. F | 69. B |
| 8. F | 39. F | 70. C |
| 9. T | 40. T | 71. D |
| 10. F | 41. T | 72. D |
| 11. T | 42. F | 73. A |
| 12. F | 43. T | 74. C |
| 13. F | 44. F | 75. D |
| 14. T | 45. F | 76. C |
| 15. T | 46. T | 77. B |
| 16. F | 47. T | 78. D |
| 17. T | 48. F | 79. D |
| 18. T | 49. F | 80. B |
| 19. F | 50. F | 81. A |
| 20. T | 51. D | 82. C |
| 21. F | 52. C | 83. A |
| 22. T | 53. A | 84. D |
| 23. T | 54. C | 85. A |
| 24. F | 55. D | 86. B |
| 25. F | 56. D | 87. A |
| 26. F | 57. B | 88. C |
| 27. T | 58. A | 89. D |
| 28. F | 59. C | 90. C |
| 29. T | 60. A | 91. A |
| 30. T | 61. D | 92. B |
| 31. T | 62. D | 93. B |

| | | |
|---|---|---|
| 94. D | 97. C | 100. D |
| 95. C | 98. A | |
| 96. A | 99. A | |

## Core Knowledge

- Optimized nutrition can improve the tolerance and response rate to radiation therapy and chemoradiation therapy, as well as improve immune status, wound healing, and complication rates. Correspondingly, optimized nutritional status reduces the chance of delays or gaps in chemoradiation treatment.

- Daily calorie requirements entail 25 to 35 kcal/kg body weight, and daily protein requirements entail 1 to 1.5 g/kg body weight. Intake of 1500 to 2000 kcal/day typically provides the daily requirements of vitamins and minerals. Daily fluid requirements generally amount to 30 to 40 mL/kg body weight.

- Megestrol acetate has been shown in four separate placebo-controlled, randomized trials to reduce weight loss during chemoradiation therapy. Specific improvements include better appetite scores and reduced anorexia. Other than edema, no major adverse effects have been reported with megestrol acetate.

- Dysphagia is a major chronic side effect of chemoradiation therapy, and its severity and duration are affected by tumor location and the specific treatment regimen used. As many as 40% of patients with head and neck cancer continued to have dysphagia 3 years after treatment.

- Xerostomia, which also exacerbates dysphagia, is the most common long-term side effect of radiation and can manifest up to 5 years after definitive treatment. A phase III trial exhibited an 83% incidence of xerostomia after 2 years when conventional radiation therapy was used. However, this incidence is significantly decreased after 2 years for those undergoing intensity-modulated radiation therapy (IMRT).

- Together with xerostomia, poor dental status can lead to caries, tooth loss, and further malnutrition in the population with head and neck cancer. More than 40% of patients with head and neck cancer were found to have fair to poor dental status at 5-year follow-up.

- Esophageal strictures after chemoradiation therapy occur in 4% to 14% of patients with head and neck cancer.

- Oral mucositis affects nearly all patients with head and neck cancer receiving radiation therapy. Up to 25% of patients treated with cycled chemotherapy alone develop mucositis, and increased severity and duration are seen with concurrent treatment. Ulcerative mucositis typically develops within 3 to 4 weeks after treatment with radiation therapy. Ulcerative mucositis induced by chemotherapy usually begins within 5 to 10 days of drug infusion.

- Taste changes usually begin after 1 week of beginning radiation therapy and worsen throughout treatment. Changes may be permanent, although recovery usually occurs within 3 to 6 months after treatment. For patients undergoing chemotherapy, salivary secretion of systemic agents often results in a sour or bitter taste alteration. Taste also is affected by salivary function and secondary infection. Poor oral hygiene further affects taste adversely. Nutritional intervention can focus on more intense flavors to prevent malnutrition.

- Labored swallowing, prolonged eating times, and the limited range of foods that can be swallowed have been shown to significantly affect relationships through social isolation.

- Aspiration rates are likely underreported in patients undergoing chemoradiation therapy, given that silent aspiration has been observed in approximately 33% of such patients. For studies examining only symptomatic patients, aspiration rates of 24% to 31% have been reported. For studies investigating all patients with radiographic imaging, higher aspiration rates of 30% to 62% have been reported.

- Preventive swallowing exercises in patients with head and neck cancer undergoing chemoradiation therapy are associated with improved swallowing-related quality of life, improved base-of tongue retraction and epiglottic inversion, larger postradiation therapy tongue muscle mass, and a shorter duration of gastrostomy dependence.

- Therapeutic interventions that may address functional or anatomical dysphagia include
  - Dietary modifications, such as thickening agents.
  - Postural strategies, such as head positioning.
  - Swallowing maneuvers, such as supraglottic swallowing or Mendelsohn maneuver.
  - Motion exercises that target strength and range of motion for the lips, tongue, and larynx.
  - Prosthetic devices, such as palatal obturators to prevent velopharyngeal insufficiency.
  - Routine swallowing therapy involvement before, during, and after treatment.

- With similar patient cohorts, the duration of percutaneous endoscopic gastrostomy (PEG) tube feeding has been found to be significantly longer than for nasogastric (NG) tube feeding. Similarly, a Cochrane Database review identified no significant difference in terms of complication rates or patient satisfaction. Prospective, randomized controlled trials have also shown that in the long term, both PEG and NG tube feedings are equally effective at maintaining body weight.

- PEG tubes have demonstrated advantages over NG tubes via improved mobility, quality of life, and the use of higher energy feedings. With appropriately selected patients, prophylactic PEG tubes have been shown to reduce mean weight loss and the rate of hospitalization during radiation therapy.

- When compared with NG tube use, PEG placement more often leads to persistent dysphagia, likely due to deconditioning of deglutition muscles and less incentive to participate in swallowing therapy. This corresponds with multiple studies showing a high rate of long-term feeding tube dependence in patients with PEG tubes.

- Patients requiring pretreatment PEG tube placement for concurrent chemoradiation therapy have been shown to require enteral feeding for an average of 6 months. A significant percentage may require PEG tube feeding for greater than 6 months. Many clinical trials report tube dependence of approximately 10% to 26% at 1 year and 5% to 14% at 2 years. Most patients eventually resume oral intake and discontinue their PEG tubes, but approximately 10% of patients with head and neck cancer require permanent enteral nutrition. This is likely lower for patients receiving single-modality treatment (e.g., radiation therapy alone).

- Prophylactic NG or PEG tube insertion should be considered for patients seen with one or more of the following symptoms:
  - Significant weight loss (greater than 5% of baseline weight in 1 month or greater than 10% in 6 months)
  - Body mass index below 18.5 kg/m$^2$
  - Dysphagia
  - Anorexia
  - Dehydration
  - Pain or any symptom interfering with the ability to eat

- NG tubes are less cosmetic, more uncomfortable, and have some risk of nasal soft tissue injury, sinusitis, and aspiration.

- Early therapeutic regimens of swallowing exercises that are designed to strengthen musculature, increase movement precision, and maintain range of motion allow for the best prevention of long-term swallowing dysfunction, even during enteral feeding. Function at 6 months after chemoradiation therapy may best predict long-term swallowing outcomes.

- Peripheral parenteral nutrition (PPN) and total parenteral nutrition (TPN) are typically less efficient and more expensive than enteral nutrition. Common risks with parenteral nutrition are infection, metabolic derangements, and an inability to meet nutritional requirements because of fluid overload.

## SUGGESTED READING

Bensinger W, Schubert M, Ang KK, Brizel D, Brown E, Eilers JG, et al. NCCN Task Force report. Prevention and management of mucositis in cancer care. J Natl Compr Canc Netw 2008;6(Suppl. 1):S1–21; quiz S22–24.

Epstein JB, Huhmann MB. Dietary and nutritional needs of patients after therapy for head and neck cancer. J Am Dent Assoc 2012;143(6): 588–92.

Findlay M, Bauer J, Brown T, et al. Evidence based practice guidelines for the nutritional management of adult patients with head and neck cancer. Sydney, Australia: Clinical Oncological Society of Australia; 2011.

Garg S, Yoo J, Winquist E. Nutritional support for head and neck cancer patients receiving radiotherapy: a systematic review. Support Care Cancer 2010;18(6):667–77.

Hutcheson KA, Lewin JS. Functional outcomes after chemoradiotherapy of laryngeal and pharyngeal cancers. Curr Oncol Rep 2012;14(2): 158–65.

Joque L, Jatoi A. Total parenteral nutrition in cancer patients: why and when? Nutr Clin Care 2005;8(2):89–92.

Raykher A, Russo L, Schattner M, Schwartz L, Scott B, Shike M. Enteral nutrition support of head and neck cancer patients. Nutr Clin Pract 2007;22(1):68–73.

Roland NJ, Paleri V, editors. Head and neck cancer: multidisciplinary management guidelines. 4th ed London: ENT UK; 2011.

Rosenthal DI, Lewin JS, Eisbruch A. Prevention and treatment of dysphagia and aspiration after chemoradiation for head and neck cancer. J Clin Oncol 2006;24(17):2636–43.

Talwar B, Findlay M. When is the optimal time for placing a gastrostomy in patients undergoing treatment for head and neck cancer? Curr Opin Support Palliat Care 2012;6(1):41–53.

# 23 Epidemiology and Biostatistics

## Questions

### TRUE/FALSE

1. When measuring the frequency of disease occurrence in an epidemic, the most appropriate measure is the case fatality rate. (T/F)

2. The probability of disease-related deaths during a specified time period is the crude mortality rate. (T/F)

3. If 17 new cases of a disease were reported in a city with a midyear population of 400,000, then the incidence rate is 4.25 per 100,000. (T/F)

4. If exposure can be reduced in a population (e.g., through a preventive program), the potential benefit is best measured by relative risk. (T/F)

5. If the absolute rate of lung cancer among smokers is 10 per 1000 per year and 1 per 1000 per year among nonsmokers, then the attributable risk of smoking is 9 per 1000 persons per year. (T/F)

6. A major limitation of cohort studies is the difficulty in determining whether the exposure or risk factor precedes the disease or outcome. (T/F)

7. Case–control studies are the design of choice for rare outcomes. (T/F)

8. Logistic regression is often used in case–control studies to examine the association between exposure and dichotomous outcome (case–control) and produces an odds ratio as the measure of association. (T/F)

9. Cross-sectional studies determine incidence, not prevalence. (T/F)

10. In experimental studies, an intent-to-treat analysis includes only patients who complete the treatment and ignores those who drop out or are excluded during the study. (T/F)

11. In case–control studies, selection bias may occur if case patients systematically recall exposures more extensively than control patients. (T/F)

12. For confounding to occur, the extraneous factor must be associated with the exposure and the outcome of interest among both exposed and unexposed individuals. (T/F)

13. A variable can be a confounder if it is a step in the causal chain of a disease. (T/F)

14. If confounding is to be controlled in a case–control study, the sample should always be restricted to those who are homogeneous with respect to the confounding factor (i.e., narrow age range). (T/F)

15. Causality should be assessed before evaluating the validity of an observed association. (T/F)

16. A simple random sample is a sample selected from a population in such a manner that all members of the population have an equal chance of being selected. (T/F)

17. A systematic sample is one obtained through the use of groups rather than individuals as the sample unit. (T/F)

18. When screening for a rare disease, investigators must use a screening test with high sensitivity. (T/F)

19. When screening for a prevalent disease (e.g., diabetes), investigators must use a screening test with high specificity. (T/F)

20. Lead-time bias is the bias that occurs when a new experimental test appears to prolong survival compared with traditional methods but, in fact, only results in an earlier diagnosis. (T/F)

21. In general, the alternative hypothesis ($H_A$) proposes that no treatment effect exists. (T/F)

22. The power of a test is the probability of rejecting the null hypothesis when it is false. (T/F)

23. Alpha ($\alpha$) represents an acceptable probability of a type I error in a statistical test. (T/F)

24. A type I error is equivalent to the false-negative rate (1 – sensitivity). (T/F)

25. For a fixed level of significance, as the sample size $(n)$ increases, the probability of making a type II error decreases and the power of the test increases. (T/F)

26. The relationship between any normal value $x$ and the corresponding normal value $z$ is given by the following equation: $z = x - \mu/\sigma$. (T/F)

27. There are $n - 1$ degrees of freedom for the test statistic $\mu$ (population mean) when $s$ (population standard deviation) is unknown. (T/F)

28. When the population standard deviation ($\sigma$) is unknown, the confidence coefficient is obtained using the Student $t$ distribution rather than the standard normal distribution. (T/F)

29. If population X has a larger standard deviation than population Y, then population X will have a smaller variance than population Y. (T/F)

30. The Student $t$ distribution is symmetric and bell-shaped, similar to the normal distribution, but has heavier tails and is therefore more prone to producing values that fall far from its mean. (T/F)

31. The strength of association and the sample size determine the magnitude of the $P$ value. (T/F)

32. The $P$ value is better than the confidence interval in separating the impact of the sample size from the strength of the association. (T/F)

33. Large $P$ values support the null hypothesis ($H_0$), whereas small $P$ values reject it. One's choice of significance level $(a)$ indicates what one considers large or small. (T/F)

34. The width of a confidence interval estimate of the population mean μ is a function of two quantities: the sample size $n$ and the population standard deviation σ. (T/F)

35. Having 95% confidence that a certain interval covers μ is a property of the method used in calculating the interval rather than a property of the pair of numbers that are calculated. (T/F)

36. A common application of the chi-square distribution is in the comparison of expected with observed frequencies. (T/F)

37. Two population proportions can be compared with the use of either the chi-square test or the two-sample $z$ test because the chi-square statistic is equal to the square of the $z$ statistic. (T/F)

38. The $t$ test is an appropriate statistical procedure when the study involves continuous data and one wishes to evaluate the difference between two population means. (T/F)

39. The basic idea underlying the simplest form of the analysis of variance (ANOVA) is that variation between observations can be viewed as having two components: between-group and within-group variation. (T/F)

40. ANOVA evaluates the equality of several population means without inflating the type I error rate. (T/F)

41. Multicollinearity is a condition in which three or more predictor variables in a multiple regression model are highly correlated. (T/F)

42. The value of the coefficient of determination can range between $-1$ and $+1$. (T/F)

43. In simple linear regression, a correlation coefficient of $-1$ indicates that no linear relationship exists between the variables $x$ and $y$. (T/F)

44. In regression analysis, the total sum of squares is the sum over all observations of the squared differences of each observation from the overall mean. (T/F)

45. The method of logistic regression models the odds ratio of a binary outcome variable as a function of predictor covariates. (T/F)

46. Censoring refers to the ability to follow all subjects until they reach the study endpoint. (T/F)

47. The survivor function S(t) is defined as the cumulative probability of survival without incurring the outcome of interest for time $t$. (T/F)

48. Kaplan-Meier plots are typically adjusted for potential differences that may exist between the study groups (e.g., age or comorbidity). (T/F)

49. The life tables approach is more useful than the Kaplan-Meier approach for small sample sizes. (T/F)

50. The hazard ratio (HR) differs from the relative risk ratio (RRR) in that the HR is cumulative over an entire study, using a defined endpoint, whereas the RRR represents instantaneous risk over the study time period or some subset thereof. (T/F)

## SINGLE BEST ANSWER

*For questions 51-75, please choose the most likely answer from the following options:*
   A. v
   B. ii, v
   C. ii, iv, v
   D. i, ii, iv, v
   E. Statements i-v are all correct
   F. Statements i-v are all incorrect

51. Which of these statements are correct?
   i. An epidemic is the spread of disease over a very wide geographical area.
   ii. An epidemic is when the mortality rate from a disease exceeds 20 per 1000 population.
   iii. An epidemic is a disease that is peculiar to a specific geographical region or population.
   iv. An epidemic is the proportion of deaths in a specified population from a certain disease in a given time period.
   v. An epidemic is when there are significantly more cases of the same disease than what would previously have been expected, in a certain population over a specified time period.

52. Which of these are among the most commonly used measures of disease frequency?
   i. Crude mortality rate
   ii. Incidence rate
   iii. Case fatality rate
   iv. Cause-specific mortality rate
   v. Prevalence

53. A decrease in prevalence may result from which of the following?
   i. An increase in incidence
   ii. A shorter disease duration due to a quicker recovery period

iii. A longer disease duration
iv. A shorter disease duration due to a quicker death
v. A decrease in incidence

54. When a new treatment prevents death but does not produce recovery, which of the following will occur?
    i. Incidence will decrease and prevalence will increase.
    ii. Prevalence will decrease.
    iii. Incidence will increase and prevalence will decrease.
    iv. Incidence will increase.
    v. Prevalence will increase.

55. The strength of association between smoking and laryngeal cancer is measured using which of the following?
    i. Population attributable fraction
    ii. Population attributable risk
    iii. Attributable risk
    iv. Cumulative incidence rate
    v. Relative risk

56. In determining whether an observed risk factor is likely to be causal, one should consider which of the following?
    i. The strength of the association
    ii. The dose–response relationship
    iii. The consistency of the association
    iv. The specificity of the causation
    v. The temporal relationship of the association

57. Which of the following characterize the incidence rate of a disease?
    i. It measures the frequency of existing cases in a population at a point in time.
    ii. It measures the number of new cases in a population over a period of time.
    iii. It is the same as the prevalence rate.
    iv. It measures the strength of association between the exposed and unexposed.
    v. It is important in the study of the probability or risk of a certain disease.

58. Which of the following statements about cohort studies are true?
    i. They cannot be prospective in nature.
    ii. Participants must be free of the outcome at the beginning of the study.
    iii. They are quicker and cheaper than case–control studies.
    iv. Sample size requirements can impede the performance of some cohort studies.
    v. They are more likely than case–control studies to meet the temporality criterion for causality.

59. Which of the following statements about case–control studies are true?
    i. They permit direct estimation of disease risk and relative risk.
    ii. They are useful for studying rare diseases.

iii. They are not subject to selection bias.
iv. They use the odds ratio as a measure of association between exposure and outcome.
v. Participants are selected at the beginning of the study on the basis of their outcome.

60. In what ways do cohort studies differ from case–control studies?
    i. Cohort studies are more suitable for studying rare diseases.
    ii. Cohort studies take longer to complete.
    iii. The control group in a cohort study is more susceptible to bias.
    iv. Cohort studies are more likely to have attrition problems.
    v. Cohort studies can determine incidence.

61. Which of the following helps determine the number of patients required to treat a specific disease in a clinical trial?
    i. The anticipated benefit
    ii. The response of the control group
    iii. The significance level
    iv. The power of the study
    v. The type II error rate

62. Which of the following can actively exclude confounding when a study is designed?
    i. Stratification
    ii. Matching
    iii. Multiple regression
    iv. Randomization
    v. Blinding

63. Which of the following are categorical variables?
    i. Birth weight
    ii. Gender
    iii. Tumor size
    iv. Social class
    v. Hair color

64. Which of the following are indicated if a distribution is said to be "negatively skewed"?
    i. It is symmetrically skewed.
    ii. It is skewed to the left.
    iii. It is symmetrical.
    iv. It is skewed to the right.
    v. It is left tailed.

65. Which of the following statements about the mean are correct?
    i. The mean is the 50th percentile on the distribution curve.
    ii. The mean is the most frequently occurring observation.
    iii. The mean is a measure of the relationship between two or more variables.
    iv. The mean is the sum of all observations.
    v. The mean is 2 standard deviations above the median.

66. Which of the following statements about the normal distribution curve are true?
    i. It is bell-shaped.

ii. It is also called the Gaussian distribution curve.

iii. It is asymmetrical about the mean.

iv. Approximately 95% of observations fall within 2 standard deviations of mean.

v. Approximately 68% of observations fall within 1 standard deviation of mean.

67. Which of the following are measures of variability?

    i. Median

    ii. Standard deviation

    iii. Mode

    iv. Range

    v. Variance

68. Which of the following statements about the standard error of the mean are true?

    i. It increases as sample size increases.

    ii. It is larger than the subject-to-subject variation in the response variable values.

    iii. It can be a positive or negative number.

    iv. It decreases as subject-to-subject variation in the response variable increases.

    v. It is the sample-to-sample variation among a set of sample means, estimating the population mean.

69. Which of the following statements about the 95% confidence interval of the population mean are true?

    i. It is wider than a 99% confidence interval.

    ii. One can be 95% confident that, in repeated samples drawn from the same population, it will give an estimated range of values that will include the unknown population mean ($\mu$).

    iii. For a single sample of $n$ measurements, one can be 95% confident that the interval will include the unknown population mean ($\mu$).

    iv. One can be 95% confident that the mean of other samples drawn from the same population will all fall within the same interval.

    v. It is calculated as $\bar{x}$ (sample mean) $\pm 196a_{\bar{x}}$ (standard error of the sample mean).

70. Which of the following statements are true if both the mean and median of a normal distribution are 210 and the standard deviation is 4?

    i. The distribution is positively skewed.

    ii. Of the values, 99.7% lie between 198 and 222.

    iii. The distribution is symmetrically skewed.

    iv. Of the values, 95% lie between 202 and 218.

    v. The center of the frequency distribution is 210.

71. Which of the following statements are true?

    i. An increase in sample size will increase the length of the confidence interval.

    ii. An increase in sample size will increase the population mean.

    iii. An increase in sample size will increase the sample standard deviation.

    iv. An increase in sample size will decrease the sample mean.

    v. An increase in sample size will decrease the length of the confidence interval without reducing the level of confidence.

72. Which of these factors influence the width of a confidence interval?

    i. Sample size $n$

    ii. The chosen confidence level

    iii. The mode

    iv. The degree of sample-to-sample variability in point estimates

    v. The degree of variability in subject-to-subject values of the response variable

73. A screening test of known sensitivity and specificity is applied to two populations X and Y. The prevalence of disease is significantly higher in population X than in population Y. Which of the following statements are true under these circumstances?

    i. The proportion of all positive tests that give false-positive results will be higher in population X than in population Y.

    ii. The proportion of all negative tests that give false-negative results will be higher in population X than in population Y.

    iii. The sensitivity will be higher in population X than in population Y.

    iv. The specificity will be higher in population Y than in population X.

    v. The proportion of all positive tests that are truly positive will be higher in population X than in population Y.

74. Which of the following statements about the correlation coefficient (regression analysis) are true?

    i. It can take on values between 0 and –1.

    ii. It is a measure of the extent to which two variables are linearly related.

    iii. It is not susceptible to sampling error.

    iv. It could be used to measure the relationship between cardiovascular disease and blood group in a case–control study.

    v. A value of 0 indicates that two variables are not related.

75. Which of the following statements about the Kaplan-Meier method are true?

    i. It cannot accommodate time-dependent variables.

    ii. It requires categorical predictors.

    iii. It is mainly descriptive.

    iv. It does not control for covariates.

    v. It is a nonparametric estimate of survival function.

## Case 23-1

In a town of 50,000 persons (27,000 males and 23,000 females), there were 1000 deaths (500 males, 500 females) in the year 2006. Of the 200 cancer cases that year, there were 30 deaths (20 males and 10 females).

76. Based on the information in Case 23-1, the crude mortality rate is

    A. 10 per 1000.

    B. 15 per 100,000.

C. 20 per 100,000.
D. 20 per 1000.
E. None of the above.

77. Based on the information in Case 23-1, the sex-specific mortality rate for females is
A. 43 per 100,000.
B. 10 per 100.
C. 10 per 10,000.
D. 22 per 1000.
E. None of the above.

78. Based on the information in Case 23-1, the cause-specific mortality rate for cancer is
A. 60 per 100,000.
B. 60 per 10,000.
C. 10%.
D. 250 per 100,000.
E. None of the above.

79. Based on the information in Case 23-1, the case fatality rate for cancer is
A. 5%.
B. 5 per 1000.
C. 15%.
D. 10 per 10,000.
E. None of the above.

80. Based on the information in Case 23-1, the proportionate mortality ratio (PMR) for cancer is
A. 30%.
B. 3 per 1000.
C. 3%.
D. 3 per 10,000.
E. None of the above.

## Case 23-2

Suppose that a researcher studied the relationship between smoking and oral cancer. The study resulted in the following data for 600 subjects:

|  | Individuals with Oral Cancer | Individuals without Oral Cancer | Total |
| --- | --- | --- | --- |
| Smokers | 200 | 41 | 241 |
| Nonsmokers | 100 | 259 | 359 |
| TOTAL | 300 | 300 | 600 |

81. The hypothetical epidemiological study outlined in Case 23-2 is an example of a(n)
A. Cohort study.
B. Interventional study.
C. Cross-sectional study.
D. Ecological study.
E. Case–control study.

82. According to Case 23-2, the relative risk of oral cancer in smokers versus nonsmokers is
A. 2.98.
B. 3.98.
C. 1.76.
D. 0.55.
E. None of the above.

83. According to Case 23-2, the attributable risk for smokers is
A. 2.98.
B. 3.98.
C. 1.76.
D. 0.55.
E. None of the above.

84. According to Case 23-2, the odds ratio is
A. 10.
B. 11.2.
C. 14.2.
D. 12.5.
E. None of the above.

85. According to Case 23-2, what is the most appropriate statistical test for determining whether a significant association exists between smoking and oral cancer?
A. Correlation analysis
B. Analysis of variance
C. Chi-square test
D. Paired t-test
E. Pooled t-test

## Case 23-3

Suppose that a researcher studied the frequency of serum cholesterol levels of 50 patients, selected at random, between the ages of 35 and 55 years:

| Cholesterol Level (mg/dL) | Frequency | Percent |
| --- | --- | --- |
| 195-199 | 3 | 6 |
| 200-204 | 7 | 14 |
| 205-209 | 13 | 26 |
| 210-214 | 19 | 38 |
| 215-219 | 6 | 12 |
| 220-224 | 2 | 4 |
| TOTAL | 50 | 100 |

86. On the basis of Case 23-3, patients with serum cholesterol levels of 210 or higher were selected for further screening. Where would these results fall?
A. Above the 54% percentile
B. Below the 20% percentile
C. Above the 38% percentile
D. Above the 46% percentile
E. None of the above

87. If one assumes that the patients in Case 23-3 are representative of the general population, what is the probability that an individual selected at random will have a serum cholesterol level of less than 215 mg/dL?
A. 12%
B. 16%
C. 88%
D. 84%
E. None of the above

88. Based on Case 23-3, if 10% of patients who take statins for a high cholesterol level experience cramping, what is the probability that the patients with a serum cholesterol level at 220 mg/dL will

experience cramping, if one assumes they are taking this medication?
- A. 2%
- B. 3%
- C. 1%
- D. 0.04%
- E. None of the above

89. If the average cholesterol level for a sample of 50 patients in Case 23-3 is 210 mg/dL, what is the probability that a sample mean less than or equal to this value would be obtained from a population whose true mean is 200 mg/dL and standard deviation is 3mg/dL?
- A. 32%
- B. 68%
- C. 28%
- D. 50%
- E. None of the above

90. Suppose the true population mean in Case 23-3 is unknown. What is the confidence interval for the population mean at a 95% confidence level?
- A. 209.18 mg/dL, 210.82 mg/dL
- B. 207.21 mg/dL, 211.32 mg/dL
- C. 200.50 mg/dL, 220.98 mg/dL
- D. 199.42 mg/dL, 221.56 mg/dL
- E. None of above

## Case 23-4

Suppose that a researcher studied the results of an HIV screening test for a group of 100,000 people:

| Test Result | HIV Status Positive (+) | Negative (−) | Total |
|---|---|---|---|
| Positive (+) | 475 | 4975 | 5450 |
| Negative (−) | 25 | 94525 | 94550 |
| | 500 | 99500 | 100000 |

HIV, Human immunodeficiency virus.
*From Agresti A, Finlay B. Statistical methods for the social sciences. 3rd ed. Upper Saddle River (NJ): Prentice Hall; 1997. p. 287.*

91. On the basis of Case 23-4, the sensitivity of the test is
- A. 90%.
- B. 95%.
- C. 87%.
- D. 9.5%.
- E. None of the above.

92. The specificity of the test in Case 23-4 is
- A. 90%.
- B. 95%.
- C. 87%.
- D. 9.5%.
- E. None of the above.

93. Based on Case 23-4, the predictive value of a positive test is
- A. 8.7%.
- B. 9.5%.
- C. 90%.
- D. 95%.
- E. None of the above.

94. Based on Case 23-4, the false-positive rate is
- A. 90%.
- B. 95%.
- C. 91%.
- D. 8%.
- E. None of the above.

95. Based on Case 23-4, the false-negative rate is
- A. 90%.
- B. 0.5%.
- C. 0.1%.
- D. 8%.
- E. None of the above.

96. Which of the following analytical models should be used to predict serum triglyceride levels in women aged 50 to 59 years from six other dietary factors?
- A. Logistic regression
- B. Multiple linear regression
- C. Simple linear regression
- D. Cox proportional hazards regression
- E. None of the above

97. Which of the following analytical models should be used to examine the relationship between warfarin dose and international normalized ratio (INR)?
- A. Logistic regression
- B. Multiple linear regression
- C. Simple linear regression
- D. Cox proportional hazards regression
- E. None of the above

98. Which of the following analytical models should be used to predict survival times in patients with laryngeal cancer, based on clinical and sociodemographic characteristics, measured at the time of diagnosis?
- A. Logistic regression
- B. Multiple linear regression
- C. Simple linear regression
- D. Cox proportional hazards regression
- E. None of the above

99. Which of the following analytical models should be used to obtain the relative risk of developing laryngeal cancer while smoking 20 or more cigarettes daily during a 10-year period, if other risk factors are controlled?
- A. Logistic regression
- B. Multiple linear regression
- C. Simple linear regression
- D. Cox proportional hazards regression
- E. None of the above

100. Which of the following analytical models should be used to describe the frequency of high diastolic blood pressure in women aged 50 to 59 years?
- A. Logistic regression
- B. Multiple linear regression
- C. Simple linear regression
- D. Cox proportional hazards regression
- E. None of the above

## Answers

| | | |
|---|---|---|
| 1. F | 35. T | 69. B |
| 2. F | 36. T | 70. C |
| 3. T | 37. T | 71. A |
| 4. F | 38. T | 72. D |
| 5. T | 39. T | 73. B |
| 6. F | 40. T | 74. B |
| 7. T | 41. F | 75. E |
| 8. T | 42. F | 76. D |
| 9. F | 43. F | 77. D |
| 10. F | 44. T | 78. A |
| 11. F | 45. T | 79. C |
| 12. T | 46. F | 80. C |
| 13. F | 47. T | 81. E |
| 14. F | 48. F | 82. A |
| 15. F | 49. F | 83. D |
| 16. T | 50. F | 84. D |
| 17. F | 51. A | 85. C |
| 18. T | 52. B | 86. D |
| 19. T | 53. C | 87. D |
| 20. T | 54. A | 88. C |
| 21. F | 55. A | 89. B |
| 22. T | 56. E | 90. A |
| 23. T | 57. B | 91. B |
| 24. F | 58. C | 92. B |
| 25. T | 59. C | 93. A |
| 26. T | 60. B | 94. C |
| 27. T | 61. E | 95. E |
| 28. T | 62. C | 96. B |
| 29. F | 63. C | 97. C |
| 30. T | 64. B | 98. D |
| 31. T | 65. F | 99. A |
| 32. F | 66. D | 100. E |
| 33. T | 67. C | |
| 34. F | 68. A | |

## Core Knowledge

### MEASURES OF MORTALITY

- The mortality rate is a measure of the number of deaths (in general or due to a specific cause, such as cause-specific mortality rate) in a population, scaled to the size of that population, per unit of time. It is usually expressed in units of death per 1000 persons per year.

- The case fatality rate represents the probability of death among diagnosed cases. It is typically used in acute rather than chronic diseases where the period from onset to death is relatively short.

- The proportionate mortality ratio (PMR) is the proportion of overall mortality that may be ascribed to a specific cause and is expressed as a percentage.

- The standardized mortality ratio (SMR) represents a proportional comparison to the numbers of deaths that would have been expected if the population had been of a standard composition in terms of age, gender, and other specified demographics.

### INVESTIGATION OF AN EPIDEMIC

- The attack rate is the cumulative incidence of infection in a group of people observed over a period of time during an epidemic.

- The term is defined as the number of exposed persons infected with the disease divided by the total number of exposed persons.

### MEASURES OF DISEASE FREQUENCY (INCIDENCE AND PREVALENCE)

- The incidence rate is the number of new cases of a disease over a specified time period divided by the population at risk of the disease in this period. It reflects the rate of disease occurrence.

- The prevalence rate is the total number of cases of disease at a given time divided by the total population at risk at a given time. It depends on the incidence and the duration of disease.

### MEASURES OF ASSOCIATION AND IMPACT (RISK)

- An important function of epidemiology is the ability to quantify the association between a risk (or protective) factor and an outcome.

- Measures can be relative or absolute.

- Relative measures give information on the strength of association between the exposure and outcome.

- The relative risk is calculated as the risk (cumulative incidence) in the exposed group divided by the risk (cumulative incidence) in the unexposed group.

- In the table below, the following formula is used: $[a/(a + b)]/[c/(c + d)]$.

- The odds ratio is the odds of disease in the exposed group divided by the odds in the unexposed group, which equals $(a/b)/(c/d)$ or $ad/cb$.

| Risk Factor | Have the Disease | Do Not Have the Disease | Total |
|---|---|---|---|
| Exposed | a | b | a + b |
| Unexposed | c | d | c + d |
| Total | a + c | b + d | a + b + c + d |

- Absolute measures give information on the frequency of disease in the exposed compared with the unexposed group, if a causal association is assumed.

- The attributable risk is the incidence in the exposed group minus the incidence in the unexposed group. This can also be expressed as the preventative fraction among the exposed.

- On a population level, the population attributable risk is an estimate of the excess risk of disease in the total study population attributable to the exposure. The population attributable fraction is the proportion of disease in the study population that is attributable to the exposure and is useful in estimating how much disease could potentially be prevented by reducing exposure to that factor.

## EPIDEMIOLOGICAL STUDIES

- Epidemiological studies can be observational or interventional. Observational studies include cohort, case–control, cross-sectional, and ecological studies. Intervention studies include randomized controlled trials (individuals) or field trials (groups).

- An intervention study is one in which an investigator randomly allocates an individual (or group) to an intervention or control group. The gold standard is a randomized controlled trial. Both groups must be similar in background characteristics. Selection bias is reduced by selecting participants through randomization and reporting bias through blinding (when the endpoint is subjective) and the use of placebos. The main method of analysis is by intention to treat (ITT). ITT analyses are done to avoid the effects of crossover and dropout, which may break the randomization to the treatment groups in a study. When designing an intervention study, investigators must decide whether they are interested in the efficacy or effectiveness of the intervention. The principal effect measures are risk and rate ratios.

- A cohort study can be retrospective or prospective in design. Participants are free of the disease at the beginning of the study and are selected on the basis of whether they are exposed to a potential risk factor. Because the incidence of disease in the exposed and unexposed groups is known, the relative risk can be calculated.

- In a case–control study, a group of case subjects and control subjects are identified on the basis of their disease status. The prevalence of or level of exposure to risk factor(s) is measured and compared with the use of the odds ratio. Although this type of study is generally less expensive and time-consuming than a cohort study, it is prone to selection and measurement bias due to difficulties in identifying suitable control subjects. It is useful for the study of rare diseases and multiple risk factors.

- A cross-sectional study is a survey of a population at a single point in time and is used to determine the prevalence of disease and risk factors in a defined population. It can measure associations between the disease and a risk factor but cannot generate causal hypotheses.

- An ecological study can be either longitudinal or cross-sectional, and populations or groups are the units of analysis rather than individuals.

## INTERPRETATION OF EPIDEMIOLOGICAL STUDY RESULTS

- Internal validity is the extent to which study results are not influenced by bias and confounding. To ensure that an observed association is causal, investigators must first exclude all other possible reasons for obtaining the result:
  - Bias can be categorized as selection bias or information bias.
  - Confounding occurs when an extraneous variable in a statistical model correlates with both the exposure and outcome. Confounding can be dealt with during the study design phase (e.g., restriction, randomization, or matching) or at the analysis phase (e.g., stratification or statistical modeling, such as multivariate regression).
  - The role of chance (random error) is dealt with by statistical methods, such as calculating a $P$ value, or a confidence interval can be used to evaluate the probability of obtaining an observed estimate by chance alone.

- The Bradford Hill criteria, otherwise known as Hill's criteria for causation, are a group of minimal conditions necessary to provide adequate evidence of a causal relationship between an incidence and a consequence, established by the English epidemiologist, Sir Austin Bradford (1897-1991) in 1965. Hill's criteria (1965) include the study design, strength of association, temporal relationship, consistency, dose–response relationship, plausibility, specificity, reversibility, coherence, and analogy.

## SAMPLING

- Random sampling is when the sample is selected in such a way that it gives each individual an equal chance of being chosen; it eliminates bias and enables the determination of the reliability of the result. Cluster random sampling involves groups rather than individuals.

- Systematic sampling involves the selection of individuals from an ordered sampling frame.

- Sampling error is the difference between the sampling result and the population characteristics.

- The standard error is the variability of the sample statistic.

## SCREENING AND DIAGNOSTIC TESTING

| | Disease Status | | |
|---|---|---|---|
| **Test Result** | **Positive (+)** | **Negative (-)** | **Total** |
| Positive (+) | a | b | a + b |
| Negative (-) | c | d | c + d |
| | a + c | b + d | a + b + c + d |

- Sensitivity is the ability of the test to give a positive result when the individual has the disease (a/(a+c)). A test with high sensitivity will have few false-negative results.

- Specificity is the ability of the test to give a negative result when the individual does not have the disease (d/(b+d)). A test with high specificity will have few false-negative results.

- The positive predictive value is the proportion of positive tests that are truly positive [a/(a+b)], and the negative predictive value is the proportion of negative tests that are truly negative [c/(c+d)].

- If the prevalence of disease is higher in one population than another, then the proportion of positive tests that are true-positive results will also be higher in this population. There will also be more false-negative results. Sensitivity and specificity are properties of the test and do not vary based on the prevalence of the disease.

## HYPOTHESIS TESTING

- Random variation means that even an unbiased sample may not represent the population as a whole. Therefore, underlying all statistical tests is a null hypothesis, ($H_0$), which is consistent with the idea that the observed difference is simply a result of random variation in the data.

- Any decision to reject $H_0$ carries a risk of being incorrect. This risk is the significance level of the test and is denoted as alpha ($\alpha$). If one tests at a 5% significance level, then there is a 5% chance that one will reject $H_0$ when it is true. This is called a type I error.

- The lowest significance level at which $H_0$ could be rejected is called the $P$ value. The $P$ value is the probability that a difference as large as that observed could occur by chance alone, that is, the smaller the $P$ value, the stronger the evidence against $H_0$.

- A type II error ($\beta$) is the probability of accepting $H_0$ when it is false.

- The power of a test ($1 - \beta$) is the probability of rejecting $H_0$ when it is false.

## DESCRIBING CLINICAL DATA

- Variables can be measured on a nominal, ordinal, ratio, or interval scale and can be broadly classified as quantitative or qualitative.

- Categorical data (e.g., count and frequency data) can be measured on all four scales, whereas continuous data can be measured on the ordinal or interval/ratio scale.

- Grouped clinical data can be described pictorially (e.g., a frequency table or histogram) or numerically (e.g., measures of central tendency [mean, median, and mode] or measures of spread [range, variance, and standard deviation]). The *mean* is the mathematical average, the *median* is the center value, the *mode* is the most commonly occurring value, *variance* is the average

squared deviation of each number from its mean, and *standard deviation* is the square root of the variance.

## STATISTICAL BUILDING BLOCKS

- A parameter is a value or characteristic associated with a population, that is, population mean ($\mu$) or population standard deviation (SD) ($\sigma$). A statistic is a value or characteristic calculated from a sample, that is, a sample mean ($\bar{x}$) or sample SD (s). Sample statistics are estimates of the corresponding population parameters.

| | Sample | Population |
|---|---|---|
| Mean | $\bar{x}$ | $\mu$ |
| Standard deviation | s | $\sigma$ |
| Standard error | $s/\sqrt{n}$ | $\sigma/\sqrt{n}$ |

- A frequency distribution is a tabulation of the frequency at which values occur in a set. It may be empirical (from a sample) or theoretical (from a population). The sampling distribution of means is the frequency distribution of the population of sample means. The central limit theorem describes the tendency of the frequency distribution to assume a normal distribution.

- The normal (Gaussian) distribution is smooth, bell-shaped, and symmetrical around the population mean ($\mu$).Of all values for a given population, 95% fall with $1.96\sigma$ of the population mean, and 99% fall within $2.58\sigma$. The relationship between any arbitrary normal value, x, and the corresponding standard normal value, z, is given by $z = x - \mu/\sigma$.

- The $t$ distribution is similar to the $z$ distribution but is sensitive to sample size and is used when the population SD ($\sigma$) is unknown. The $t$ distribution has heavier tails than the normal distribution, meaning that it is more prone to producing values that fall far from its mean. The ratio $t = (\bar{x} - \mu)/s/\sqrt{n}$ measures by how many standard errors the sample mean differs from the certified value.

## CONFIDENCE INTERVALS

- Because the value of a sample statistic will vary between samples, confidence intervals are useful in defining the interval within which the true population is likely to fall.

- The width of a confidence interval will depend on both the level of confidence that the interval will encompass the unknown population value and the standard error of the estimate (i.e., the degree of sample-to-sample variation), which, in turn, depends on the level of individual variation in the population and the sample size *(n)*.

- For a normal distribution, the 95% confidence interval estimate of the population mean ($\mu$) is calculated as $\bar{x} \pm 1.96\ \sigma_{\bar{x}}$ (where $\sigma_{\bar{x}}$ is the standard error of the estimate). In practice, the population SD ($\sigma$) is rarely known, and the sample SD (s) is used to estimate $\sigma$.

This additional source of variability is accounted for with the use of the Student $t$ distribution rather than the normal distribution and has $n - 1$ degrees of freedom.

## TESTS OF STATISTICAL SIGNIFICANCE

- Differences between groups are indicated with categorical or continuous data or analysis of variance (ANOVA).
  - Regarding categorical data, when the data are in the form of counts (i.e., frequency data), the chi-square test can be used to test differences in population proportions.
  - Regarding continuous data, when a study involves only two groups with interval/ratio data, the $t$ test can be used to evaluate the significance of the difference between two population means.
  - ANOVA examines the significance of group differences between two or more groups. The F test statistic is equal to variation due to treatment divided by experimental error, which is equal to the mean square for treatments divided by the mean square for error (MST/MSE).
- Relationships can be analyzed with various statistical methods.
  - Correlation and regression analyses evaluate associations involving continuous or interval/ratio data.
  - The correlation coefficient *(r)* indicates the extent to which two variables are related. A value of –1 indicates a perfect negative linear relationship, +1 indicates a perfect positive relationship, and 0 indicates that the variables are unrelated.
  - The coefficient of determination *($r^2$)* measures the proportion of variation in one variable that can be explained by the variation in the other. When $r^2 = 1$, all of the variation in the dependent variable *(y)* is attributable to its linear relationship with the independent variable *(x)*.
  - The objective of regression analysis is to derive a linear equation that best fits a set of data pairs $(x_i, y_i)$ that can predict values of $y$ for given values of $x$. The best fitting line is one in which the sum of the squared distance of all the data is y = a + bx, where *a* is equal to the intercept (the value of $y$ when $x = 0$) and *b* is equal to the slope. The slope is the change in the average value of $y$ for every one unit change in $x$. Multiple linear regression differs from simple linear regression in that rather than having one covariate, the equation has multiple predictor variables.
  - Logistic regression is useful for evaluating the risk of a binary outcome variable, which can take on only two possible values. The odds of the outcome (P/1 – P) are reported rather than the probability (P).

## SURVIVAL ANALYSIS

- Survival analysis is used to examine the risk of a binary outcome variable (i.e., event or failure).
- The survivor function S(t) is the probability of being alive at a particular time $t$.
- The median survival is defined as the point during follow-up in which 50% of the study population has died.
- Censoring is when a subject leaves the study before incurring the outcome of interest (i.e., dropout, loss to follow-up, enrolled at different times, study ends at predetermined time point, death before outcome of interest [when outcome of interest is not death]).
- The Kaplan-Meier (KM) method allows subjects to contribute information to the survivor function S(t) as long as they remain in the study and to stop contributing when they are censored. Changes to S(t) occur only when a failure occurs (i.e., subjects who drop out in between events are removed when the next failure occurs). Plots of the KM estimated survivor function reflect observed differences for different groups of subjects with respect to follow-up time. KM plots represent unadjusted study data.
- The Cox proportional hazards model fits separate logistic models for each failure time. The follow-up time is held constant for all subjects at the time point of each comparison. The model yields a measure of risk called the *hazard ratio* (HR). Because HRs are calculated by averaging instantaneous risks throughout the study period, the HR represents a summary of relative risk of death during follow-up. The HR is the derivative or instantaneous slope of S(t). While S(t) represents overall survival, the HR represents the instantaneous risk of mortality, or the mortality rate.

## SUGGESTED READING

Agresti A, Finlay B. Statistical methods for the social sciences. 4th ed. Upper Saddle River (NJ): Prentice Hall; 2009.

Clark TG, Bradburn MJ, Love SB, Altman DG. Survival analysis part I: Basic concepts and first analyses. Br J Cancer 2003;89(2):232–8.

Curado MP, Hashibe M. Recent changes in the epidemiology of head and neck cancer. Curr Opin Oncol 2009;21(3):194–200.

Essex-Sorlia D. Medical biostatistics and epidemiology: examination & board review. East Norwalk (CT): Appleton and Lange; 1995.

Grimes DA, Schulz KF. The Lancet epidemiology series. Lancet 2002:359.

Hebel JR, McCarter RJ. A study guide to epidemiology and biostatistics. 7th ed. Burlington (MA): Jones and Bartlett; 2012.

Kestenbaum B. Epidemiology and biostatistics: an introduction to clinical research. New York: Springer; 2009.

Kleinbaum DG, Klein M. Survival analysis: a self-learning text (statistics for biology and health). 2nd ed. New York: Springer; 2005.

Knapp RG, Miller MC. Clinical epidemiology and biostatistics. The national medical series for independent study. Media (PA): Harwal; 1992.

Mehanna H, Paleri V, West CML, Nutting C. Head and neck cancer—part 1: epidemiology, presentation, and prevention. BMJ 2010;341:c4684.

# Index

Page numbers followed by f indicate figures; t, tables; e, online content.

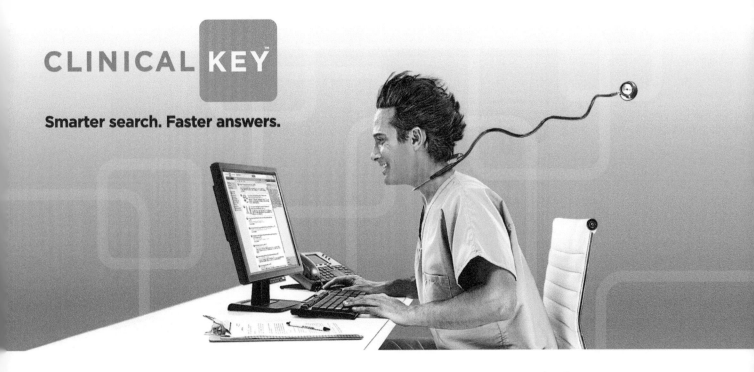

**CLINICAL KEY**™

Smarter search. Faster answers.

# Smarter, Faster Search for Better Patient Care

**Unlike a conventional search engine, ClinicalKey is specifically designed to serve doctors by providing three core components:**

**1 Comprehensive Content**

The most current, evidence-based answers available for every medical and surgical specialty.

**2 Trusted Answers**

Content supplied by Elsevier, the world's leading provider of health and science information.

**3 Unrivaled Speed to Answer**

Faster, more relevant clinical answers, so you can spend less time searching and more time caring for patients.

**Start searching with ClinicalKey today!**
Visit *ClinicalKey.com* for more information and subscription options.

ELSEVIER

Printed and bound by CPI Group (UK) Ltd, Croydon, CR0 4YY

08/05/2025

01864791-0001